Personal Project Pursuit

Goals, Action, and Human Flourishing

Personal Project Pursuit

Goals, Action, and Human Flourishing

Edited by

Brian R. Little
Carleton University and Harvard University

Katariina Salmela-Aro
University of Helsinki and University of Jyväskylä

Susan D. Phillips
Carleton University

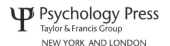

Psychology Press
Taylor & Francis Group
NEW YORK AND LONDON

First published 2007 by Lawrence Erlbaum Associates, Inc., Publishers

Published 2014 by Psychology Press
711 Third Avenue, New York, NY 10017

and by Psychology Press
27 Church Road, Hove, East Sussex, BN3 2FA

Psychology Press is an imprint of the Taylor & Francis Group, an informa business

Cover design by Kathryn Houghtaling

Library of Congress Cataloging-in-Publication Data

    p. cm.
Includes index.
ISBN : 978-0-8058-5486-2 (pbk)

2006
—dc22   2006000000
                                                      CIP

Contents

About the Contributors

Monika Brandstätter, MA, began studying psychology in her native Austria at the University of Salzburg. During her studies, she was selected to participate in an international student exchange program and traveled to Carleton University, Canada, where Dr. Brian Little introduced her to personal projects analysis (PPA). Her work in Dr. Little's Social Ecology Laboratory led to a thesis on gender differences in project stability and subjective well-being and to a Magistra degree in psychology summa cum laude (Salzburg). After graduation she was awarded a fellowship to enter graduate studies at the University of Victoria, Canada. Working with Dr. Christopher Lalonde in the Lifespan Development Program, she applied her training in PPA to studies of self-continuity and identity formation. Her thesis research combined Little's PPA methodology with Lalonde's Self-Continuity Interview to explore the ways in which personal projects function to support abstract conceptions of the self. Following the completion of her master's degree, Brandstätter accepted a training position as a clinical psychologist at the Roseneck Hospital, Center for Behavioral Medicine, in Prien am Chiemsee, Germany.

Neil C. Chambers completed his early studies in linguistics and modern languages at Dalhousie University (Halifax, Canada) and Brown University (Providence, RI). His graduate work focused on comparative verbal aspect and included studies in Russia and China. After 10 years of employment with the government of Canada, he returned to university to complete his PhD in psychology (personality) under the tutelage of

Dr. Brian Little at Carleton University. His dissertation brought together his two academic careers by focusing on individual differences in time perspective and phrasing in the personal projects of the young and the elderly. Chambers is now managing a foreign intelligence training center in Ottawa, Canada. He has coauthored several book chapters on PPA.

Andrew J. Elliot received his PhD at the University of Wisconsin–Madison in 1994, and is currently a professor of psychology at the University of Rochester. Elliot has produced approximately 80 scholarly publications, received research grants from both public and private agencies, and been awarded four different early- and midcareer awards for his research contributions (including the American Psychological Association Distinguished Scientific Award for Early Career Contribution to Psychology). His research areas include achievement and affiliation motivation; approach and avoidance motivation; goals, motives, the self, and behavioral regulation; subjective well-being; and parent, teacher, and cultural influences on motivation and regulation. Elliot is a fellow at both the Society for Personality and Social Psychology and the American Psychological Association. He is a former associate editor at the *Journal of Personality* and a current associate editor at *Personality and Social Psychology Bulletin.*

Ron Friedman is a doctoral candidate in the University of Rochester's social psychology program, specializing in human motivation. His research focuses on the role of nonconscious environmental cues in motivation and performance within achievement contexts. Friedman graduated from Brooklyn College with a BA in political science and managed numerous political campaigns before abandoning his post as chief of staff to a U.S. congressman to fulfill his lifelong ambition of conducting hierarchical linear regressions in underlit, windowless rooms. He is the proud owner of a Yamaha Vino scooter and collects pets.

Alexandra M. Freund is a professor of psychology at the University of Zurich, Switzerland. Her primary focus is on the development of motivational processes in adulthood. Freund completed her doctoral studies at the Centre for Lifespan Development, Max Planck Institute for Human Development, Berlin in 1993 on self-definition in old age. This was followed by a postdoctoral fellowship at Stanford University. In 2002, she returned to Berlin as a research scientist at the Max Planck Institute, where, together with Paul B. Baltes, she initiated and codirected the project "Personal Goals in Lifespan Development." In 2003, she was a faculty member at Northwestern University (Evanston, IL) before taking her current position at Zurich. In 2000, Freund was elected founding member of the Young Academy of Sciences, Germany, where she continues to be involved in multiple interdisciplinary projects.

Travis L. Gee is a research fellow at the Centre of National Research on Disability and Rehabilitation Medicine at the University of Queensland, Australia, and a consulting psychologist on a part-time basis. He taught psychology at the University of New England in Australia for several years following the completion of his PhD in Dr. Brian Little's Social Ecology Laboratory at Carleton University, Canada, where he has also taught research methods and statistics as well as theories of personality. His methods and statistics positions also include a number of years as a lecturer at the University of Ottawa. As chair of the editorial board of *Counselling Australia* and coeditor of the new online journal *Counselling, Psychotherapy and Health,* he has received an outstanding contribution award from the Australian Counselling Association, for which he is also an occasional policy writer. Gee's honors include two advisory positions on the Curriculum Development Committee and the overseeing Academic Committee of the Australian Institute of Professional Counsellors. His contributions to disability research include ongoing work on the Personal Projects System Rating Scale, which he has managed to sneak into some ongoing research projects in Australia with some soon-to-be-published success.

Adam M. Grant is a doctoral candidate in organizational psychology at the University of Michigan. His research, supported by a National Science Foundation fellowship and presented in an article forthcoming in the *Academy of Management Review,* focuses on designing work contexts to motivate employees to care about making a positive difference in other people's lives and examining how this motivation makes a difference in employees' lives. His specific areas of interest include work motivation, job design, prosocial behavior, personal projects, and well-being. Grant graduated from Harvard University with a BA magna cum laude with highest honors in psychology and was elected to the Phi Beta Kappa honor society. He also earned an American Academy of Political and Social Science fellowship for exceptional academic accomplishments, concern for improving social conditions, and extraordinary potential for becoming an outstanding social scientist. While working at Let's Go Publications, he set numerous company records for advertising sales and earned the Manager of the Year award for leadership, commitment, and business acumen. In high school, he was an All-State and All-

American springboard diver; he still enjoys hurling himself into somersaults, twists, and occasional crash landings, and has served as a springboard diving instructor for the past 10 years. He also performs as a professional magician.

Maryann F. Joseph is a PhD candidate in clinical psychology at McGill University in Montreal, Canada, where she is pursuing a social ecological approach to health psychology. With support from a prestigious Canada Graduate Scholarship, she is examining intriguing applications to respiratory illness and chronic pain. By the time she entered her doctoral studies, Joseph was already a personal projects enthusiast. She had been a member of Dr. Brian Little's Social Ecology Laboratory at Carleton University, where she received her BA Honours in psychology, earning the Governor General's medal for highest graduating average and the Queen's Jubilee medal for distinguished community service and outstanding achievement. Her undergraduate thesis, which focused on the relation of "free traits" to health and well-being, was awarded the annual prize by the Canadian Psychological Association for the best thesis in psychology. Joseph anticipates pursuing a lifelong intellectual career project of psychology as well as a continued commitment to community service. Nevertheless, this singer-songwriter admits to occasional diversions with images of indie-folk-rock stardom and indulgences in a variety of idiosyncratic restorative projects.

Christopher E. Lalonde completed his PhD in developmental psychology at the University of British Columbia. Prior to this he was a Research Associate in Community Child Health at the British Columbia Research Institute for Children's and Women's Health. He joined the Lifespan Development Area in the Department of Psychology at the University of Victoria in 1998 and is now Associate Professor and area coordinator. Lalonde's research interests include social-cognitive development in middle childhood and cultural influences on identity formation in adolescence. In particular, his work focuses on changes in reasoning about matters of selfhood and the abilities of young persons to maintain a sense of personal continuity across the profound changes that occur during the transition from childhood to adulthood. This work has two main facets. The first concerns the normal course of development and various ways in which developmental and cultural forces intersect to influence the course of identity formation. The second focuses on the consequences of failures in this developmental process that may account for the dramatic increase in suicide risk that attends the teenage years. As a visiting scholar at the University of Queensland, he is currently studying rates of suicide among indigenous youth in both Canada and Australia.

Len Lecci is a professor of psychology and licensed clinical psychologist at the University of North Carolina–Wilmington. He received his PhD in 1995 from Arizona State University and completed an internship through Harvard Medical School. His current research interests include motivational and perceptual underpinnings of health concerns (hypochondriasis), decision making in the context of health settings, and the effects of individual differences in bias on juror decision making. Lecci has had National Science Foundation funding for his research on hypochondriasis and normative experiences of health fear, and this research culminated in a U.S. congressional briefing on terrorism and disaster response before the House Science Committee. He is currently the Director of Clinical Services at Memory Assessment and Research Services, a technology transfer initiative through the University of North Carolina–Wilmington that focuses on innovations in the early detection of dementia. Lecci has published in journals such as the *Journal of Personality and Social Psychology, Law and Human Behavior, Health Psychology, Journal of Abnormal Psychology,* and *Cognition and Emotion.* In 2005, Lecci was awarded the University of North Carolina–Wilmington's Distinguished Teaching Professorship Award and The Board of Trustees Teaching Excellence Award.

Brian R. Little is a Distinguished Research Professor Emeritus in the Department of Psychology at Carleton University and Associate of the Department of Psychology at Harvard University. He received his PhD at the University of California at Berkeley and has taught at Oxford, Carleton, and Harvard Universities. He was in the inaugural group of Fellows at the Radcliffe Institute for Advanced Study at Harvard and has lectured in personality psychology and in advanced human assessment at Harvard for several years. He has received awards both for his research and teaching, and has given two G. Stanley Hall lectures for the American Psychological Association. Little has been an active member of the Society for the Study of Human Development and serves on the editorial board of its journal. In 2005, he was also elected as a member-at-large of the board of the Association for Research in Personality. The developer of PPA, he has had a career-long project of integrating diverse perspectives in personality and developmental science. His core projects are to remain married to his wife, Professor Susan Phillips, and to eventually play professional basketball with any team that will take him.

Ian McGregor, after studying philosophy and comparative religion at a seminary and three universities in Ottawa, Canada, completed a BSc in Human Biology (Guelph, 1988), a BA and MA in personality psychology (Carleton, 1992, 1994). His PhD in social-personality psychology (Waterloo, 1998), which earned the international J. S. Tanaka Award for best dissertation in the field of personality psychology. Since a brief postdoctoral fellowship at Northwestern University, McGregor has been an assistant and associate professor at York University in Toronto. His research on uncertainty, self-identity, and zealous extremism is funded by the Social Sciences and Humanities Research Council of Canada.

Amy H. Peterman received her PhD in clinical psychology from the University of Pittsburgh, then completed a postdoctoral fellowship in psychosocial oncology at Rush-Presbyterian-St. Luke's Medical Center (RPSLMC) in Chicago. After spending another year as a junior faculty member at RPSLMC, she moved to Evanston Hospital and Northwestern University Medical School where she spent 8 years conducting research on quality of life, coping, and goal interference and attainment in people with cancer and chronic neurological conditions. She was also an active psychotherapist specializing in this area. Recently, Peterman moved to the University of North Carolina at Charlotte where she is an associate professor of psychology and teaches in the newly initiated PhD program in health psychology. Her research into the personal project pursuit of people with cancer will continue in this new venue. If asked to name her most meaningful project, she would list "nurturing relationships with my husband, my 5-year-old daughter, my 2-year-old son, and our two cats."

Susan D. Phillips is a professor and director of the School of Public Policy and Administration at Carleton University in Ottawa, Canada. She is also a Senior Academic Fellow with the Canada School of Public Service and Senior Research Scholar with the Centre for Voluntary Sector Research and Development, located in Ottawa. Phillips has published extensively in the areas of citizen engagement, social movements, public policy and the nonprofit sector, and urban governance. She has served as an Associate Editor of *Canadian Public Policy*, an editor of *How Ottawa Spends* (an annual review of public policy), and a member of the editorial board of the *Philanthropist*. Her interest in PPA began with its application in studying women's social movement organizations for her doctoral dissertation in political science. That interest continues not only to be lived vicariously through her husband, Brian R. Little, but in joint research with him on public sector management and volunteerism. Their joint research on gender and management using PPA has been funded by the Social Sciences and Humanities Research Council of Canada and on volunteerism by the Canada Volunteerism Initiative. Needless to say, "mine," "yours," and "our" projects have a particular resonance in her household.

Michaela Riediger received her PhD in psychology in 2001 at the Free University Berlin, under the mentorship of Professors Alexandra Freund and Paul Baltes. She is currently a research scientist at the Center for Lifespan Development of the Max Planck Institute for Human Development, Berlin, Germany. Her work focuses on the investigation of developmental-regulatory functions of intentional and nonintentional motivational processes in various phases of adulthood.

Katariina Salmela-Aro is a professor of psychology at the Department of Psychology, University of Jyväskylä, Finland. She received her PhD in personal projects and subjective well-being from the University of Helsinki, Finland, and was a postdoctoral fellow at the Max Planck Institute in Berlin, Germany. Salmela-Aro belongs to the Academy of Finland's Centre of Excellence in Motivation and Learning, and is a fellow at the Helsinki University Collegium for Advanced Studies in Finland and at the Centre for Human Development and Well-Being at the City University of London. She is an associate editor of the *European Psychologist* and *Psykologia*. Her main interest focuses on motivation and well-being during life transitions.

Kennon M. Sheldon is a professor of social and personality psychology at the University of Missouri–Columbia. His primary research interests center on goals, motivation, psychological well-being, creativity, personality theory, and the resolution of social dilemmas. He is also active in the positive psychology movement, having received a $30,000 Templeton Prize in 2002 for his contributions to this emerging field. Sheldon has published two books in the last 3 years: *Motivating Health: Applying Self-Determination Theory in the Clinic* (Yale University Press, 2003, with Geoff Williams and Thomas Joiner), and *Optimal Human Being: An Integrated Multilevel Perspective* (Lawrence Erlbaum Associates, 2004). Sheldon is married with three children, and pursues stained-glass making, backpacking, river-running, and tennis in his spare time.

Bettina S. Wiese received her diploma in psychology from the University of Marburg, Germany, in 1994. Until 1999, she was a doctoral student at the Center for Lifespan Development, Max Planck Institute for Human Development, Berlin. In 1995, she received the Georg-Sieber Award for Applied Psychology. After completing her PhD on goal structures in the work and family domains at the Free University of Berlin in 1999, she worked for 2 years as a research scientist at the Darmstadt University of Technology, Germany, where she was a member of an interdisciplinary research group on product development and marketing. Between 2001 and 2005, she had a senior research scientist position in industrial and organizational psychology at the University of Koblenz-Landau, Germany. In 2005, Wiese accepted her current position as an assistant professor of applied psychology at the University of Zurich, Switzerland. Her main research interests concern processes of successful self-regulation in adulthood with a focus on proactive career development as well as the interplay of work and family.

Preface

The chapters in this volume examine the nature of personal goals and personal projects and how they contribute to well-being. The volume explores both the internal and external dynamics of personal project pursuit and should be of interest to researchers in personality and developmental science as well as in applied fields concerned with human flourishing.

The volume was originally intended to bring into convergence two research perspectives that had run along parallel lines for several years. One of these perspectives, personal projects analysis (Little, 1983), was developed within the field of personality psychology. Personal projects are extended sets of personally salient action, and are a constitutive feature of everyday lives, ranging from the annoying tasks of any given Tuesday to the overarching commitments of a lifetime. They were proposed as an integrative unit of analysis for studying individuals in context, and empirical studies over two decades have demonstrated that the content, structure, and dynamics of personal projects are intimately linked to human well-being (Little, 1989, 1999).

The other perspective, the study of personal goals, emerged primarily from developmental psychology (e.g., Salmela-Aro, 1992). Whereas personal projects research was largely based in North America, much of the personal goals research drew on the long and distinguished tradition of goal research in Europe (e.g., Heckhausen, 1989/1991; Heckhausen & Heckhausen, in press) although it has more recently assumed an important place in North American personality psychology. In a series of international workshops and symposia, we began to explore the linkages between these two research traditions. This volume contains chapters that emerged from these intellectual exchanges in Ottawa, Helsinki, and Berlin.

As we began to read and critique each other's research it soon became clear that, apart from some terminological subtleties and different intellectual lineages, research programs on personal projects and on goals are largely exploring the same phenomena, albeit from slightly different angles. Essentially, personal projects are goal-directed actions in context, and so the study of personal goals and project pursuit are examining overlapping aspects of the same temporally extended phenomenon. Personal projects have an internal face: the content, structure and dynamics of goals and aspirations. They also have an external face: the social ecological context in which pursuits are enacted, fostered, or frustrated. The chapters of this volume are organized primarily around these two divisions—the internal and external faces of projects or goals—although we recognize, and indeed emphasize throughout, that they are intimately linked.

Part I sets the stage for the volume by introducing the theoretical background of personal projects research and providing a guide to its methodology. Although there now exist several reviews of this perspective (Little, 1987, 1993) the two chapters of this section make a distinctive contribution. Little (chap. 1), provides a selective, idiosyncratic account of how personal projects analysis came into being. This chapter takes the reader through the different academic behavior settings, from the early 1970s to the present, that prompted the development of personal projects as units of analysis. It traces the roots of personal projects to Murray's personology, to Kelly's personal construct theory, and to social ecological concerns, particularly in a life span context. It also provides a comparative analysis of goals, projects, and other analytic units and argues that each has a distinctive role to play in studying human personality and development. Little and Gee (chap. 2) present the first published introduction to personal project analysis (PPA) methodology. Although not intended to be a formal manual, the chapter takes the reader through the process of research decisions that need to be addressed when doing PPA and is designed to help individuals unfamiliar with the methodology to adapt it for their particular research needs. A central theme of the chapter is the modular and flexible nature of the methodology. PPA is not a fixed test; rather, it provides a flexible framework for and strong encouragement of creative methodological explorations of personal projects.

In Part II the internal dynamics of goal formulation and project inception are examined. Elliot and Friedman (chap. 3) start with one of the most fundamental features of goal pursuit, whether it involves approaching or avoiding a goal object, and present a comprehensive hierarchical model of approach and avoidance with an emphasis on how these forces play out in the pursuit of personal goals. Riediger (chap. 4) tackles the fact that, during their daily lives, individuals are pursuing multiple goals and projects, some of which may be in conflict. She reviews key methodological issues in examining how goal interference and facilitation have an impact on well-being across the life span. Chambers (chap. 5) explores how the linguistic features of how we talk about our projects influence their successful or unsuccessful pursuit. The final chapter in Part II, by McGregor (chap. 6), examines the roots of passionate project pursuit, proposing that the origins of such pursuits are largely compensatory convictions occasioned by existential uncertainty. Together, these chapters illustrate the competing demands that characterize the internal dynamics of project pursuit. They also inform us, sometimes implicitly, sometimes explicitly, about how the internal dynamics of project pursuit can be sustained and can contribute to human flourishing. We learn about the value of engaging approach rather than avoidance goals, promoting facilitation among potentially competing goals, phrasing projects as direct actions rather than oblique possibilities, and having sufficient existential certainty that one's passionate projects engender flourishing rather than fanaticism.

Part III presents chapters that place relatively more emphasis on the outer ecology within which goals and projects are pursued and that identify how this ecology enables and constrains the processes and outcomes of goal and project pursuit. The part begins at the dyadic level, proceeds through organizations, and concludes with broader life-span pursuits in sociocultural perspective. Salmela-Aro and Little (chap. 7) examine how personal projects both affect and reflect interpersonal relationships, reviewing different approaches to understanding the relational aspects of project pursuit, and their contributions to human well-being. Grant, Little, and Phillips (chap. 8) focus on projects in the workplace. They distinguish the project from the traditional task and job units of work that are typically studied in organizational research, and discuss the utility of projects in predicting, understanding, explaining, and enhancing well-being in organizational settings. Freund (chap.

9) takes a life span perspective on goal pursuit, exploring how the interplay of personal goals and age-related expectations affects the course of individual development. The final chapter in Part III, by Brandstätter and Lalonde (chap. 10), investigates the link between personal projects and the construction of individual and cultural identities, utilizing personal projects as a vehicle for explaining variations in individual and cultural continuity and change. Together, these chapters accentuate the role that social ecologies play in shaping the nature, forms, and outcomes of personal projects. They highlight the importance of interpersonal relationships, organizational contexts, societal expectations, and cultural narratives in affecting the pursuit of personal projects. They also suggest several pathways for orchestrating the external social ecological contexts of project pursuit to enable and enhance human flourishing: forming mutually supportive projects with others, redesigning projects rather than jobs in the workplace, integrating personal projects with cultural and social expectations, and promoting continuity in core cultural projects.

Whereas the previous two parts emphasized the internal and external dynamics of project pursuit with reference to their implications for well-being, Part IV focuses squarely on the role of project pursuit in human well-being. Wiese (chap. 11) challenges the presumption that successful personal goal pursuit is conducive to well-being, identifying several moderating variables that strengthen and weaken this relationship. Peterman and Lecci (chap. 12) review the relevance of personal projects to health and illness, examining how projects can be hindered by, but also leveraged to ameliorate maladaptive health beliefs. Sheldon (chap. 13) considers how integration of personal goals with multiple levels of personality—psychological needs, traits, identities, social relations, and culture—may enhance human well-being. Little and Joseph (chap. 14) propose that "acting out of character," behaving in discord with one's biological, socially learned, or idiosyncratic natures in the service of core personal projects, may sustain meaning but exact costs for well-being. Together, these chapters underscore the breadth and depth of linkages between personal projects and human well-being. They show how personal projects can serve to both illuminate and enhance the varieties of human flourishing, from psychological well-being to physical health. These chapters also make a more subtle point: The sustainable pursuit of personal projects is contingent on the vitality of the contexts within which lives develop, an area that moves us, ready or not, into the domain of philosophical analysis.

In Part V, the final part, Little and Grant (chap. 15) provide a retrospective account of the central themes of the volume. Prospectively, they discuss the relevance of the volume to contemporary research in psychology and related areas. They conclude with an analysis of human flourishing and how it is related to the sustainable pursuit of core projects. In a reflexive mode, they discuss the sustainable pursuit of PPA and related methodologies in helping us understand the human predicament.

ACKNOWLEDGMENTS

We would like to acknowledge the support of those who contributed in imp0ortant ways to the project culminating in this book.

We wish to acknowledge the generative influence of Jari-Erik Nurmi, University of Jyväskylä, whose enthusiasm for bringing together personal projects and goal researchers was critical to the inception of this project. Only the vagaries of project conflict and temporal ecology prevented him from being a coeditor of the book.

We would also like to acknowledge the exceptional research assistance of Deanna Whelan at Carleton University, whose superb combination of technical and social skills were critical to our being able to say "Project completed."

Jennifer Thake and Tania Morrison provided enthusiastic support just when it was needed. Adam Grand was unstinting in his assistance at all stages of the book. The Social Sciences and Humanities Research Council of Canada provided assistance when the study of personal projects was a strange new creature and we are grateful for their support over the years.

We also acknowledge and appreciate the institutional support received from Carleton University, Harvard University and the Radcliffe Institute for Advanced Study, and the University of Helsinki and University of Jyväskylä.

To the authors of the chapters of *Personal Project Pursuit* we extend our warm thanks for their collegiality and for their patience with demanding editors.

Finally, we would like to thank the participants in the studies that are reported in this book. As the reader will see, we accord them a central role in the process of creative research. Literally, without their commitment and cooperation we would have had nothing to write about.

To all, here's to your core projects and their sustainable pursuit. Cheers!

REFERENCES

Heckhausen, H. (1991). *Motivation and action* (P. K. Leppman, Trans.). New York: Springer. (Original work published 1989)

Heckhausen, J. & Heckhausen, H. (in press). Motivation and action. New York: Cambridge University Press.

Little, B. R. (1983). Personal projects: A rationale and method for investigation. *Environment and Behavior, 15,* 273–309.

Little, B. R. (1987). Personal projects and fuzzy selves: Aspects of self-identity in adolescence. In T. Honess & K. Yardley (Eds.), *Self and identity: Perspectives across the life span* (pp. 230–245). London: Routledge & Kegan Paul.

Little, B. R. (1989). Personal projects analysis: Trivial pursuits, magnificent obsessions and the search for coherence. In D. M. Buss & N. Cantor (Eds.), *Personality psychology: Recent trends and emerging directions* (pp. 15–31). New York: Springer-Verlag.

Little, B. R. (1993). Personal projects and the distributed self: Aspects of a conative psychology. In J. M. Suls (Ed.), *The self in social perspective: Psychological perspectives on the self* (Vol. 4, pp. 157–185). Hillsdale, NJ: Lawrence Erlbaum Associates.

Little, B. R. (1999). Personality and motivation: Personal action and the conative evolution. In L. A. Pervin & O. P. John (Eds.), *Handbook of personality: Theory and research* (2nd ed., pp. 501–524). New York: Guilford.

Salmela-Aro, K. (1992). Struggling with self: The personal projects of students seeking psychological counseling. *Scandinavian Journal of Psychology, 33,* 330–338.

I

Personal Project Pursuit: Theoretical and Methodological Foundations

1

Prompt and Circumstance: The Generative Contexts of Personal Projects Analysis

Brian R. Little

I want to discuss the circumstances that prompted the development of personal projects analysis as a line of inquiry and how these influences shaped this book. In a sense I want to examine the personal projects underlying personal projects, but how best to go about this? I could summarize the theoretical and empirical articles written over the past three decades, but that would be redundant with published reviews on how the concept of personal projects applies to areas such as personality and environment (Little, 1983, 1987b, 2000a), life-span development (Little, 1987a, 1999a), studies of the self and identity (Little, 1993), and clinical diagnosis and counseling (Little & Chambers, 2000, 2004). Alternatively, I could reconstruct a chronology of the orderly sequence through which the concept, beginning in the late 1960s, developed over the years, framing it as the inexorable progression of a compelling logic. However, that would be misleading. In reality, as with many protracted intellectual endeavors, the development of projects analysis and the coming together of this volume were, in many ways, the products of fortuitous prompts, chance encounters, productive misunderstandings, and inchoate ideas wrestled into coherence, sometimes decades after their initial impetus. So another type of introduction is required, one that has not been written before but that provides a sequential and reasonably coherent account of the personal projects perspective.[1]

What follows, therefore, is a highly selective recounting of the generative contexts that shaped the development of personal projects analysis and consequently this volume. Because the contexts that stimulate and sustain projects are a core focus of the personal projects approach to studying lives, this seems an appropriately reflexive way to proceed (Bannister, 1966). Also, my students inform me that this way of telling the story gives them an inside feel for what our research is all about. Writing the chapter from this perspective also allows me to acknowledge influences that have shaped my research over the years. These include fortuitous events, evocative institutions, and stimulating individuals. Both goodwill and good luck figure in the story.[2]

The chapter is in two sections. The opening section is an idiosyncratic account of the roots of the personal projects perspective in which I revisit the scholarly settings and generative contexts that stimulated its core concepts. Although there is a certain degree of arbitrariness and potential distortion in reconstructing the early influences on my work, particularly errors of omission, I have tried to render the account with fidelity. The second section gathers up these cumulative concepts and gives them a more formal treatment. I define and lay out the central notions of the personal projects perspective and the social ecological framework that, together, inform aspects of this book. I give particular attention to an enduring theme throughout my work over the years and developed again in many of the following chapters—how personal projects play a pivotal role in human well-being and flourishing. I also note

---

[1]It may be helpful at the outset to clarify our use and variations of terms referring to personal projects, personal projects analysis, and personal projects perspective. We see *personal projects* as the unit of analysis in our research. Occasionally, the term *projects* is used, particularly when talking about project pursuit or project conflict and in these cases *personal* is implicit. We have traditionally used the term *personal projects analysis* (PPA) to refer to our methodology. However, in this volume we occasionally use the term as a more generic one for both theoretical and methodological considerations regarding personal projects. We reserve the abbreviation PPA for strictly methodological aspects of our work. We also use the terms *personal projects perspective* and *project analytic perspective* when addressing theoretical issues where we are drawing comparisons with other major theoretical perspectives such as psychodynamic or trait perspectives. Our goal is to use terms precisely without being prolix. Additional terminological issues are introduced and clarified as needed.

[2]Of course, I have much more to tell about my life but that must wait for a more suitably intimate venue.

briefly the similarities and differences between personal projects and related units of analysis in personality and developmental science and other areas of research and practice. Finally, I stand back and, from a more synoptic vantage point, discern some patterns that have become clearer as the projects perspective has been adopted and adapted by others. In conclusion, I suggest some consequences that this still moving image has both for the study of lives and for attempts to enhance their vitality.

PERSONAL PROJECTS AS ANALYTIC UNITS: ROOTS, ROUTES, AND RANDOMNESS

The origins of research and theory on personal projects go back more than 30 years and involve several different intellectual influences. Some of these arose directly from my experiences in various scholarly institutions and behavior settings. Others were carried from setting to setting as enduring personal preferences, the most compelling of which has been an irrepressible desire to connect, link, and integrate diverse forms of inquiry: to rub ideas together and, particularly with highly combustible students, to create sparks and see what ensues.

Classical Personology: Snow Flurries, Murray, and Synoptic Visions

C. P. Snow's (1959) published Rede lecture on "The Two Cultures" had a major impact on me as an undergraduate in the early 1960s. Snow, a chemist and novelist, concluded that a growing gap between scientists and humanists was becoming unbridgeable and that the implications for society were ominous. I was struck by Snow's argument for the tension between the sciences and the humanities but even more by the acrimony that greeted the argument. After a few flurries of disagreement there was a blizzard of *ad hominem* abuse directed back at Snow, who was seen by some (e.g., Leavis, 1963) as unfit to pronounce on such matters: lacking, it was alleged, distinction in either domain. This seemed much more than an academic disagreement. It reflected fundamental differences in orientation, in committed preferences, in ideology, in preferred modes of knowing and communicating, and in core beliefs about the quality of life and lives. As I had strong interests in both the sciences and the humanities, I vacillated between them before eventually discovering psychology. I was hopeful that this could be a field in which the two cultures might be bridged and creative synergies between the sciences and the humanities might be achieved (Little, 1972, 2005).[3]

One day in the spring of 1961, I chanced upon a rather tattered copy of Henry A. Murray's (1938) *Explorations in Personality* in a shop in Victoria, British Columbia, and bought it for 25 cents. I was intrigued by how Murray's Psychological Clinic at Harvard had been engaged in the interdisciplinary analysis of human personality that directly met some of the challenges posed by Snow. In essence, Murray's vision was for a psychology that looked at individual personality from the perspective of many different researchers, working separately, who then came together in diagnostic councils or assessment panels and attempted to create an integrative picture of the person. It was the diversity of backgrounds of those who contributed to this assessment that was remarkable. They came from the entire spectrum of the academic and artistic community. Indeed, in the preface to the volume, Murray (1938) acknowledged both this diversity and the difficulties in finding a common language: "It is true that we never completely succeeded in merging our separate Ideologies. How could such a thing come to pass in a group composed of poets, physicists, sociologists, anthropologists, criminologists, physicians ...?" (p. xi). That he aspired at all to bring these different specialists to the table was audacious, although not surprising considering Murray's professional background. After undergraduate study in history, Murray went into medicine, practiced surgery, took a PhD in biochemistry, and achieved fame as a literary scholar, particularly for his research on Herman Melville. Here, clearly, was a person driving projects designed to confront and survive Snow storms. I would later come to believe bridging between the disciplines would require more than the bringing together of different specialists. It would require, as Murray's illustrious colleague at Harvard, Gordon Allport (1937, 1958) argued, appropriate units of analysis that facilitate interdisciplinary analysis. Nevertheless, Murray's integrative vision for what he called personology was to infuse my research for decades.[4]

---

[3]It was, of course, true that psychology itself was divided into a similar conflict of cultures between those adopting scientific and humanist orientations. Indeed, my earliest empirical research was on precisely those orientations (Little, 1972, 2005).

[4]Some contemporary scholars use the term *personality science* rather than personology. Both are characterized, as is cognitive science, by an intellectual reach extending from the life sciences to historical and narrative perspectives (Cervone & Mischel, 2002; Little, 2005).

Murray became best known for his multiform assessment approach, his weaving of Jungian unconscious themes into the field of personality and for the measurement of needs and corresponding environmental "press" in the study of motivation. Although this was fascinating, there was another aspect of his work that intrigued me more. Like Allport, Murray was uncomfortable with the reactive model that the stimulus–response theory of the day espoused. Instead, he posited that much of our behavior comprises what he called *serials,* temporally extended enterprises that typically involve acting on a concern, possibly setting it aside and returning to it until it was completed or abandoned. These sets of behavior make sense only through understanding the internally generated aspirations guiding their enactment. He described the nature of these stimulus-free pursuits as *proactive.*[5] Murray's concept of serials prompted me to speculate on how we might assess and explore these extended sets of personally salient action. However, that prompt lay dormant for a decade until I wrote my first article on a method for assessing "personal projects" (Little, 1983). That article began with an explicit acknowledgment of serials as a generative concept that had been essentially uncharted because, unlike many of Murray's other constructs, it lacked a compelling assessment instrument through which it could be explored.

Although I first met personology through reading Murray, my later exposure would be more direct, as a graduate student at the University of California at Berkeley. Here, at the Institute for Personality Assessment and Research (IPAR), the personological tradition was being vigorously extended under the leadership of Donald MacKinnon. This Harvard–Berkeley axis of personology would subsequently play a key role in the development of personal projects research, albeit one that unfolded in a rather peculiar and unexpected series of fortunate events.[6]

---

[5] The *Oxford English Dictionary* does not cite an earlier use of the term *proactive.* It is possible that Murray may have coined a term that became so popular as to be almost hackneyed within a few decades.

[6] The axis also included the Office of Strategic Services where, under Murray's direction, the Harvard Psychology Clinic procedures were adapted and expanded to include procedures for selecting individuals who would have the characteristics necessary to survive behind enemy lines in World War II. Robinson (1992) wrote an exceptionally rich history of Murray's life and the institutions he created.

George Kelly and the Partially Prepared Mind

In a fascinating article, Bandura (1982) examined the role that chance could play in the course of life development and on its relative neglect in psychological theories. He also explicitly discussed its relevance to the trajectory of academic careers, noting that two people, who just happened to sit next to each other at the convention where he first presented this idea, ended up getting married (to each other). The sequence of events leading to the unfolding of the personal projects perspective amply supports the influence of chance and fortuity in scholarly inquiry (see also Campbell, 1981).

At the time I was applying to graduate school I was convinced that neuropsychology was the route for me and I had been lucky enough, as an undergraduate at the University of Victoria in Canada, to be a research assistant in one of the first clinical neuropsychology laboratories focused primarily on children. I was attracted by the fun of helping design and build the equipment and calibrate the instruments for neuropsychological assessment and by the elegance of experimentation that the field required. That clinical neuropsychology could contribute to the amelioration of human suffering also mattered a lot. One day I was looking for the *Stereotaxic Atlas of the Brain* in the college library when I pulled down a misshelved copy of George Kelly's (1955) *Psychology of Personal Constructs*. It was a massive two-volume work on human personality. Having been at least partially prompted for "personality psychology" by reading Murray, I thought I would take a quick skim through Kelly. About 5 hours later and rather stiff from sitting squat-legged on the library floor, I was hooked. Kelly wrote as if he were sitting on the floor alongside me, chatting amicably with a fellow scientist, a stance that happened to reflect exactly Kelly's core assumption about the everyday people he studied (Bannister, 1966; Kelly, 1955).

Kelly's writing style was engaging and his content was iconoclastic. He held that most personality, clinical, and motivational theories were based on untenable assumptions. They assumed that people are primarily passive creatures, buffeted about by the vicissitudes of reinforcement or the prodding of unconscious forces. Kelly took a different view, which, although in the spirit of Allport and Murray, was more radical. He saw each person as a lay scientist who erects and tests hypotheses, revises them in the light of experience, and generally engages life in an anticipatory instead of reactive mode. The means through which individuals experience their worlds are personal constructs, essentially conceptual templates or goggles through which people idiosyncratically view the constantly changing contexts of daily life. Even emotional concerns could be addressed through invoking an individual's personal construct system: Anxiety is becoming aware that an event is outside the range of convenience of one's constructs; guilt is awareness of being dislodged from a core role construct; and hostility is the attempt to extort validation for a construct or hypothesis one already suspects has been disconfirmed.

My discovering Kelly as I did was most certainly a chance encounter, albeit one I was moved to pursue by having read Murray. Pasteur's dictum about chance favoring the prepared mind, or in my case the partially prompted one, continued to ring true, as another serendipitous event soon followed. Norah Carlsen, a faculty member, was looking for a research assistant to help her complete her doctoral dissertation on cognitive complexity as measured by Kelly's repertory grid technique. This time I was fully Pasteurized. I quickly devoured everything I could on measuring people's personal constructs, established contact with Kelly, began doing nonparametric factor analyses by hand, received copies of his Ohio State students' dissertations, and realized I was becoming a true personal construct theorist. I was also experiencing true cognitive dissonance because, while I was in the process of becoming a committed Kellian, I was busing to Berkeley to study brains.

Berkeley: Persons, Places, and Passion

Just a few days after I arrived at the University of California in 1964, the free speech movement began and a new era of activism was unleashed. It had a subtle and enduring influence on me. The campus radicals were viewed by some faculty (none, so far as I knew, in the Department of Psychology) as merely engaged in Oedipal struggles with the university patriarchy, a view I thought patently absurd. I became even more strongly committed to the solicitous but sophisticated Kellian stance toward explaining human conduct. This approach begins by giving initial credence to individuals' personal accounts of what they are doing. The eventual course of inquiry may well discover inconsistencies, distortions, and self-delusion, but attempts to directly solicit accounts of why students did not want to be "folded, mutilated, or bent" like mistreated computer cards seemed more constructive than dismissing their dissent as the mere eruption of primitive unconscious processes. Once again, just as with the reaction to Snow's two cultures argument, I realized that academic institutions and human personalities could collide with incredible force. Along with the political ferment, there was a confluence of intellectual forces that shaped the personal projects perspective in ways that, I realize in retrospect, were pivotal. Despite a lingering affinity for neuropsychology, and particularly the elegance of experimentation, both my commitment to a personal construct psychology and my reactions to the events swirling around the Berkeley campus inclined me toward personality psychology. I managed to convince the department to allow me to switch areas from Group A (experimental) to Group B (personality, social, developmental, and clinical psychology). I began to get firsthand exposure to both personality psychology and what would come to be called social ecology. Kenneth Craik, whose reputation as a creative young faculty member spread rapidly among the graduate students, not only offered the first graduate course in environmental psychology, but also through his affiliation with IPAR, introduced us to the West Coast version of the personological tradition. Craik exposed us to the vital relation between human conduct and its physical context, and to an appreciation of how both our natural and built environments had potentially profound and largely unexplored impacts on human well-being.

Although I had minimal direct contact with IPAR, I was assigned to be a teaching assistant for its Director, Donald MacKinnon, who as a student and colleague of Murray's had brought to Berkeley the same goal of integrative, synoptic inquiry as Murray had pursued at Harvard. I was exposed to both formal and anecdotal accounts of the challenges of studying exceptionally creative artists, scientists, and architects. IPAR's pioneering work on creativity and human flourishing was both scientifically rigorous and socially significant and it raised some fundamental issues about the nature and sustainability of audacious human pursuits (Barron, 1963).

I was particularly taken by the classic study of architects by IPAR staff (MacKinnon, 1962). The subjects in this study were "certified" creative individuals, those who had met stringent international standards for outstanding achievement in the design and completion of architectural works of enduring significance. They were invited to Berkeley to be studied with the diversity of methods that had become part of the Harvard–Berkeley assessment approach. There was an ingenious research design component to the IPAR study. One of two control groups comprised architects who practiced in the same firms as the highly creative architects. This provided a control for such factors as the type of firm, general socioeconomic status, and features of the city in which the practice was located. By the use of participant pseudonyms, assessors at IPAR were unaware of whether they were studying highly creative or not as creative individuals. The pattern of results was instructive. Highly creative architects were big picture people, socially skilled when required, but essentially asocial. They were complex, open to both positive and negative emotions and willing to express them. They were often, in fact, a royal pain.

Whereas the IPAR scholars were particularly interested in the ways in which highly creative individuals managed to balance the internal pressures and contradictions of their personalities, I was more interested in their relation to the control group of architects, who were more detail oriented, conscientious, and agreeable and were less chimerical than their creative peers. What fascinated me was the question of whether the creative projects that led to fame for the firm (or, at least, for its principals) could ever have been accomplished without the contributions and personality characteristics of both the creatives and the controls. The social ecology of creative projects in firms might turn out to be something similar to the dynamics of families, and I thought that would make an intriguing field study. However, that would have meant going to where the creative people were actually pursuing their projects, rather than paying their way to come to Berkeley.[7]

It was also clear that although IPAR was Murrayan to the core, it was the more psychodynamic insights of the personological perspective and the use of consensual judgments by assessment panels that received the greatest attention, not the serial-pursuing proactive person that would later figure in research on personal projects. The generative context of the Berkeley end of the Harvard–Berkeley axis, then, raised more questions than answers for me. However, the questions generated sparks for decades and continue to do so to this day.

Berkeley's psychology department afforded me the freedom to plot a highly individualistic course of study and research in which I tried to conjoin Kellian constructivism with a personological assessment orientation. This resulted in what I hoped was a constructive alternative to personal construct theory in which individuals were seen not as panoptic scientists, but as psychospecialists with channelized cognitive, affective, expressive, and behavioral orientations (Little, 1968, 1972). This

---

[7]I later found out that Craik had been doing precisely such a study as a participant observer in a San Francisco Bay Area architecture firm.

perspective, which I termed *specialization theory*, also allowed me to return to the Snow storms that had intrigued me as an undergraduate. At its most fundamental level, specialization theory postulated that differential orientation toward person and things underlay the antagonisms between scholars in the humanities and the sciences (Little, 1968, 1972, 2005). I was also getting empirical evidence that person and thing orientation were orthogonal constructs. Generalists (high on both) were shown to be more creative than those with other orientations. They could flexibly shift between construing persons and things and complex arrays of both in a personalistic or a physicalistic manner (Little, 1968, 1976a, 1976b).

Essentially what emerged from my training at Berkeley was an appreciation of the integrative power of the personological tradition and the necessity of incorporating contextual, social ecological features into the study of personality. More important still was a focus on human excellence, creativity, and flourishing and how these are related to features of both persons and the contexts in which their daily actions unfold. This was elegantly captured by one of the most creative of the researchers studying creativity at IPAR, Frank Barron, who, in the first chapter of his book, *Creativity and Psychological Health*, (Barron, 1963) wrote:

> A quick glance at a good psychological library is sufficient to indicate that psychologists have traditionally been much more interested in psychological illness than in psychological health ... . Just after World War II, however, a group of psychologists at the University of California, in reviewing what during the war they had learned at first hand of heroic reactions to terrible stress, decided that it was high time that psychology should take a look at the positive side of human nature and concern itself with unusual vitality in human beings rather than with disease. (pp. 1–2)

This view was very much part of the *Zeitgeist* of Berkeley in those days, as it is of the positive psychology movement today (Seligman & Csikszentmihalyi, 2000). It had two direct impacts on me. First, it convinced me not to become a clinical psychologist. Second, it stimulated me to develop concepts and instruments that could explain the sources of meaning that animate human lives. In short, I wanted to explore how people could muddle through as well as fall apart; how they could flourish as well as flounder.

Theodore R. Sarbin was already a legend at Berkeley in the 1960s and I was deeply fortunate to fall under his influence. He encouraged me to keep on with a constructivist Kellian perspective, not dissimilar to his own, and urged me to remember that human personality could be fruitfully conceived as role performance. It was literally decades later that I realized how those subtle Sarbinian promptings on the performative aspects of project pursuit would play out. Sarbin, recently returned from a sabbatical at Oxford University, also encouraged me to consider spending time at Oxford to work on sorting out some of the questions with which I was grappling at the time. I was particularly concerned with finding a unit of analysis that would incorporate both the microlevel concerns of daily life and the overarching issues of personal and societal flourishing.

I left Berkeley with my Kellian constructivism intact but with very strong contextualist and personological leanings. I was convinced that our pursuits, be they utterly mundane or boldly creative, are channeled through two systems of constraints and affordances: those arising from our internal personal systems and those arising from the social ecological systems of daily life. I needed time and space in which to construct a framework for a dynamic theory that would allow me to integrate these seemingly contrastive views. Well, that sounds rather grandiose. What I really needed was to escape the passionate intensity (and stimulus overload) of Berkeley and find a space for reflection. I needed what I would later come to call a restorative niche.

Oxford: Social and Statistical Interactions

Again, fortuitously, I was able to spend several years at Oxford University, an environment equally stimulating but rather less frenetic than Berkeley. I studied, and subsequently tutored and lectured in the Department of Experimental Psychology, where I affiliated with Michael Argyle's Social Skills Laboratory. Argyle's group was breaking new ground by looking at social behavior, including neurotic behavior, as involving learned and potentially trainable social skills rather than as the playing out of deeper forces that would require psychodynamic therapy (e.g., Argyle, 1969). Social skills analysis focused on the microlevel aspects of social interaction, such as displaying appropriate eye contact and taking turns in social exchanges, and presumed that, if the minutiae of skilled social performance could be identified, individuals could be trained to interact more effectively. Argyle often talked about social skills by invoking an automobile driving metaphor. People who some might consider neurotic were—like bad drivers—essentially lacking basic social skills. In their case, the deficit was not in driving off the road, but in putting off other people. They did not know when to signal, how to brake evenly, or how to merge with interpersonal traffic, and thus others found them odd, disturbing, and occasionally frightening. By identifying, typically with videotape analysis, the social performances that seemed problematic, people could be trained in these basic skills. The plight of sad and lonely lives might thereby be lessened or lifted. Social skills training proved to be highly successful and was rapidly incorporated into diverse fields of applied psychology (e.g., Argyle, Bryant, & Trower, 1974).

As at Berkeley, I played a rather peripheral and even somewhat contrarian role in the Social Skills group, although rituals of afternoon tea and warm collegiality made even a contrarian role extremely pleasant. I was encouraged to maintain my allegiance to both Kellian and Murrayan convictions and challenged to show their relevance to advancing the social skills program. When I was asked to present my views at the weekly colloquia I took Argyle's driving skills metaphor in a different direction, or rather, to a different level of analysis. Although I was intrigued by the varieties of social ineptitude and the clashes of interpersonal gears, I wanted to know the answer to another question: Where were people trying to get to in their interpersonal journeys? They may learn perfectly well how to coordinate the micromechanisms of social interaction, but be utterly lost with respect to a destination. Where were they going, and why? In essence, although I did not formally label it as such until 2 years later (Little, 1972), I wanted to know what their personal projects were. This middle level of analysis, between the microlevel exploration of social skills and the macrolevel design of flourishing communities, was a territory that intrigued me greatly and I began to crystallize my thinking about it during those years.

In the early 1970s, the Social Skills program formed a close collaborative relationship with Rom Harré, who, as a distinguished philosopher of science, was developing a challenging and controversial reconstruction of the philosophical foundations of social psychology. He was writing convincingly of the need to seek explanations of social conduct in the accounts individuals give of their reasons for action. He was a passionate advocate of "treating people for *scientific purposes* as if they were human beings" (Harré & Secord, 1972, p. 6), a conviction most congenial to a committed Canadian Kellian. This view of social creatures as agents and as collaborative partners convinced me that my more humble attempts to reconceptualize personality psychology along similar lines were not totally idiotic.

There was another influence operating at Oxford in the late 1960s and early 1970s that shaped the development of personal projects analysis. Part of the growing consensus among the Social Skills group was that much of social behavior could be attributed to the particular situation in which individuals were interacting rather than to the putative stable traits of personality they brought with them to the encounter. There was much excitement over the publication of Walter Mischel's (1968) *Personality and Assessment.* Mischel had been a student of Kelly's, and his attack on the inability of trait measures to predict social behavior was consistent with my growing interest in how situations "pulled" for various standard interpersonal responses irrespective of stable individual differences. It was also consistent, of course, with the Kellian view that individuals were actively construing their contexts and shifting their behaviors accordingly, rather than mindlessly manifesting their fixed traits.

I used Kellian repertory grids to explore this issue by asking individuals to rate what microlevel social behaviors they would enact in different social situations and then partitioned variance into that attributable to environments, to individuals, and to their interaction. In the terms of the day, the question was whether P(ersons), E(nvironments) or P × E interactions would account for most of the variance. The evidence provided strongest support for E effects and for P × E interactions (Argyle & Little, 1972). Argyle and I were very much aware that it would be easy to make the results come out in favor of P or E simply by making the individuals or environments studied more or less homogeneous. Getting middle-aged Druid triplets to appraise their social conduct when (a) contemplating in the forest, (b) being set on by damsels in a pub, or (c) just hanging out at Stonehenge would almost certainly yield a strong environmental effect. So sampling a diversity of respondents as well as situations seemed an essential next step. We were convinced also that these results would be influenced by culture, particularly when comparing Anglo-American individualist respondents with those from more collectivist cultures in which situations and formal roles were recognized as key determinants of one's actions. By using the same grid technique with students in Japan and England we were able to show that this was indeed the case. Japanese students were more likely to report having their microlevel social interactions influenced by the situation than were their English counterparts (Argyle, Shimoda, & Little, 1978).

In publishing these two articles, I found myself part of what ended up being the Great Trait Debate that dominated much of personality psychology for a decade. I had divided loyalties and was personally happy that a Kellian technique could show that both "Berkeley persons" and

"Oxford situations" needed to be taken into account when exploring people's behavior. In my tutorials I made sure the students read Mischel, but that they also read Craik's (1969) review of Mischel's book, entitled "Personality Unvanquished," in which the countervailing strengths of the personological paradigm were articulated. In response, my students urged me to read Oxford analytic philosophy in which similar issues were being debated in the subfields of the philosophy of action and moral philosophy. I did so, and much of my subsequent and continuing work on personal projects was shaped by an awareness and appreciation of parallel developments in classics and philosophy (e.g., Davidson, 1980; Lomasky, 1984; Nussbaum, 1994; Williams, 1981).

The study of abstract statistical interactions, partitioning variance into sources due to persons and situations, particularly in contrast with the observation of "live" people in social interactions, seemed problematic on two counts. First, there was a methodological concern. There was an arbitrariness regarding the type of situations that were being examined. We needed a more systematic way of determining the contextual encounters in which people were actually engaged. In essence, we needed samples of daily conduct and a rationale for the evocation or elicitation of those samples. We certainly needed a winnowing device that would enable us to sample a manageable but meaningful set of these contextual encounters (see Little & Gee, chap. 2, this volume).

Second, there was a more philosophical issue concerning where the causal lelers, if indeed they were causal, would be located when explaining the daily comings and goings of individuals. I could hear the echoes of both the Murrayan and Kellian influences clearly: The locus of explanation was to be found at the level of the individual person. The convergence of internal processes and external influences, of constructs and contexts, required a new unit of analysis. It would start by soliciting information at the individual, idiographic level, but then allow personality researchers to inductively aggregate the findings fro   that level to deal with equally important normative or nomothetic inquiries. As researchers gradually accumulated information about what people were up to, what they thought and felt about their pursuits, we would formulate theoretical propositions that would then help explain and anticipate empirical observations as yet unmet. The new unit would conjoin personal features and contextual features. The person features would range from relatively fixed traits and propensities to dynamically shifting personal constructs and goals; the contextual features would range from microlevel shifty eyes and shuffling feet to macrolevel pubs and public hearings. These "carrier units" would, in themselves, contain elements of persons and situations and would comprise goal-directed action in context. They would, in short, be personal projects (Little, 1972, 1976b, 1983), and I suspected that they would be a critical factor in determining whether lives were going well or miserably, whether they were cruising along or grinding to a halt.

Canada, Carleton, and the Social Ecology of Circumstance

In 1972, the late Peter Gzowski, a much loved Canadian journalist and radio host, held a contest to find the best Canadian equivalent of the American phrase, "As American as apple pie." The winning response, submitted by listener Heather Scott, was "As Canadian as possible under the circumstances." As a Canadian, I thought it splendid. It pithily summarized the perspicacity one needed when sleeping next to an elephant and it was an insightful comment on the interdependency of identity and circumstance.

It was precisely the blend of possibility and circumstance in the mid-1970s that animated my return home to Canada, identity in hand, for an extended period. Carleton University in Ottawa, the nation's capital, provided an inviting context in which personal projects analysis could develop and be integrated into a larger framework with implications for public policy, particularly in the areas of environmental, developmental, and health policy. As a new faculty member in developmental psychology, I started up the Social Ecology Laboratory (SEL) where we studied people in context so that pure research and policy-relevant research would develop in tandem.[8] Carleton's SEL was for years the center of research on personal projects, its methodological developments, and its applied pursuits. Much of this research is contained in the dozens of theses and dissertations completed by a committed and creative group of SELmates. Many of these studies are

---

[8]The term *social ecology* has referred to various intellectual enterprises over the years. Environmental psychology, ecological psychology and social and community psychology all were flourishing in the early 1970s and each explored key aspects of the impact of contextual systems on personal systems (Little, 1976a). At Carleton we were influenced by the social ecological framework of Moos (e.g., Moos & Insel, 1974), which took the most synoptic view of contextual influences, including aspects of the physical environment (both natural and built) as well as organizational, social, and cultural forces and their dynamic and reciprocal impact on people's pursuits. We also emphasized that biological process within individuals might also be regarded as part of the social ecological forces impacting them, requiring integration with external forces for the effective adaptation by the individual (Little, 1999b).

referred to in this volume and have been summarized extensively elsewhere (Little, 2000a, 2000c).[9]

From the outset, the SEL was concerned with conceptualizing and appraising subjective well-being and the quality of lives in a life-span developmental context (e.g., Little, 1988; Little & Ryan, 1979; Palys & Little, 1983). My students, colleagues, and I developed a social ecological framework for examining how biological, cultural, and environmental systems of influence impinge on the individual. The individual's core adaptive task was the integration and resolution of these disparate and, at times, competing demands (Little & Ryan, 1979). We assumed that adaptation was strongly influenced by age, cohort effects, and historical circumstance. Our programmatic research started with a simple social ecological path model depicted as Figure 1.1, but was expanded and revised, as we will see, in the light of research results and the need for new integrative concepts that addressed emerging theoretical problems. As shown in Figure 1.1, our initial research focused on well-being and competency as outcome measures, with both critically influenced by the content, structure, dynamics, and impact of personal projects. Benefits accruing to the project pursuer included both intrinsic pleasure with the project process and the sense of achievement when it was completed. Benefits to others and the surrounding eco-setting would derive from the accomplished project and the satisfied pursuer. Of course, to

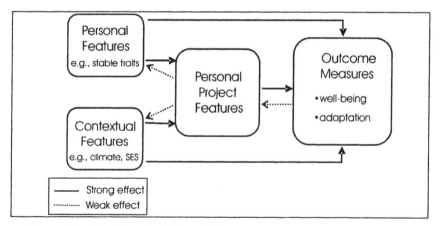

Figure 1.1.   Social ecological model.

[9]Summaries are also available on the Web at http://www.brianrlittle.com/research/index.htm under the heading "Annotated Bibliography."

the extent that project pursuit was unsuccessful or the project harmful or malevolent, at least one person, perhaps many, might be diminished.

We also included blocks of measurable variables that were expected to contribute to human well-being. Thus, person factors (e.g., traits, competencies, and other personal propensities) and environmental factors (e.g., the social, physical, and economic features of daily life) were posited as having direct effects on well-being and quality of life as well as indirect effects by operating through personal projects.

The SEL had a strong methodological focus. As well as developing modules for the study of personal projects (see Little & Gee, chap. 2, this volume), we developed measures for appraising quality of life, including measures of emotional, social, and physical well-being (Little, 1988). Although in the early stages of our research we regarded personal project features as predictors of well-being and flourishing, we gradually came to regard the status of one's project pursuits in themselves as constitutive of well-being (see also Omodei & Wearing, 1990).

We were committed to doing research that might enhance the quality of lives of people in diverse contexts. Many of our studies in the early days of that lab were on groups that formed small social ecologies, such as Newfoundland outport children, new Indochinese refugees to Canada, and even members of the (then) all-male Royal Canadian Mounted Police. We believed that studying such groups and whether they foundered, floundered, or flourished required microcontextual features to be taken into account. However, instead of having diverse researchers pooling their collaborative insights, as in the classic Harvard–Berkeley approach, we took a different approach. We developed appraisal dimensions for personal projects that drew on constructs used by scholars in many fields including sociology, linguistics, and economics. For example, respondents would generate their ongoing personal projects and appraise the extent to which they involved other people (and whom, specifically), or the extent to which their projects required English language skills, or the extent to which a given project conflicted with that of one's spouse. Many standard and ad hoc dimensions were developed for modular use in PPA; that is, they could be plugged in as needed to suit the research question. Our aspiration, from an applied perspective, was to make the cumulative stored holdings of this research available to policy analysts who would be able to determine which kinds of projects or appraisal dimensions were most conducive to flourishing among particular groups such as recent immigrants, older people in rural regions, or single parents living in cities.

At a theoretical level, personality psychology in the late 1970s was still in a state of disarray, with trait psychologists and situationists engaged in crossfire with little prospect of anything other than continued divisiveness in the field. In 1981, I organized a small retreat-like conference at a remote location in Canada's Gaspé Peninsula in which some of the key protagonists of the trait debate were brought together. Social policy analysts who were concerned with human development and quality-of-life issues also joined us. The hope again was to highlight some bridging concepts that might allow for commerce between factions—this time researchers who had a common interest in human personality but who were using seemingly incommensurate units of analysis.

One of the most promising of the emerging bridging units discussed and debated was that of the *act trend* (e.g., Buss & Craik, 1983). Craik, one of the participants, demonstrated how traits could be viewed as acts engaged in by individuals that were construed by self and others as prototypical of certain categories of trait concepts (e.g., the act of "cheering loudly at a hockey game" may be seen as prototypical of the trait of extraversion). However, these acts could also be seen as the contextual press of a situation or behavior setting (most fans cheer at hockey games). They could also be seen as a means through which a personal project could be accomplished (e.g., "show support for Katriona in her chosen sport"; Buss & Craik, 1983; Craik, 2000). It seemed evident that theorists of different orientations could benefit by adopting acts as units that provide for a common focus, although whether these alternative accounts were truly commensurable remains hotly disputed. At the very least, as I put it in a review chapter that was partially based on themes emerging from the retreat, theorists of different orientations were finally able "to get their acts, together" (Little, 1987b, p. 234).

At about the same time as some reconciliatory progress between trait and situational psychology was occurring through the study of acts and act trends, my own work on personal projects was being adopted and adapted by a new generation of highly creative researchers, particularly in the work of Cantor on "life tasks" and of Emmons on "personal strivings," each of which is discussed in a later section. Personal projects and related constructs comprised, as did acts, an integrative function, albeit at a somewhat higher level of molarity. The common element was a focus on action, and because each unit of analysis was explicitly based on the elicitation of idiosyncratic sets of action engaged in by individuals, I called these collectively *personal action construct* (PAC) units (Little, 1989). PAC units were conceived to be legitimate challengers to the growing influence of Big Five trait units (Hooker & McAdams, 2003; Little, 1987b, 1989).

My colleagues at Carleton over the years were generous in encouraging and shaping the course of personal projects analysis. In another context this will be acknowledged individually, but for purposes of this brief intellectual history, I must single out Lloyd Strickland, whose insights into the similarities among activity theory, action theory, and the emerging projects approach stimulated me to look beyond the Anglo/American/Canadian context of my research and examine its linkages with perspectives emanating from Europe. It just so happened that at the same time, a few people in Europe were doing the same thing in reverse (Salmela-Aro, 1992; Salmela-Aro & Nurmi, 1996).

To Helsinki and Back: Pursuing Personal Projects Analysis Abroad

I like to think that chance encounters in libraries play a continuing role in the evolution of personal projects theory and research. Just as I had accidentally discovered Kelly's work, Salmela-Aro, our coeditor and then an undergraduate student in ecology, discovered my 1983 *Environment and Behavior* article by chance in the architecture library at the University of Helsinki. Later, as a graduate student in psychology, she remembered the article and went on to adapt PPA methodology for her own research on developmental transitions in adolescents. Under the guidance of her doctoral advisor Nurmi, Salmela-Aro published a series of studies that drew attention both to the method of personal projects and its relevance to life-span developmental psychology (e.g., Salmela-Aro, 1992). I served as external examiner for the incipient Dr. Salmela-Aro in 1996. Although the Finnish term for an external examiner is the rather more ominous sounding "Opponent," there was clearly little to oppose. Indeed, it was clear that PPA could help illuminate developmental issues, particularly when studied longitudinally, and it, in turn, could be enriched by the concepts drawn from action and activity theory. When the first Symposium on Personal Projects was held in Ottawa in 1996, it featured the work of Salmela-Aro and the contributions of others in personality, social, and motivational psychology who had also adapted aspects of the methodology, including several of the authors of chapters in this volume (Elliot, Gee, Lecci, McGregor, and Sheldon).

I returned to Finland in 2001, when the Department of Psychology from the University of Helsinki invited a group of researchers to the second Symposium on Personal Projects. Besides the Finnish group of Nurmi, Salmela-Aro, and their students, there were researchers from the Max Planck Institute on Human Development in Berlin. Their research, deeply indebted to the work of Paul and Margaret Baltes (e.g., Baltes & Baltes, 1990), showed how the insights of a life-span developmental psychology could both inform and be informed by consideration of the "personal goals" and projects that people were pursuing at different points in their lives, particularly in periods of transition. This volume contains chapters by three of those scholars (Freund, Riediger, and Wiese).

On the last morning of the Helsinki Personal Projects Conference, the two "senior" scholars, Nurmi and myself, who respectively represented the European and North American perspectives, led an informal session that provided, without us realizing it at the time, the germ of this book. We were literally sketching the similarities among action theory, activity theory, goal theory, and personal projects analysis, and it was clear that there were potential synergies, points of contrast, and matters of considerable intellectual itch that needed scratching. Of particular interest to me was the strong life-span developmental focus of the European researchers. Despite the explicit life-span orientation of our own social ecological framework, PAC units had been explored primarily in the field of personality and social psychology.

One issue that needed to be worked out was terminological. Many researchers, including those at the Max Planck Institute, were studying personal goals. Are these essentially interchangeable with personal projects? Although the methodologies these researchers were using had been drawn from the early PPA research or from similar work on strivings, life tasks, or current concerns, clarification was needed on whether goal and project constructs are essentially interchangeable. I address this issue in the final section.

Soon after returning from Helsinki, it became clear that the time was ripe to put together a volume in which publications on project pursuit, now accelerating at a fast rate, might be gathered together. At the same time, and independently of our work, the study of goals and goal pursuit was flourishing in diverse areas of psychology and several important works had appeared that featured goal units (e.g., Ford, 1987; Karoly, 1993; Pervin, 1989). Still, there seemed something distinctive about what we were doing in the study of personal projects and, in between my first and second visits to Finland, I was granted a wonderful opportunity to engage in explorations in personality from a unique vantage point. I was invited to visit one of the earliest generative contexts of personal projects—except this time it was decidedly not tattered and did not cost me 25 cents.

Harvard, Radcliffe, and Coming Full Circle: Random Trips Back to the Roots

In 2000, I was selected to be in the first group of Fellows at the newly formed Radcliffe Institute for Advanced Study at Harvard University. The Fellows came from disciplines as diverse as anthropology and astronomy and included practicing artists and novelists as well as more traditional scholars. The variety of disciplines represented at the Institute was uncannily like that convened by Murray a few decades earlier and a few blocks away. The Institute was the ideal setting for someone long fascinated with building bridges between the arts and sciences (Little, 2005). It also provided an idyllic setting in which I could reflect on what we had learned about personal projects and social ecology over the past couple of decades. In particular, I was concerned with showing the mutual relevance of personal projects analysis and contemporary research in moral, ethical, and economic philosophy. The common element in these fields was the question of the quality of life, happiness, well-being, and, in its fullest expression, human flourishing. In my Fellows Lecture that year I proposed that my framework offered a novel perspective on these perennial questions of how to live well (Little, 2000b).

Each Fellow's presentation was followed the next day by a lunch at which there was lively and challenging commentary and questioning. I was fully prepared for one question: To what extent did I feel that psychologists had any special claim to prescribing how one ought to live one's life. My response was that as scientists, we could not adjudicate forms of the good. However we could provide a sophisticated evidentiary base that would inform those who do adjudicate such matters. I was not prepared, however, for some unexpected sparks. Given the diversity of talents gathered around the table, I casually mentioned some growing evidence from different researchers that novelists seem to have a shorter life span than those working in the visual or plastic arts and then speculated on how the sheer physicality of project pursuit in these areas might be intriguing to explore. I might have expected the novelists to be worried, perhaps even upset, but it was the sculptors and painters who got most exercised. They felt they deserved to win the early termination award! After all, they worked daily with toxic materials and often endured oppressive physical demands. They were at least as ready to die for their craft as those who only sit and type.

My home base while at the Radcliffe Institute was in the Henry A. Murray Center, which provided access to some of the archival treasures of the field of personality and developmental psychology, including Murray's own raw data from his monumental *Explorations in Personality*. The boxes were literally 10 strides away and I felt a strong connection with the intellectual tradition that first kindled my excitement in psychology 40 years earlier. It was exciting to discover, for example, that Murray had asked his participants about their "life goals" and the data were sitting in boxes unanalyzed because no framework for such analysis had then been developed. There was only one thing missing, and that was a group of students with whom to share the adventure.

Serendipity struck again, albeit in an unfortunate way for Professor Ellen Langer in the Psychology Department at Harvard. Halfway through my tenure at the Radcliffe Institute, I received a message that Ellen had slipped on some ice, smashed up her leg, and would have to cancel her undergraduate course in social psychology. The call came for an immediate replacement, and someone suggested me. The possibility of teaching in the department where Murray and Allport had created the foundations of academic personality psychology was very tempting and the Institute allowed me to teach while still attending to my Fellowship functions. Although I had taught social psychology for a number of years, I felt this offered an opportunity to bring in the personological tradition through its own back door. I warned the students that this would be a very different kind of social psychology course, but they came anyway. An unfortunate slip for Professor Langer was a most fortuitous trip for me back to the very roots of the tradition I had identified with so early in my career.

It turns out that Harvard needed someone to teach personality psychology the following term, and I was again fortunate to be in the right generative context at precisely the right moment. I began to teach personality each spring term, together with undergraduate and graduate courses in advanced methods in assessment and research design. I was also very fortunate to have a number of students express interest in the study of personal projects and, under the leadership of Adam Grant, we formed the Harvard Area Personal Projects Interest (HAPPI) group, comprising mainly Harvard undergraduate and graduate students in psychology. Although the group is now dispersed across many institutions, it continues to serve as a generative context in its own right, influencing the way we think about personal projects and expanding the areas in which it is being imaginatively applied.[10]

In my classes and with the HAPPI group I would challenge the students to have a go at the theoretical assumptions and methodological approach taken by personal projects analysis. One of the issues about which some students were concerned was what they took to be the tacit and erroneous assumption that people are consciously aware of all of their projects. In a department currently famous for studies of implicit attitudes, ironic processes, and "thin slices" of behavior, the thick textures of personal projects appeared literally too self-conscious and in need of integration with recent work on the experimental analysis of motivated goal pursuit. Although from the start there had been room for such influences on project pursuit, they had never been systematically explored and I agreed they should be. In turn, I think I convinced some of the students that an excellent starting point for the study of the individual life course was the solicitation of accounts by individuals of what they thought they were doing at present and in the future. The fruits of these exchanges are reflected in some of the chapters in this volume.

THE CUMULATIVE YIELD OF GENERATIVE CONTEXTS: PERSONAL PROJECTS AND SOCIAL ECOLOGY

The cumulative yield of these rather diverse generative contexts gave rise to a personal projects framework for theory, assessment, research, and application, as well as a more comprehensive social ecological framework, within which personal projects have a pivotal role.

Personal Projects: Integrative Middle-Level Units of Analysis

To guide us in this discussion, it is useful to offer a formal definition of personal projects and then to examine each term: Personal projects are extended sets of personally salient action in context.

---

[10]We also had members from the Harvard Business School and a PhD student from MIT's Media Lab. I am delighted to say that a recent addition to the HAPPI group is Ai-Li S. Chin, a student of Murray's during the heyday of the Harvard Psychological Clinic, whose insights on personal projects and aging will, I hope, stimulate another generation of students.

- Extended: Personal projects are not momentary behaviors, but pursuits that are typically extended temporally and spatially. Although they may be conceived, enacted, and completed in one uninterrupted sequence, this is rare. Projects are, like Murray's serials, actions that are extended—typically for hours, sometimes days, occasionally for decades.
- Sets: Personal projects are rarely a single action, but a group of interrelated ones. The connections among such functionally related actions might not be obvious to the outside viewer.
- Personally salient: The person pursuing the project is the definer of the project and therefore a Kellian approach to inquiry is required to discern the project that links the disparate actions of which it is comprised. Among the limitless array of possible actions in daily life, personal projects are those that stand out as particularly salient and idiosyncratically noteworthy. Their function is to attain, maintain, or avoid a state of affairs foreseen by the individual and to integrate the disparate demands impinging on persons.
- Action: Projects typically involve interactive commerce with the world outside the individual. Unlike mere behavior, however, project action is intentional, volitional, and conative; projects are the ends we are pursuing, as well as being the means to other ends.
- In context: Personal projects are enacted in a social ecology comprising physical, social, cultural, and historical contexts. Moreover, projects may create such contexts both as individual and collective pursuits.

The realization that contexts and projects are interdependent provides a natural segue to summarizing and emphasizing how each of the intellectual generative contexts I have been part of over the years has shaped the development of personal projects.

Linkages With Generative Contexts

Each of the generative contexts described earlier has contributed to the definition and subsequent elaboration of personal projects as units of analysis.

The personological tradition of Murray is reflected in the conception of personal projects as temporally extended sets of action. The integrative aspirations of that tradition are also given particular attention: Personal projects involve cognitive, affective, conative, and behavioral aspects of human conduct. The project of "caring for my mother," for example, may be a set of actions that we think about frequently, feel joyous or sad about at times, and strive to carry out through behavioral acts that will impact her. Indeed, the personal project as an analytic unit has been adopted by researchers and practitioners working from diverse explanatory frameworks, from the phenomenological link of projects with self (Little, 1993) to the Skinnerean analysis of projects in terms of the rewards and punishments associated with them at present and in the anticipated future (Ogilvie & Rose, 1995). Personal projects have also been adopted by researchers in diverse fields beyond psychology, including geography, political science, marketing, education, gerontology, and particularly in the occupational therapy and rehabilitation fields. The personological tradition's embracing of both biological and cultural sources of human motivation and conduct is also explicitly part of the project analytic perspective, represented by what we call the *biogenic* and *sociogenic* aspects of human natures; that is, those originating, respectively, from biologically rooted sources and those originating from social and cultural sources (see Little & Joseph, chap. 14, this volume).

The Kellian roots of personal projects are readily apparent and inspired my view of the *idiogenic* aspects of human natures, that is, actions generated by idiosyncratic construal and commitment. Another Kellian influence is the emphasis on the systemic nature of personal projects. With very rare exceptions, individuals are engaged with a set of personal projects that form a personal project system. That system may be one of mutually facilitating pursuits, a protracted exercise in project conflict and frustration, or essentially independent pursuits carried out in relative isolation from each other but still subject to the potential tensions created by a systemic force field. The dynamic balancing and management of project systems is produced and directed by individuals themselves; sometimes creatively, sometimes catastrophically, for self and others.

The Berkeley personological tradition has had several impacts on our research program over the years. First, we used assessment instruments that had been used at IPAR, such as Gough's California Psychological Inventory and his Adjective Check List, to measure stable aspects of personality that would be shown to predict aspects of project pursuit. Second, we incorporated IPAR's emphasis on creative achievement and vitality into our research framework, particularly its joint focus on the positive and the negative, the lighter and darker sides of human nature.

However, Berkeley's most comprehensive influence was the emphasis on the environmental aspects of the personological tradition. Theoretically, we postulated that personal projects arise as a result of the demands of both internal and environmental pressures, with the latter involving micro-, meso-, and macrolevel systems of influence (Little & Ryan, 1979). Thus the project of "caring for my mother" may entail the management of internal factors such as emotional ambivalence conjoined with genuine love (e.g., Emmons & King, 1988). However, it also requires management of the microlevel subtleties of the mother's mood and memory loss and the middle distance frustrations of the time pressures involved in visiting her. These, in turn, are embedded in macro societal and cultural forces that determine who is expected, if anyone, to care for a frail elderly person in need (Bronfenbrenner, 1979; Little & Ryan, 1979).

The social skills context, particularly with its emphasis on the capacity of individuals to change their patterns of social interaction, is directly reflected in what I refer to as the *tractability* of personal projects. Unlike most traits, personal projects can be changed. Either informally or through professional consultation, one can learn to reformulate one's projects, to scale down the overly ambitious ones, take on more estimable undertakings, attract greater support for important projects, or attune the system as a whole to be more sustainable. Similarly, one can create environments that generate both worthy and attainable project possibilities and that can forestall or mitigate unnecessary project conflict.

The dual focus on individual happiness and the larger social good and on singular projects and the social ecology was a constituent feature of the SEL at Carleton. Research using personal projects was aimed at understanding not only individuals, but also organizational and cultural phenomena such as women's groups and other voluntary associations, aboriginal communities, and large public-sector organizations (e.g., Little, 2000b; Phillips, 1992; Phillips, Little, & Goodine, 1997).

Although aware of the development of action and activity theory, as mentioned earlier, the direct sharing of experiences and research issues with colleagues in Finland and Germany reinforced the importance of life-span shifts in project pursuit and of looking at projects as the carriers of transitions across the life course. I saw particular value in linking research on personal projects with Baltes' selection–optimization–compensation model of development (e.g., Baltes & Baltes, 1990) and with Nurmi's (1992) research program on personal goals, future extension, and developmental transitions. Both of these linkages are given considerable attention in this book.

Finally, the return to the roots of personology and the adoption of personal projects by some of the students at Harvard provided a symbolic symmetry to the development of the projects perspective. What ended up being personal projects analysis had been originally prompted by Murray's call for a dynamic, temporally sensitive unit of analysis and by his enthusiastic advocacy for interdisciplinary collaboration. Revisiting the history of the development of personal projects analysis with the students at Harvard has been invigorating. It has reinforced my sense, shared by some others, that personality psychology is going through a period of remarkable growth and renewal and that a personality science is on the way to becoming an exciting core at the heart of university curricula (Little, 2005; Mischel, 2004).

However, there was an ironic twist in the students' arguments that a fully adequate project analytic perspective would need to address issues of unconscious processes, tacit goals, and implicit projects. In his preface to *Explorations in Personality,* Murray (1938) "confessed" that in exploring personality at the Harvard Psychological Clinic:

> We became so bent upon the search for covert springs of fantasy and action that we slighted necessarily some of the more obvious and common phases of behavior. This has resulted in a certain distortion which may seem great to those whose vivid experiences are limited to what is outwardly perceived and public, to what is rational and consciously intended. (p. xii)

Murray's tone suggests he was not particularly worried about this "certain distortion" and that those theorists capable of truly vivid experience will gladly sacrifice the study of mundane intentional pursuits for the mysteries of the deep. It is therefore ironic that Murray's rather neglected concept of *serials,* outwardly perceived action guided by consciously formulated goals, was the initial prompt underlying the study of personal projects. There is a further irony in that some of my students clearly felt that a tip back in the original Murrayan direction of covert, preconscious, and irrational sources of personality might be a wise move. As attested to by other chapters in this volume, the case can be made that both inner experience and outbound pursuits have key roles to play in an integrative personality and developmental science.

RELATION TO OTHER UNITS OF ANALYSIS:
PAC UNITS, GOAL UNITS, AND THE FOCUS
OF CONVENIENCE

It is important to recognize that the development of personal projects as analytic units proceeded over three decades. During this period, other units waxed, waned, and waxed again, trait units being the clearest example. In the next sections, I explore how personal projects relate to these alternative units of analysis. Personal constructs, not surprisingly, are the first port of call.

From Personal Constructs to Personal Projects

At the start of this chapter I suggested that the development of personal projects analysis was not simply the unfolding of an inexorable logic, but was partially the result of the fortuitous prompts and circumstances discussed in this chapter. However, there was an assumptive framework and methodological logic that did explicitly guide the project analytic perspective: Kelly's personal construct theory.

Although widely circulated since 1978 in draft form, the original detailed treatment of personal projects was not published until 1983. During its initial development I was exploring how to conjoin Kelly's method for studying inner systems with environmental planning methods for studying ecosystems. I was aware that Sartre had centered much of his existentialist philosophy on the concept of *le projet* and that projects were frequently invoked both in the engineering project management literature and in general political and social discourse. By qualifying it with the term *personal,* however, I was explicitly and directly extending the line of argument of personal construct theory to more rigorously incorporate the social, physical, and cultural contexts of lives.

For Kelly, all human processes are "channelized" by the personal constructs we erect to anticipate events. Hence our degrees of freedom in daily life are contingent on our capacity for flexible construal. However, the nature of the environment in personal construct theory was left relatively unexplored. Personal constructs tasted like Murrayan serials but without the fortifying ingredient of context. I tried to argue (not convincingly to some Kellians) that canalizations of the environment also played a critical role in the shaping of our lives (Little, 1972). By adopting personal projects as analytic units we could maintain a Kellian emphasis on internal constructive processes, but also explore the contextual forces that shape the course of action. Both internal and external systems were canal zones in development across the life course. Both could serve to satisfy or stultify our needs and desires, set limits on aspirations, or stimulate paths of audacious accomplishment. Both seemed necessary for a plausible theory of personality and human development.

I took something else from Kelly, who delighted in upending people's expectations. He began his *Nebraska Symposium on Motivation* chapter with this challenge: "There is something you all should know at the outset of this paper: I have no use for the concept of motivation" (Kelly, 1962, p. 83). He followed this up with several alternative titles for the distinguished lecture series including "What Is Everybody up to These Days" and "The Nebraska Symposium on *What Now*" (p. 83). Kelly's assumption was that humans, as active agents, are already in motion and that we need to understand the directions in which they are headed rather than how their motivational engines get turned on and revved up. I found this Georgian cutting of the Gordian knot of motivation a seductive if not totally compelling move. Looking back at his Nebraska Symposium article after many years, I realize how his alternative titles were eerily prescient of what personal project researchers are up to today. Alternatively, they may simply demonstrate how generative ideas insidiously slip into our adaptive unconscious, making us happily oblivious to how they influenced what we think is our own theorizing.

Given this intellectual provenance, it came as a genuine surprise to me when some researchers viewed personal projects research as being primarily a contribution to motivational psychology. Although delighted with the recognition of my work having some impact, it was rather like getting sustained applause for one's elbows. At first, I just did not get it. I did see personal projects as providing greater opportunity than either personal constructs or traits to examine conative and volitional aspects of human pursuit. This is true. Like Kelly, however, my assumption was that the conative, cognitive, affective, and behavioral aspects of human conduct were intertwined and that, to capture this interconnectedness, it would be helpful to extend the range of convenience of personal constructs to include action and context—in other words to work with personal projects as the focal unit. Functionally, personal projects are adaptive ways to integrate diverse biogenic and sociogenic demands through idiogenic choice and action. Motivation was implied by, indeed constitutive of, such choice and action. However, as with Kelly, it is not my focus. Rather, that focal concern is personal action in context.

While I was developing personal projects as units that could integrate the Kellian and contextual perspectives, it turned out that other theorists were working along very similar lines. The time was ripe for the emergence of new units of analysis that would address issues for which conventional units were not well suited.

Klinger's (1975, 1977) concept of *current concerns,* for example, was an important new unit of analysis that emerged independently, but roughly contemporaneously with personal projects analysis. Current concerns are launched when commitments are made and they guide attention, both explicitly and unconsciously, to cues that are associated with such commitments. Klinger's work was particularly strong in encouraging both questionnaire-type studies and experimental methods to examine processes relating to personality and clinical issues. The linkages between personal projects and current concerns have been recently reviewed (Little & Chambers, 2000, 2004). As current concerns directed attention to the subtle internal dynamics of goal pursuit, other units were emerging that placed more of an emphasis on personal action.

PAC Units: Personal Projects, Personal Strivings, and Life Tasks

Shortly after the publication of the 1983 paper on personal projects, the methodology was adapted for use in two highly influential and productive research programs. Cantor's unit of "life tasks" was designed to examine how daily pursuits reflected normative, age-graded societal expectations (Cantor & Kihlstrom, 1987; Cantor, Norem, Niedenthal, Langston, & Brower, 1987). In Cantor's early research, individuals were given the standard personal projects procedure and then asked to align as many projects as they could with normative life tasks for their particular setting. For example, university students were postulated as having life tasks such as becoming independent from parents, making friends, and doing well academically. The students' appraisals of these life tasks and the subtleties of their timing were reliably linked to successful adaptation and the transition through university (e.g., Cantor & Fleeson, 1994; Cantor et al., 1987; Zirkel & Cantor, 1990).

Emmons (1986) adapted aspects of both personal projects and current concerns research and methodology to develop his concept of personal strivings. *Personal strivings* are what one is typically trying to do in daily pursuits. Again, an extremely productive research program developed around this unit, with appraisals of one's strivings predicting both psychological and physical well-being and providing a distinctive approach to some of the overarching concerns of human lives (Emmons, 1999).

By the late 1980s, personal projects, life tasks, and personal strivings were beginning to be recognized as a new and distinctive family of analytic units for personality and developmental research, sharing a focus on personal action. I called these units of analysis PAC units (Little, 1989). Their distinctive features become clear when compared with two other analytic units that were enjoying rising popularity in the 1980s, trait and narrative units. Relative to trait units, PAC units are middle-level units of analysis, phrased in the idiosyncratic language of the person being assessed. They are sensitive to contextual features and are explicitly regarded as dynamic rather than static units. If traits are more concerned with the "having" side of personality, PAC units are concerned with what people are doing in daily life (Cantor, 1990). Narrative units, those derived from life stories, share a number of features with PAC units, but are particularly effective at capturing the self-reflective and coherence-making accounts that focus on the "being" aspects of personal identity (Little, 2001; McAdams, 1993; Runyan, 1982; Sarbin, 1986).

Calling PAC units "middle level" demands further explication about different levels of research in personality psychology (Hooker, 2002; Little, 1987b; McAdams & Emmons, 1995). McAdams (1995, 1996) suggested a three-level structure to the field, with trait units at the first level, personal concerns (PAC units, in my terms) at the second level, and narrative units at the top. I suggested that some clarity might be given to McAdams's hierarchical model by looking at it as a building with three tiers, with the second level having PAC units as the central load-bearing unit (Little, 1996). In conferences during those years I would present a "House of Personality" in which the three tiers were depicted as floors in a complex edifice housing personality psychologists and their close relatives. A special variant of that graph, created for a festschrift given in honor of Theodore Sarbin in Berkeley, appears in Figure 1.2.

It should be emphasized that I do not see the house as representing different levels of personality; rather, I see it as graphically portraying the different levels of analysis employed by psychologists studying personality and development. There is an important difference. Researchers form close epistemic communities that may often be isolated from

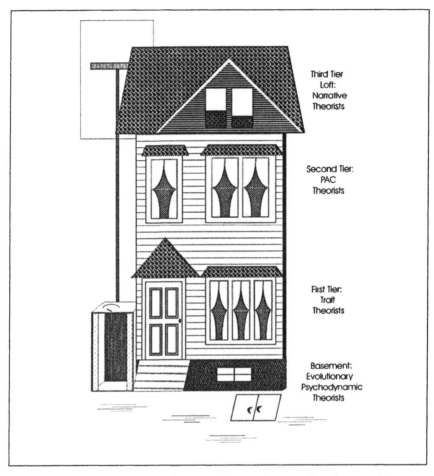

Figure 1.2. "The House of Personality" in honor of Sarbin's uplifting discourse.

one another even though they are ultimately concerned with understanding the same complex phenomenon. Alternative metaphors of the relationship between different types of personality psychologists that were being discussed in those days included villages, five-ring circuses, and war zones. In contrast to these, the House was meant to deal with the issue that is the dominant theme of this chapter: the ways in which scientists, at all levels of the structure, could communicate with one another. In philosophical terms, the House is an epistemological visual aid, not an ontological proposition.

I felt the house metaphor helped situate the different approaches to personality that were influential in the field and, in the spirit of advocacy for the folks on the second floor, I thought it displayed some of the benefits of adopting PAC units. For example, the second-floor researchers were within easy reach of constructs drawn from both trait theorists on the first floor and narrative theorists on the top floor. They are influenced by traits and constitute a fundamental element of life narratives. I also felt it important to put in a basement, perhaps more a root cellar, where both evolutionary and psychodynamic theorists could be seen carrying out their distinctive work.

When Sarbin heard that I had put him up in the loft he requested that we at least provide an elevator for him! I immediately complied, realizing that this was not just a whimsical personal touch, but also a wise metaphor for collegial communication. By using constructs that allow us to connect with and enter into the domain of researchers on different levels we can literally elevate our discourse. I admit to contriving to get entrance to the outside elevator only from the second floor, but my colleagues would not let me get away with that, even metaphorically.

Unpacking PAC Units: Single or Triple Visions? In a detailed and thoughtful analysis of the emergence of PAC units, Krahé (1992) concluded, "it has become clear that there is a significant degree of both conceptual and methodological overlap between personal strivings, life tasks, and personal projects that raises the question of the distinctive qualities of each approach" (p. 191).

This is an important question, and it will be helpful, in answering it, to invoke again Kelly's concept of the "focus and range of convenience" of explanatory constructs. The focus of convenience is where a construct has its highest fidelity and acuity; the range of convenience is the extent of phenomena to which the construct might effectively be deployed. I believe that each of these PAC units has a somewhat different range and focus of convenience, although personal projects has a broader range of convenience than other PAC units. The range of convenience of PAC units could be seen as aligned along a spectrum, at one end of which are constructs focused on internal processes and self-regulatory tendencies and at the other end with external affordances and constraints.

Personal strivings, under this view, are located more toward the internal end of the PAC spectrum; life tasks are located more on the external end. Personal projects occupy a middle position. Although there are environmental contexts within which strivings are enacted, these are given less attention than the internal, motivational, and self-defining features of the strivings. Such external concerns fall within the range of convenience of the construct but are not its focus. Similarly, although there are internal, self-regulatory aspects to life-task pursuit, the locus of tasks is primarily external; the sanctions for being on time with them or undertaking them in the correct order, and of one's relative success in completing them are all primarily matters of cultural and social expectations and life-course developmental pressures (J. Heckhausen, 1999).

Personal projects are middle-level units both vertically (as are all PAC units) when viewed as a house of personality, but also horizontally along the continuum of other PAC units. Personal projects are designed to elicit the ongoing goals and actions of individuals without priming or selecting for their typicality regarding the self or their normative matching of societal expectations. To be sure, there is some overlap in the content of personal projects with other PAC units. We regularly see personal projects generated by respondents that could be regarded as personal strivings or life tasks (or personal goals, current concerns, self-guides, or even evolutionary tactics). Indeed, two of the standard rating dimensions of personal projects, self-identity (to what extent this project is "really" you—a personal trademark) and others' view (to what extent this project is seen as important by other people), are ways of accessing features very similar to strivings and life tasks.

In noting the proliferation of projects, tasks, and strivings as units of analysis, Krahé (1992) was essentially asking whether a generic unit with an extensive range of convenience may provide for greater parsimony. She suggested that goals might be such a unifying concept, if such were needed. My own position is that we need the triple vision afforded by each of these units, if only because their foci of convenience allow a more detailed and differentiated analysis of particular types of research issues. However, it is helpful, theoretically, to employ units such as personal projects that have a focus of convenience at the tipping point between internal, self-regulatory processes and external ecological forces and that can serve as a point of convergence and integration for other PAC units (Little, 1996).

Goal Units: Helsinki Redux

Remember Helsinki? I mentioned that at our Personal Projects Conference where we grappled with the terms personal projects and personal goals. Are these simply different names for the same concept or are goals, like tasks and strivings, differentiable from projects in ways that matter? Although adopting or adapting personal project methodology, some of the European researchers at the Helsinki conference as well as some of the authors in this volume have a preference for the term personal goals and see them as theoretical equivalents to personal projects. Certainly the goal concept has had a very long and illustrious history in psychology, both in experimental psychology and in social, cognitive, and organizational psychology (Austin & Vancouver, 1996; Carver & Scheier, 1998; H. Heckhausen, 1989/1991; Higgins & Sorrentino, 1986; Pervin, 1989) and with increasing frequency the term personal goals has been widely adopted. So, it is appropriate to examine personal projects and personal goals in terms of their range and foci of convenience. I should forewarn that I take a rather distinctive view on this, but felt it inappropriate to force that view on the other authors of this volume. Consequently, both personal goals and projects are used throughout the volume without detailed explication of reasons for preferring one term to the other. Indeed, in many cases the terms are truly interchangeable.

However, I do believe there are some subtle differences that are important. At the risk of being tendentious, let me put it bluntly: Personal projects are not goals, and even when the modifier of *personal* is added to goals, something important differentiates the two terms. The difference turns on the concept of action. Personal projects are extended sets of personally salient action, and such action has both an inner face and an outer face. It is the inner face of action that is most closely related to goals. Indeed most projects are carried out to achieve goals, although frequently they are multigoal pursuits (Little, 1983; Palys & Little, 1983). However, projects are also expressive enactments with an outer face that is typically part of the public domain. This extension of the range of personal projects from inchoate wishes and wants to action in and on contexts is reflected in the two major divisions of this volume: internal and external aspects of project pursuit. It is true that if we invoke, as some authors do, the term goal pursuit, we can enter into the domain of action and extend the range of convenience of the goal construct. The question remains, however, whether there are subtle differences between goal and project pursuit. I suggest there are, and one rather surprising source of agreement comes from the field of robotics.

In an intriguing critique of contemporary research on interactions between humans and robots, Clancey (2004) took issue with the notion of robot collaborators. He did this by detailed examination of the minutiae of humans interacting during terrestrial exploration on the moon and in the Canadian High Arctic. In the light of his field data on how humans interact during exploration, he suggested that "we find a better fit in the language of activity and coordinated action; not the language of goals, problem solving, and tasks" (p. 9). He argued that even two scientist-explorers may not have a collaborative relationship. They may simply be "two people working on personal projects interwoven in time and place" (p. 9). He argued, as have others, that projects do not necessarily have a fixed endpoint and they are essentially creative acts, explorations that may turn in unexpected directions.

Given this view, it is not surprising that Clancey (2004) was skeptical about the capacity of robots to be collaborators. "Here lies the rub: Without consciousness, a robot cannot have a *project*. Projects are an essential aspect of identity, of the experience of being a person, an entity with a history, with ambition, with creative concerns" (p. 11). Unlike people, he argued, "a machine without a sense of self cannot have a project, for it cannot conceive 'what I am doing now'" (p. 11). In short, because robots cannot have personal projects they cannot have joint projects and therefore cannot collaborate.

It is somewhat ironic that it is in the study of robotics that we find one of the most compelling statements about the identity-bearing, passion-engendering aspects of personal project pursuit, as well as an explicit repudiation of goals because they are insufficient to convey a vital distinction between persons and things.

Social Ecological Framework: Persons, Environments, Projects, and Flourishing

Personal projects as analytic units are nested within a larger social ecological framework for personality and developmental science. The basic model was introduced earlier in the chapter, but I would like to show how it has been expanded over the years (Little, 2000a). Essentially the revised social ecological model differentiates between relatively stable and relatively dynamic features of both persons and environments, and provides more depth to both the influences of personal projects and the nature of the outcomes predicted by the model. This revision is presented as Figure 1.3.

The outcome measures now explicitly refer to concepts that involve a broadened conception of human flourishing that includes not only emotional, social, and physical well-being, but also a sense of meaning

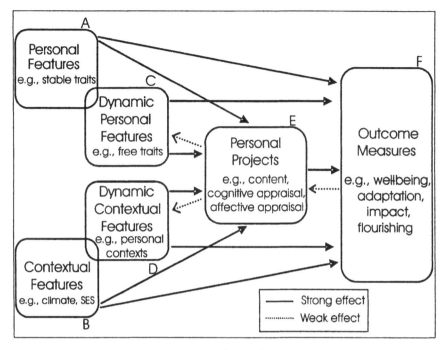

Figure 1.3.   Revised social ecological model.

in one's pursuits (e.g., McGregor & Little, 1998) and having positive effects on one's ecosystem through valued and creative action. It should be emphasized that flourishing is an essentially contestable construct and I have taken one of several defensible stands on how it might be defined theoretically (see, e.g., Paul, Miller, & Paul, 1999). By adopting a view that specifies a positive effect on one's contexts as a constituent element of flourishing, I avoid the conceptual difficulties of having happy, healthy, and wise psychopaths qualify as leading flourishing lives. Does one need both a sense of meaning and happiness in one's pursuits to be regarded as flourishing? Although not shown in Figure 1.3, this is contingent on life-stage and contextual issues (McGregor & Little, 1998). At different stages of life, one may need to trade off some of the elements of well-being and flourishing.

The expanded social ecological model proposes that there are five major sources of influence on human flourishing. First, relatively stable person features and, second, relatively stable environmental features are posited as having direct effects on flourishing as well as indirect influences through their impact on personal projects. These represent, respectively, the traditional personological P variables—particularly traits such as the Big Five (John, 1990)—as well as the more Berkeley-influenced E variables. As we have come to anticipate, P × E interactions, although not graphed, are expected to be frequent.

Personal projects, as in the earlier model, are depicted as having direct effects on human flourishing. In the early work of the SEL, we identified five major factors derivable from measures of personal project appraisals (see Little & Gee, chap. 2, this volume) that influenced flourishing: project meaning, structure, community, efficacy, and (inversely) stress. Because of the addition of new affective dimensions to PPA in recent years, a revised five-factor model appears to capture the influence of personal project dimensions more effectively: meaning, manageability, support, positive affect, and negative affect. As will be seen in chapter 2, the model presented here is a considerable simplification of the measured variables that emanate from the Personal Projects box. Conceptually, however, it reflects a summary of the research yield to date. Individuals experience well-being to the extent that they are engaged in personal projects that they appraise as estimable, meaningful undertakings, that are manageable, that are both supported by and redound to the benefit of others, and that are positive and rewarding.

It may be fairly asked if we might have expected anything other than these results. Could human flourishing be linked to the pursuit of projects that were meaningless, chaotic, socially disengaged, and essentially horrid? This would stretch credulity, admittedly. However, the combination of the personal project and social ecological models allows us to ask far more nuanced questions when we link project pursuit both to the stable person features and to the contextual or environmental features of the model. What categories of projects generate the positive appraisals, and how do stable traits interact with the appraisal of different types of projects to predict flourishing? We know, for example, that extraverts tend to report higher subjective well-being, but we have shown that this is largely mediated by being engaged in interpersonal rather than academic and work projects (Little, Lecci, & Watkinson, 1992). We know, too, that enjoyment of projects is a moderately good predictor of subjective well-being, but we have also shown something not as obvious: Enjoyment of projects is correlated substantially with conscientiousness (Little et al., 1992). We have shown that project appraisals are intimately linked to appraisals of one's work climate, but only for women (Phillips et al., 1997).

The model shows bidirectional arrows between personal projects and flourishing, so we expect that a life full of positive projects will confer a sense of well-being that, in turn, will enhance the likelihood of accruing more such projects. In a meta-analysis of the relation between personal project appraisals and well-being (Wilson, 1990), the best predictors were perceived efficacy and control (under the manageability factor), lack of stress (under negative affect), and enjoyment (under positive affect).

The social ecological model, as mentioned, treats both stable person features and stable environmental features as influences on human flourishing. For example, there is fairly compelling evidence that extraversion and neuroticism have strong relations with subjective well-being (Costa & McCrae, 1980) and conscientiousness with academic and organizational achievement (Costa & McCrae, 1992). Similarly, there is strong evidence that environmental features can be extremely positive or deeply toxic (Frost, 2003). In one revision of the model, I included two further sets of influences that reflect the earlier influences of Murray's personological tradition and of Sarbin's emphasis on the performative aspects of role behavior (Little, 2000a). These are shown in Figure 1.3 as personal contexts and as free traits, and both are intimately linked to the personal projects that individuals are pursuing.

Murray distinguished between the alpha and beta press of situations, with the former being the physical reality of an environment or situation and the latter being the subjective interpretation of the person confronted by that context. These correspond respectively to the stable environmental context and the personal context blocks of the model. Both are important in influencing human flourishing, but it is the subjectively construed personal context that I posit has the greater influence because this is the context as perceived to be relevant to the person's current goals and ongoing projects (Little, 2000a).

Sarbin (1986, 1996) articulated the essential function that roles play in human personality and, indeed, he argued that in many important respects role enactments are constitutive of what we mean by an individual's personality. Although Sarbin warned against the reification of traits of personality and would be uncomfortable with Box A in Figure 1.3, his conception of role performance can be linked to current models of fixed traits (e.g., Costa & McCrae, 1994) by considering the part played in everyday human conduct by what I have called free traits. One chapter of this volume (Little & Joseph, chap. 14, this volume) is devoted to this, but I briefly sketch the central notion here as well.

Although an individual may well be genetically disposed to traits such as introversion or hostility, there are occasions in which one's personal projects, roles, and commitments may enjoin that person to act out of character. Others may construe such project or role-induced patterns of behavior as indicative of fixed traits characteristic of the individual; however, they could be more accurately considered free traits, culturally scripted sets of acts that are strategically adopted by individuals to advance their personal projects. Both personal contexts and free traits have links with well-being and flourishing, although this relation may be rather complex. To construe a situation as salutary, when it clearly is not, may provide the positive spin that enables an individual to persist in what otherwise may be a terribly disappointing, if not debilitating environment. The personal context may facilitate "muddling through" but over time the "real" environment may exact its toll. Similarly, an agreeable person who has to act disagreeably to advance a core project may incur psychological and physical costs. Thus one aspect of human flourishing—the successful completion of an important project—may be achieved at the cost of one's psychological well-being and physical health.

In short, I approach the study of personality and of human development through two interdependent frameworks. The personal projects framework focuses on the ways in which individuals integrate the diverse demands impinging on them from inner biological needs to outer forces. The broader social ecological framework, within which projects are a pivotal component, accords significance to features of one's life that exist independently of our construal of them that may unexpectedly sneak up and delight or devastate us.[11]

FLOURISHING AS THE SUSTAINABLE PURSUIT OF CORE PROJECTS

Looking back over the development of the personal project and social ecological frameworks, there is a discernable patter by which various

---

[11]This raises an issue that goes beyond the scope of this chapter but that I believe is of central importance for differentiating a social ecological model of well-being from a goal-oriented model. The former, notwithstanding the central role of personal projects as ways of shaping lives, does not advance the proposition that the well-lived life is one that involves only the prudential pursuit of goals, even core goals. Focal pursuit of goals and projects may often blind us to peripheral matters that may actually be better for us or contribute, without our having a preconception of its capacity to do so, to our own flourishing. Philosophically, this issue has received lively and sophisticated treatment in a technical work (Larmore, 1999) and in a volume addressed to a somewhat broader audience (Ogilvy, 1995).

concepts, issues, preferences, and commitments have been retained, albeit in modified form throughout their development. My early research was primarily concerned with methodological issues that would allow a resolution of the person–environment debate and would show some fidelity both to the personological tradition and the Kellian constructivist tradition. The concern with social justice, with helping people shape more meaningful lives, led me and my collaborators to use outcome measures in our research that assess not only personal happiness and subjective well-being, but also a broadened conception of human flourishing. We were concerned to show that personal projects may contribute to happiness but also to a sense of meaning in one's life (Little, 1998; McGregor & Little, 1998; McGregor, McAdams, & Little, in press) and that project pursuit might redound to the greater good, for example, in volunteering activities, even when the primary goal for the project pursuer was self-fulfillment (Phillips, Little, & Goodine, 2002). Part of the integrative passions underlying my work made me sensitive to questions of quality of life and flourishing that would be found in other disciplines, particularly ethical and legal philosophy and increasingly economic theory (Easterlin, 2003; Frey & Stutzer 2002) in which questions of happiness have become matters of serious concern. For example, Lomasky (1984, 1987) drew on a conception of personal projects in constructing a theory of human rights. Similarly, Williams (1981) developed the concept of *ground projects,* those pursuits without which a person might seriously consider whether to continue living. These, and similar philosophical treatments of factors that influence human flourishing (e.g., Paul et al., 1999) provide a rich space for interdisciplinary research deeply resonant with the ameliorative issues that were central to the emergence of classical personality psychology (Little, 2005; Nicholson, 2003).

The approach to human flourishing that animates this volume can be captured in a single sentence: Human flourishing is contingent on the sustainable pursuit of individuals' core projects. By core projects, we mean projects that are central to the individual's project system as a whole. Core projects are those that are most resistant to change, most extensively connected with other projects, and intrinsically valued by the person as pursuits without which the meaning of one's life would become compromised. By sustainable pursuit we mean that both internal and external factors facilitate the pursuit of the project. Depending on whether the project has a delineable conclusion, such factors will help advance the project toward its successful achievement. To the extent that it is an interminable project (e.g., "caring for my children's needs") these factors will be lifelong sustaining resources.

We revisit this issue of core projects and sustainability in the final chapter of this volume, but it is helpful here to stress that one of the key factors in sustainability of a person's core projects is that both internal and external systems must maintain their integrity and potency throughout the course of the pursuit. This means that projects that accomplish goals of the individual, but in the process compromise the contextual support elements, are not sustainable in the long run. Moreover, there is a vital interdependency between the viability of the person's core projects and the generative contexts within which they are pursued. If a relationship, organization, or state cannot provide sustenance to the core projects and aspirations of people, both individually and collectively, then those contexts will lose their generative power and be at risk for displacement by other forces that may be only too happy to nurture the deepest aspirations of project pursuers. In short, the generative contexts within which people pursue their most cherished goals and core projects stimulate project pursuit and provide the environments in which they may be successfully accomplished or maintained. They provide both prompts and circumstances, reminders of what matters to us and contexts that allow us to be as much like ourselves as humanly possible. In educational settings, truly generative contexts attract curious, generative students. They ask us to tell them stories about our projects and then urge us to tell others. Indeed, this chapter represents, in part, the discharging of a long-standing promissory note to my students and colleagues to tell the story of how personal projects analysis came about. "So, is it finished?" they ask. "Can it ever be?" is my honest response.

REFERENCES

Allport, G. W. (1937). *Personality: A psychological interpretation.* New York: Holt, Rinehart & Winston.

Allport, G. W. (1958). What units shall we employ? In G. Lindzey (Ed.), *Assessment of human motivation* (pp. 239–260). New York: Holt, Rinehart & Winston.

Argyle, M. (1969). *Social interaction.* London: Methuen.

Argyle, M., Bryant, B., & Trower, P. (1974). Social skills training and psychotherapy: A comparative study. *Psychological Medicine, 4,* 435–443.

Argyle, M., & Little, B. R. (1972). Do personality traits apply to social behavior? *Journal of the Theory of Social Behavior, 2,* 1–35.

Argyle, M., Shimoda, K., & Little, B. R. (1978). Variance due to persons and situations in England and Japan. *British Journal of Social and Clinical Psychology, 17,* 335–337.

Austin, J. T., & Vancouver, J. B. (1996). Goal constructs in psychology: Structure, process, and content. *Psychological Bulletin, 120,* 338–375.

Baltes, P. B., & Baltes, M. M. (Eds.). (1990). Psychological perspectives on successful aging: The model of selective optimization with compensation. In P. B. Baltes & M. M. Baltes (Eds.), *Successful aging: Perspectives from the behavioral sciences* (pp. 1–34). New York: Cambridge University Press.

Bandura, A. (1982). The psychology of chance encounters and life paths. *American Psychologist, 37,* 747–755.

Bannister, D. (1966). Psychology as an exercise in paradox. *Bulletin of the British Psychological Society, 63,* 21–26.

Barron, F. (1963). *Creativity and psychological health: Origins of personality vitality and creative freedom.* Princeton, NJ: Van Nostrand.

Bronfenbrenner, U. (1979). *The ecology of human development.* Cambridge, MA: Harvard University Press.

Buss, D. M., & Craik, K. H. (1983). The act frequency approach to personality. *Psychological Review, 90,* 105–126.

Campbell, D. T. (1981). Perspective on a scholarly career. In M. B. Brewer & B. E. Collins (Eds.), *Scientific inquiry and the social sciences: A volume in honor of Donald T. Campbell* (pp. 454–501). San Francisco: Jossey-Bass.

Cantor, N. (1990). From thought to behavior: "Having" and "doing" in the study of personality and cognition. *American Psychologist, 45,* 735–750.

Cantor, N., & Fleeson, W. (1994). Social intelligence and intelligent goal pursuit: A cognitive slice of motivation. In W. Spaulding (Ed.), *Nebraska symposium on motivation* (Vol. 41, pp. 125–180). Lincoln: University of Nebraska Press.

Cantor, N., & Kihlstrom, J. K. (1987). *Personality and social intelligence.* Englewood Cliffs, NJ: Prentice-Hall.

Cantor, N., Norem, J. K., Niedenthal, P. M., Langston, C. A., & Brower, A. M. (1987). Life tasks, self-concept ideals, and cognitive strategies in a life transition. *Journal of Personality and Social Psychology, 53,* 1178–1191.

Carver, C. S., & Scheier, M. F. (1998). *On the self-regulation of behavior.* New York: Cambridge University Press.

Cervone, D., & Mischel, W. (Eds.). (2002). *Advances in personality science.* New York: Guilford.

Clancey, W. J. (2004). Roles for agent assistants in field science: Understanding personal projects and collaboration. *IEEE Transactions on Systems, Man and Cybernetics—Part C: Applications and Reviews, 34*(2), 1–12.

Costa, P. T., & McCrae, R. R. (1980). Influence of extraversion and neuroticism on subjective well-being: Happy and unhappy people. *Journal of Personality and Social Psychology, 38,* 668–678.

Costa, P. T., & McCrae, R. R. (1992). *NEO PI-R professional manual.* Odessa, FL: Psychological Assessment Resources.

Costa, P. T., & McCrae, R. R. (1994). Set like plaster? Evidence for the stability of adult personality. In T. Heatherton & J. L. Weinberger (Eds.), *Can personality change?* (pp. 21–40). Washington, DC: American Psychological Association.

Craik, K. H. (1969). Personality unvanquished. *Contemporary Psychology, 14,* 147–148.

Craik, K. H. (2000). The lived day of an individual: A person–environment perspective. In W. B. Walsh, K. H. Craik, & R. H. Price (Eds.), *Person–environment psychology: New direction and perspectives* (2nd ed., pp. 233–266). Mahwah, NJ: Lawrence Erlbaum Associates, Inc.

Davidson, D. (1980). *Essays on actions and events.* New York: Oxford University Press.

Easterlin, R. A. (2003). Explaining happiness. *Proceedings of the National Academy of Science of the United States of America, 100,* 11176–11183.

Emmons, R. A. (1986). Personal strivings: An approach to personality and subjective well-being. *Journal of Personality and Social Psychology, 51,* 1058–1068.

Emmons, R. A. (1999). *The psychology of ultimate concerns: Motivation and spirituality in personality.* New York: Guilford.

Emmons, R. A., & King, L. A. (1988). Conflict among personal strivings: Immediate and long-term implications for psychological and physical well-being. *Journal of Personality and Social Psychology, 54,* 1040–1048.

Ford, D. H. (1987). *Humans as self-constructing living systems: A developmental perspective on behavior and personality.* Hillsdale, NJ: Lawrence Erlbaum Associates.

Frey, B., & Stutzer, A. (2002). What can economists learn from happiness research? *Journal of Economic Literature, 40,* 402–435.

Frost, P. J. (2003). Toxic *emotions at work: How compassionate managers handle pain and conflict.* Boston: Harvard Business School Press.

Harré, R., & Secord, P. F. (1972). *The explanation of social behavior.* Lanham, MD: Rowman & Littlefield.

Heckhausen, H. (1991). *Motivation and action* (P. K. Leppman, Trans.). New York: Springer. (Original work published 1989)

Heckhausen, J. (1999). *Developmental regulation in adulthood: Age-normative and sociostructural constraints as adaptive challenges.* New York: Cambridge University Press.

Higgins, E. T., & Sorrentino, R. M. (Eds.). (1986). *Handbook of motivation and cognition.* New York: Guilford.

Hooker, K. (2002). New directions for research in personality and aging: A comprehensive model for linking levels, structures, and processes. *Journal of Research in Personality, 36,* 318–334.

Hooker, K., & McAdams, D. (2003). Personality reconsidered: A new agenda for aging research. *Journal of Gerontology: Psychological Sciences, 58B,* P296–P304.

John, O. P. (1990). The "Big Five" factor taxonomy: Dimensions of personality in the natural language and in questionnaires. In L. A. Pervin (Ed.), *Handbook of personality theory and research* (pp. 66–100). New York: Guilford.

Karoly, P. (1993). Mechanisms of self-regulation: A systems view. *Annual Review of Psychology, 44,* 23–52.

Kelly, G. A. (1955). *The psychology of personal constructs.* New York: Norton.

Kelly, G. A. (1962). Europe's matrix of decision. In M. R. Jones (Ed.), *Nebraska symposium on motivation* (pp. 83–123). Lincoln: University of Nebraska Press.

Klinger, E. (1975). Consequences of commitment to and disengagement from incentives. *Psychological Review, 82,* 1–25.

Klinger, E. (1977). *Meaning and void: Inner experience and the incentives in people's lives.* Minneapolis: University of Minnesota Press.

Krahé, B. (1992). *Personality and social psychology: Toward a synthesis.* London: Sage.

Larmore, C. (1999). The idea of a life plan. In E. F. Paul, F. D. Miller, & J. Paul (Eds.), *Human flourishing* (pp. 96–112). Cambridge, UK: Cambridge University Press.

Leavis, F. R. (1963). *Two cultures? The significance of C. P. Snow, with a new pref. for the American reader and an essay on Sir Charles Snow's Rede lecture by Michael Yudkin.* New York: Pantheon.

Little, B. R. (1968). Psychospecializaton: Functions of differential orientation toward persons and things [Abstract]. *Bulletin of the British Psychological Society, 21,* 113.

Little, B. R. (1972). Psychological man as scientist, humanist and specialist. *Journal of Experimental Research in Personality, 6,* 95–118.
Little, B. R. (1976a). *Personal systems and specialization.* Unpublished doctorial dissertation, University of California at Berkeley, Berkeley, CA.
Little, B. R. (1976b). Specialization and the varieties of environmental experience: Empirical studies within the personality paradigm. In S. Wapner, S. B. Cohen, & B. Kaplan (Eds.), *Experiencing the environment* (pp. 81–116). New York: Plenum.
Little, B. R. (1983). Personal projects: A rationale and method for investigation. *Environment and Behavior, 15,* 273–309.
Little, B. R. (1987a). Personal projects and fuzzy selves: Aspects of self-identity in adolescence. In T. Honess & K. Yardley (Eds.), *Self and identity: Perspectives across the life span* (pp. 230–245). London: Routledge & Kegan Paul.
Little, B. R. (1987b). Personality and the environment. In D. Stokols & I. Altman (Eds.), *Handbook of environmental psychology* (pp. 205–244). New York: Wiley.
Little, B. R. (1988). *Personal projects analysis: Theory, method and research.* Ottawa, ON, Canada: Social Sciences and Humanities Research Council of Canada.
Little, B. R. (1989). Personal projects analysis: Trivial pursuits, magnificent obsessions, and the search for coherence. In D. M. Buss & N. Cantor (Eds.), *Personality psychology: Recent trends and emerging directions* (pp. 15–31). New York: Springer-Verlag.
Little, B. R. (1993). Personal projects and the distributed self: Aspects of a conative psychology. In J. Suls (Ed.), *Psychological perspectives on the self* (Vol. 4, pp. 157–181). Hillsdale, NJ: Lawrence Erlbaum Associates.
Little, B. R. (1996). Free traits, personal projects and idio-tapes: Three tiers for personality research. *Psychological Inquiry, 8,* 340–344.
Little, B. R. (1998). Personal project pursuit: Dimensions and dynamics of personal meaning. In P. T. P. Wong & P. S. Fry (Eds.), *The human quest for meaning: A handbook of psychological research and clinical applications* (pp. 193–212). Mahwah, NJ: Lawrence Erlbaum Associates.
Little, B. R. (1999a). Personality and motivation: Personal action and the conative evolution. In L. A. Pervin & O. P. John (Eds.), *Handbook of personality theory and research* (2nd ed., pp. 501–524). New York: Guilford.
Little, B. R. (1999b). Personal projects and social ecology: Themes and variation across the life span. In J. Brandtstadter & R. M. Lerner (Eds.), *Action and self-development: Theory and research through the life span* (pp. 197–221). Thousand Oaks, CA: Sage.
Little, B. R. (2000a). Free traits and personal contexts: Expanding a social ecological model of well-being. In W. B. Walsh, K. H. Craik, & R. Price (Eds.), *Person environment psychology* (2nd ed., pp. 87–116). New York: Guilford.
Little, B. R. (2000b, November). *Personal projects and free traits: Lives, liberties and the happiness of pursuit.* Radcliffe Fellows Lecture presented at the Radcliffe Institute for Advanced Study at Harvard University, Cambridge, MA.
Little, B. R. (2000c). Persons, contexts and personal projects: Assumptive themes of a methodological transactionalism. In S. Wapner, J. Demick, T. Yamamoto, & H. Minami (Eds.), *Theoretical perspectives in environment–behavior research* (pp. 79–88). New York: Plenum.
Little, B. R. (2001). Personality psychology: Havings, doings and beings in contexts. In J. S. Halonen & S. F. Davis (Eds.), *The many faces of psychological research in the 21st century.* Retrieved May 1, 2005 from http://www.brianrlittle.com/articles/havings_doings_beings.htm
Little, B. R. (2005). Personality science and personal projects: Six impossible things before breakfast. *Journal of Research in Personality, 39,* 4–21.

Little, B. R., & Chambers, N. C. (2000). Analyse des projets personnels: Un cadre intégratif pour la psychologie clinique et le counselling [Personal projects analysis: An integrative framework for clinical and counseling psychology]. *Revue Québécoise de Psychologie, 21,* 153–190.

Little, B. R., & Chambers, N. C. (2004). Personal project pursuit: On human doings and well beings. In M. Cox & E. Klinger (Eds.), *Handbook of motivational counseling: Concepts, approaches and assessment* (pp. 65–82). Chichester, UK: Wiley.

Little, B. R., Lecci, L., & Watkinson, B. (1992). Personality and personal projects: Linking Big Five and PAC units of analysis. *Journal of Personality, 60,* 501–525.

Little, B. R., & Ryan, T. J. (1979). A social ecological model of development. In K. Ishwaran (Ed.), *Childhood and adolescence in Canada* (pp. 273–301). Toronto: McGraw-Hill Ryerson.

Lomasky, L. E. (1984). Personal projects as the foundation for basic rights. *Social Philosophy and Policy, 1,* 35–55.

Lomasky, L. E. (1987). *Persons, rights and the moral community.* New York: Oxford University Press.

MacKinnon, D. W. (1962). The nature and nurture of creative talent. *American Psychologist, 17,* 484–495.

McAdams, D. P. (1993). *The stories we live by: Personal myths and the making of the self.* New York: Morrow.

McAdams, D. P. (1995). What do we know when we know a person? *Journal of Personality, 63,* 365–396.

McAdams, D. P. (1996). Personality, modernity, and the storied self: A contemporary framework for studying persons. *Psychological Inquiry, 7,* 295–321.

McAdams, D. P., & Emmons, R. A. (Eds.). (1995). Levels of domains in personality [Special issue]. *Journal of Personality, 63*(3).

McGregor, I., & Little, B. R. (1998). Personal projects, happiness, and meaning: On doing well and being yourself. *Journal of Personality and Social Psychology, 74,* 494–512.

McGregor, I., McAdams, D. P., & Little, B. R. (in press). *Personal projects, life-stories, and well-being: The benefits of acting and being true to one's traits.*

Mischel, W. (1968). *Personality and assessment.* New York: Wiley.

Mischel, W. (2004). Toward an integrative science of the person. *Annual Review of Psychology, 55,* 1–22.

Moos, R. H., & Insel, P. M. (1974). *Issues in social ecology: Human milieus.* Palo Alto, CA: National Press Books.

Murray, H. A. (1938). *Explorations in personality.* New York: Oxford University Press.

Nicholson, I. A. M. (2003). *Inventing personality: Gordon Allport and the science of selfhood.* Washington: American Psychological Association.

Nurmi, J.-E. (1992). Age differences in adult life goals, concerns, and their temporal extension: A life course approach to future-oriented motivation. *International Journal of Behavioral Development, 15,* 487–508.

Nussbaum, M. C. (1994). *The therapy of desire: Theory and practice in Hellenistic ethics.* Princeton, NJ: Princeton University Press.

Ogilvie, M. D., & Rose, K. M. (1995). Self-with-other representations and a taxonomy of motives: Two approaches to studying persons. *Journal of Personality, 63,* 633–679.

Ogilvy, J. (1995). *Living without a goal.* New York: Doubleday.

Omodei, M. M., & Wearing, A. J. (1990). Need satisfaction and involvement in personal projects: Toward an integrative model of subjective well-being. *Journal of Personality and Social Psychology, 59,* 762–769.

Palys, T. S., & Little, B. R. (1983). Perceived life satisfaction and the organization of personal project systems. *Journal of Personality and Social Psychology, 44,* 1221–1230.

Paul, E. F., Miller, F. D., Jr., & Paul, J. (Eds.). (1999). *Human flourishing.* Cambridge, UK: Cambridge University Press.

Pervin, L. A. (Ed.). (1989). *Goal concepts in personality and social psychology.* Hillsdale, NJ: Lawrence Erlbaum Associates.

Phillips, S. D. (1992). Projects, pressure and perceptions of effectiveness: An organizational analysis of national Canadian women's groups (Doctoral dissertation, Carleton University, 1990). *Dissertation Abstracts International, 52*(11-A), 4075.

Phillips, S. D., Little, B. R., & Goodine, L. A. (1997). Reconsidering gender and public administration: Five steps beyond conventional research. *Canadian Journal of Public Administration, 40,* 563–581.

Phillips, S. D., Little, B. R., & Goodine, L. A. (2002). *University students as volunteers.* Toronto: Canadian Centre for Philanthropy.

Robinson, F. G. (1992). *Love's story told: A life of Henry A. Murray.* Cambridge, MA: Harvard University Press.

Runyan, W. M. (1982). *Life histories and psychobiography.* New York: Oxford University Press.

Salmela-Aro, K. (1992). Struggling with self: The personal projects of students seeking psychological counselling. *Scandinavian Journal of Psychology, 33,* 330–338.

Salmela-Aro, K., & Nurmi, J.-E. (1996). Depressive symptoms and personal project appraisals: A cross-lagged longitudinal study. *Personality and Individual Differences, 21,* 373–381.

Sarbin, T. R. (Ed.). (1986). *Narrative psychology: The stored nature of human conduct.* New York: Praeger.

Sarbin, T. R. (1996, August). *The poetics of identity.* Henry Murray Award Address presented at the annual meeting of the American Psychological Association, New York.

Seligman, M., & Csikszentmihalyi, M. (2000). Positive psychology: An introduction. *American Psychologist, 55,* 5–14.

Snow, C. P. (1959). *The two cultures and the scientific revolution.* Cambridge, UK: Cambridge University Press.

Williams, B. (1981). *Moral luck.* Cambridge, UK: Cambridge University Press.

Wilson, D. A. (1990). *Personal project dimensions and perceived life satisfaction: A quantitative synthesis.* Unpublished master's thesis, Carleton University, Ottawa, Ontario, Canada.

Zirkel, S., & Cantor, N. (1990). Personal construal of life tasks: Those who struggle for independence. *Journal of Personality and Social Psychology, 58,* 172–185.

2

The Methodology
of Personal Projects Analysis:
Four Modules and a Funnel

Brian R. Little and Travis L. Gee

Chapter 1 is essentially about why to do personal projects analysis (PPA); this chapter is more about how to do it. It is not, however, meant to be a comprehensive, step-by-step manual on PPA, but a systematic introduction to its components and the rationale for their creation. To accomplish this, we therefore give an occasional "word to the 'whys?'" to justify choices made in developing the methodology. Because PPA has been adopted and adapted by others for exploring units of analysis such as personal goals and personal action constructs, we intend this chapter to reflect and provide guidance to their concerns as well.

Our methodological views may easily be taken as somewhat contrarian, because we favor a destandardization of some components of assessment. This is done through allowing personally salient and ecologically representative idiosyncratic units to be assessed along a set of dimensions that are explicitly modular and adaptable. These dimensions tap into the thoughts, feelings, and actions of respondents, information about which is carried by the unit, the personal project. This allows joint access to idiographic and nomothetic levels of analysis, therein increasing the fidelity of measurement within individuals without significant costs to comparability across individuals. However, we oppose the contrarian label, and prefer to see our assessment philosophy as more complementary because we do not eschew other forms of assessment in favor of it (Little, 2005).

It should be emphasized that PPA is not a test or a set of tests. It is an open-source methodology, more Linux-like and modular than proprietary and fixed. It is a suite of what might be called "plug and pray" assessment modules operating like a computer system board. New components can be seamlessly integrated in the hope that they will provide what the researcher designed them to provide. Of course, retention and use of these modules cannot be justified by "faith validity" alone. As described later, such decisions are based on successful demonstration of psychometric properties such as construct validity and predictive utility, as well as on criteria unique to the methodology.[1] PPA was designed from the outset to encourage both adaptation of standard modules to facilitate comparative inquiry and creation of new ones that would provide greater sensitivity for the particular problem being studied. In these respects, it differs from some of the traditional approaches to human assessment, particularly orthodox trait assessment. We adopt trait assessment in the broader social ecological framework within which projects analysis is embedded (Little, 1999a, 2000a; Little & Ryan, 1979). However, this chapter occasionally highlights the contrast between these alternative ways of assessing human development and personality (see Little, Lecci, & Watkinson, 1992).

Over the years we have digitally stored a great deal of data gathered from personal projects assessment with diverse groups of individuals. Many of these observations are linked to information collected on both stable and dynamic features of persons and their contexts, as well as to both "hard" and "soft" indicators of well-being, adaptive behavior, and

---

[1]Twelve specific criteria have guided the development of PPA and have been dealt with in detail elsewhere (Little, 1999b, 2000b). These criteria are regarded as propaedeutic to more conventional psychometric criteria. Briefly noted, they propose that units of analysis for human assessment be reflexive, personally salient, evocative, ecologically representative, temporally sensitive, relevant to "social indicators," systemic, middle-level, modular, conjointly idiographic and normative, integrative, and directly applicable. Although several of these assessment criteria are alluded to throughout this chapter and volume, elucidation of the criteria is not our primary goal. Rather, we present, for the first time, a guide that takes the reader through the actual process of doing PPA and provides the research decisions involved in that process.

flourishing (see Little, chap. 1, this volume). Together these comprise the social ecological assessment data bank (SEAbank).[2]

In essence, PPA asks individuals to provide a listing of their personal projects, select a subset that they will focus on, and rate each of these selected projects on a set of dimensions that have theoretical significance, practical utility, or both. Respondents may then complete additional modules that assess the impact, hierarchical structure, and contextual nature of their personal projects.[3]

The resulting data comprise a set of indexes that can be examined and explored at the individual level (person-centered measurement) or at the level of normative, comparative analysis (variable-centered measurement).[4] For example, a group of individuals can rate their idiosyncratic projects on dimensions such as how stressful they are and how much they feel they are in control of each project. These appraisals of stress and control can be correlated within the single case (across an individual's projects). This is one variant of person-centered measurement and can be augmented by idiosyncratic information contained in the PPA, such as the actual project descriptions and open-ended information about where and with whom projects are undertaken. Variable-centered measurement is obtained by calculating the average score for each person on each relevant dimension or index. The resulting vector score can be used much like orthodox individual difference measures; for example, the mean score on project control can be treated for analytic and predictive purposes in the same way as a score on a test of locus of control. Note that, although both levels of measurement in PPA involve the use of appraisal dimensions, the relation between these dimensions may or may not correspond when one examines them at different levels.[5]

---

[2]Access to SEAbank can be arranged by contacting the first author at blittle@fas.harvard.edu

[3]The "listing" of projects and completion of modules have been typically done through completion of written forms. However, recent advances in PPA have involved oral interviews and both computer and Web-enhanced versions.

[4]It is important to clarify that we are referring here to a distinction of long-standing significance in the history of personality assessment: that which contrasts assessment focused on the individual, sometimes referred to as an idiographic approach, with that focused on relations between variables measured across individuals. More recent distinctions between person- and variable-centered analyses have arisen in discussion of hierarchical modeling and associated psychometric concerns. Although related, these need to be differentiated. Our view is that both forms of individual and variable-level measurement are appropriate intellectual enterprises.

[5]This may give rise to problems and paradoxes when attempting to generalize across levels of analysis. Thus ecological fallacies and individual differences fallacies have been invoked, each of which is a variation on Simpson's (1951) paradox. We have discussed these issues elsewhere (Gee, 1999; Little, 1987c, 2005).

For example, the person-centered strategy may reveal a moderately strong positive relation between control and stress for a given individual. We could then drill down to see which particular projects were carrying this relation, perhaps discovering that a number of recreational pursuits were being pursued precisely because they involved relinquishing control to experience the pleasure of discovery. On the other hand, the variable-centered strategy may reveal a very strong negative relation between stress and control. Such results may appear paradoxical, and we consider aspects of this statistical issue in the final section. For now, we wish simply to emphasize that PPA was explicitly designed to facilitate two approaches to measurement with honored traditions in the field of personality: person-centered, idiographic analysis, and more variable-centered, normative analysis.

Although most of the core components of PPA methodology have been used since the late 1970s, the methodology has been adapted over the years in ways that allow particular research problems to be explored. For expository purposes in this chapter we can regard the original methodology and its basic modules as the major themes of a personal projects suite and the different adaptations that have accrued along the way as variations on those themes. Although beyond the scope of this chapter, the development of PPA has been accompanied, from the outset, with alternative approaches to the statistical treatment of the data it generates. We briefly and selectively discuss some of these issues in Appendix A.

This chapter takes us through each of the four basic elements or modules of PPA: project elicitation, project appraisal, hierarchical analysis (connecting projects to reasons why they are undertaken and to the concrete acts through which they are accomplished), and cross-impact assessment. Before examining the conjoining of themes and variations in each of these modules, we need to attend to the funnel.

FUNNELING: THE PROBLEM OF WINNOWING IN PSYCHOLOGICAL ASSESSMENT

By adopting an approach to human assessment that takes the Kellian credulous approach seriously, at least at the start of the assessment process, we approach our participants as having singular insights about their concerns and pursuits. In short, we view them as specialists, experts in their own life space (Little, 1968, 1972, 1976). As a purely intellectual exercise, most people could generate an almost limitless number of goals, commitments, preferences, tasks, comforts, and joys in their lives. Both they and we would be overwhelmed at the task of explicating them. As the emperor is reputed to have said of Mozart's music in the movie *Amadeus,* "there are too many notes." We need to provide a funnel, a winnowing device that allows the person's most salient concerns and pursuits to be elicited and articulated in coherent fashion, such that we, like Mozart, select the right notes.

Such adaptive winnowing is also a constituent feature of daily life. We selectively attend to a subset of possible projects through which we compose our days. Personal projects, both as everyday strategies for living and as assessment units, provide precisely that funneling function. Consistent with our theoretical aspirations, the winnowing enables us to access and integrate diverse aspects of human cognition, conation, affect, and action. Underlying each step is the assumption that the processes used by the respondent in funneling are those that they use in everyday life, which we prefer to the alternative of multiplying entities unnecessarily by assuming that respondents have somehow evolved a different set of processes for completing surveys than for other, more naturally occurring functions (Little, 1972).

FOUR ASSESSMENT MODULES FOR PERSONAL PROJECTS ANALYSIS: ELICITATION, APPRAISAL, HIERARCHY, AND IMPACT

For each of these modules we provide the basic technique and variations on it, and discuss the types of data that are generated. Although research design issues are not a focus of this chapter, we offer, when appropriate, selective examples of implications of PPA for different strategies of research and intervention. The version of PPA that follows is meant primarily for use with university students, although with appropriate changes we have used it extensively with large and diverse community samples as well. The example is also based on the computer-assisted version of PPA, which allows rapid transfer of project data provided by respondents from module to module.[6] Examples of print versions appear as appendices in Little (1983, 1993). To aid discussion of each module, we introduce them separately. Both in printed and computer versions, PPA is presented as a continuous and linked series of

---

[6]An electronic version of PPA can be accessed at http://www.brianrlittle.com, and it can also be downloaded for printing.

modular components, although some modules may be excluded in any particular administration of PPA, depending on the purpose and focus of research.

The Personal Project Elicitation Module: What's Up?

The initial module in PPA is formally called the personal project elicitation module; more informally we refer to it as the project dump in the sense that respondents are encouraged to generate their planned or on-going projects without constraint. As illustrated in Table 2.1, the module begins with a brief description of personal projects, together with examples, and respondents are given 10 to 15 minutes to write down (or type for electronic versions) their own personal projects.[7] It is, in essence, a somewhat more formal way of asking a person what in everyday discourse would be phrased as "What's up?"

Simply looking at the list of projects generated in the dump provides rich information both about the respondent and the context within which that person is living. Here are examples of personal projects generated by different respondents that are stored in SEAbank:

- Lose 10 pounds.
- Be a better Druid.
- Maybe apologizing to my brother.
- Become more extraverted.
- Figure out how to pay rent.
- Continue to "grow" as a person.
- Organize a neighborhood watch program.
- Tell my sister to get rid of her sickening boyfriend.
- Help my husband get through Christmas.
- Finish renovating Mom's basement.

Clearly, personal projects comprise a considerable array of activities and aspirations, ranging from the mundane tasks of Monday morning to the consuming passions of a lifetime. In the examples just given, the first project listed is (within a few pounds) the most frequent project listed over the years. The second one is truly idiosyncratic. Some of the projects are concrete and instantly achievable; others are phrased so as to

---

[7]These instructions are slightly modified from the original (Little, 1983) version to generate a broader range of personal projects.

TABLE 2.1

The Project Elicitation Instructions (Electronic Version)

Personal Projects Analysis

We are interested in studying the kinds of activities and concerns that people have over the course of their lives. We call these personal projects. All of us have a number of personal projects at any given time that we think about, plan for, carry out and sometimes (though not always) complete.

Some projects may be focused on achievement ("Getting my degree") others on the process ("Enjoying a night out with friends"); they may be things we choose to do or things we have to do; they may be things we are working towards or things we are trying to avoid. Projects may be related to any aspect of your daily life, university, work, home, your self, relationships, leisure and community, among others. Please think of projects in this broad way.

Some Examples of Personal Projects:
- Pass my psychology course
- Cut down on junk food
- Play with my cat
- Clean my apartment
- Try not to make my parents mad
- Clarify my religious beliefs
- Exercise more often
- Go to Europe this summer
- Be a better parent
- Break off with Robert
- Climb the Matterhorn
- Understand Suzanne better
- Find a part-time job
- Stop putting off studying until the last minute

We are also interested in finding out what you think and how you feel about these personal projects and activities, how important or stressful they are, and so on.

Project Elicitation

To start, please take 10-15 minutes and type in the following cells as many personal projects and activities you can that you are currently engaged in or considering

Project #	Project Description
1	
2	
3	
˅	˅
15	

be interminable. Some projects are individualistic and self-focused pursuits; others are done strictly for the sake of others. The listing of personal projects represents what people think they are doing in their lives. In fact, if asked carefully, we can find out the salient projects they are not currently pursuing in their lives as well (Hotson & Little, 2000).

There are a number of analyses that can be done with the original project dump, each generating a score, an index, or set of indexes that can be used at the idiographic level by clinicians or personologists for more intensive probing or as variables or vector scores for standard normative level research.

Variations on the Elicitation Module

The original PPA was a printed package to be filled in by hand (Little, 1983, 1993). We have developed computer and Web-based versions in recent years, the latter of which can increase dramatically the number of respondents and enhance both efficiency and flexibility in administration. However, for clinical and intensive research designs we recommend a project-oriented interview in which the instructions are read and the respondent can either have responses audio- or video-recorded or complete the standard PPA in written form with the interviewer offering clarification as needed (e.g., Goodine, 2000; Phillips, Little, & Goodine, 1996, 1997). What is lost in standardization in the interview format is gained in respondents offering spontaneous comments and elaborations on current projects and the contexts surrounding them. A further variation on this more open-ended approach to project elicitation is to have the person simply tell a short story about each project, for example, about its significance in his or her life.

Indexes Derived From the Personal Project Elicitation Module

Project Load and Phrasing Level. The sheer number of projects generated by a respondent can be informative. The average number of projects listed in the standard elicitation procedure taking 10 minutes is approximately 15. When respondents are allowed to take the PPA package home with them and return it over a weekend, the range has been from 1 project to 368. From a clinical perspective, extremes of overload (e.g., 30 or more projects) or underload (3 or less) elicited during a standard project dump may have diagnostic significance. However, it is important to take project "chunking" or phrasing level into account. That is, some individuals may choose to list large projects (e.g., complete my BA); others may focus on smaller scale pursuits (e.g., finish my term paper) that could be regarded as a component of the larger project. In research on the phrasing level of projects we have distinguished between the *ecological load* of a project (e.g., "complete my BA" would be rated as having a higher load than "complete my term paper" as it involves a greater cost of time and other resources) and the *linguistic complexity* of the project (e.g., "have coffee with Dad" would be rated toward the simple end on this dimension, whereas "attempt to integrate the demands of my Dad and my own desire for independence" would be scored as complex). A comprehensive treatment of the measurement and correlates of the phrasing level of projects appear in MacDiarmid (1990).

Content and Category Analyses of Personal Projects. The projects listed in the dump can be categorized in various ways, and then the number of projects in a given category or the proportion of total projects generated in different categories can be used as indexes for either normative (between subject) or idiographic (within subjects) analysis. Our earliest version categorized projects according to the different domains of activity to which the project was linked. These appear in Table 2.2 together with relevant examples. High degrees of interjudge agreement have been achieved with these categories.

With the computer and Web versions of PPA, we provide a module in which respondents can do their own categorizing. This allows a project like "help fix up Deanna's den" to be categorized as an interpersonal or a maintenance project depending on whether the primary focus of the project pursuer is on Deanna or her den.

It is important to note that each of these categories can be broken down into subcategories depending on the sample being studied and the particular research question being explored. For example, with adolescents the category of interpersonal projects was further broken down into boyfriend/girlfriend and sexual categories because of the frequency with which they were generated (Little, 1987b).

Comprehensive taxonomies for categorizing goals have been developed (Chulef, Read, & Walsh, 2001) and can be adapted for use with personal projects. Throughout this book, alternative systems for content analyzing personal projects or goals are proposed and their reliability and utility demonstrated. Elliot and Friedman (chap. 3, this volume)

TABLE 2.2
Personal Project Categories with Examples

Project Categories	Examples
Interpersonal	Get along better with Jane Impress my stats tutor Get revenge on Jonathon
Academic	Complete my thesis Pass high school Get more out of math class
Work	Get a promotion Finish my inventory Keep the boss from finding out what I did Tuesday
Intrapersonal	Raise my consciousness Be more extraverted Find inner peace
Recreational/Leisure	Go to Vanuatu for a week Go fishing Watch better quality TV shows
Health	Lose ten pounds Go to gym regularly Try to start riding my bike more
Maintenance	Mow the lawn Pay the bills Wash the dog
Other	Complete this questionnaire for experimental credit

demonstrate highly reliable coding of the extent to which a person lists approach or avoidance goals. Chambers (chap. 5, this volume) developed a linguistically sophisticated procedure of category analysis in which tense, mode, and aspect are incorporated and he shows how these subtle aspects of project phrasing predict relevant outcome measures (e.g., the "try to" before "start riding my bike more" would not bode well for the success of that project).

One of the most interesting category systems for examining personal projects was created by Ogilvie and his colleagues (e.g., Ogilvie & Rose, 1995; Ogilvie, Rose, & Heppen, 2001). They took traditional constructs from operant conditioning and developed a taxonomy that captures the motivational basis of project pursuit. The acronym PACK captures these different project motives that are based on the desire to *keep* or *acquire* positive experiences or to *prevent* or *cure* negative experiences. Again, both interrater reliability and utility in predicting a range of outcome variables are high, adding evidence for the value of exploring project content.

Diversity and Balance in Project Pursuits. Another index that can be derived from the project elicitation module is the extent to which a number of different categories of projects are being pursued in contrast to being engaged in projects in only a few domains. This can be done by counting the number of different categories of projects, and can be refined by making differentiations within particular domains of interest. Christiansen (1996) made a detailed and compelling case for balanced project pursuit as essential to health and well-being.[8]

Practical and Technical Considerations in Content and Category Analysis

There are some practical issues concerning category analysis of personal projects that should be raised here. These questions also address issues relating to the exact elicitation instructions to use, the number of projects to generate, and the examples that are used in the PPA instructions.

The difference between person-centered and variable-centered assessment, as mentioned earlier, is crucial to decision making about adapting PPA for research or applied activities. Retention of all of the projects generated during the project dump is desirable for category analysis in the case of person-centered assessment. Even in variable-focused research it is desirable to have a sufficient number of projects to generate potential exemplars of most of the categories that are of theoretical interest.

Domain Funneling: Strategic Winnowing of Project Categories. Beyond the natural winnowing provided by having individuals generate their salient projects, we also encourage another funneling. Some researchers are interested in examining projects within particular domains and elicit projects within those domains only. For example, Phillips et al. (1996, 1997) were particularly interested in work projects and how they impacted nonwork projects, and respondents were given space in which to generate two separate lists. Similarly, Dowden (2004) explored the

---

[8]However, it should be pointed out that Christiansen's case for balance is particularly centered on the need to avoid undue conflict between projects, a topic that is explicitly explored under the impact module discussed in a later section.

projects of entrepreneurs and restricted his elicitation procedure to various categories of pursuit in the entrepreneurial domain. This funneled elicitation procedure increases the power of detecting relations within the domain of interest (e.g., work or health projects), although it sacrifices the possibility of establishing the representativeness of that project category in the overall project system of the individual. It might also increase the likelihood of eliciting projects that, although made salient by the instructions, are actually less reflective of the ongoing pursuits of the respondent. As in all assessment-based research, there are trade-offs to be calculated between bandwidth and fidelity, as well as estimation of the power lost but insight gained, from the intensive study of the complete project system of a small group of individuals.

Use of Examples: Appropriate Priming and Due Diligence. It may be fairly asked whether the provision of examples of projects may unduly influence the kinds of projects generated by respondents. The alternative is simply to describe what we mean by a personal project, goal, striving, or life task, and have individuals generate their own list without the benefit of examples (see also Cantor, 1994; Emmons, 1986). Early calibration research on this question (Little, 1988) showed that the proportion of projects in different categories in the examples did not produce similar proportions of projects in the project dump. However, this is a matter requiring more attention. The trade-off here is that not using examples may lead to a truncation in elicitation of the types of projects we are interested in exploring. This in turn could restrict the range from which we are sampling and so limit our ability to detect important relations. For example, with older participants, we have found that projects were sometimes conceived of as larger scale tasks (e.g., fix the backyard fence). However, when we gave age-appropriate examples from the full range of the categories in Table 2.2, respondents were more likely to generate a diversity of projects, including pursuits of a more subtle or intrapersonal nature.

Continuing research on the sensitivity and utility of various elicitation formats is required both for psychometric and substantive reasons.[9] For now, our best estimate is that giving examples from a diversity

---

[9]Indeed, some of the most exciting research with goal and personal action construct (PAC) units is taking place at the level of elicitation of such units through priming procedures (including subliminal priming) as reflected by Freund (chap. 9, this volume) and Sheldon (chap. 13, this volume). Little (1987a), in a primer on PPA for counselors and clinicians, suggested a priming procedure in which individuals would revisit their project list and add other possible projects that they would like to engage in but are not, and deep priming, which involved having individuals list in a free associative and unconstrained fashion any desired projects and

of domains generates reliable and robust data. If the data were unduly influenced by the use of examples in the elicitation module, we would not expect such results. Providing examples, therefore, may have some influence, but not an undue influence on the projects generated in PPA, particularly if they represent a diversity of types of project.

The Personal Project Appraisal Module: How's It Going?

Once the person has generated a set of personal projects we proceed to the personal project appraisal module. This comprises a set of dimensions based both on theoretical and applied considerations on which individuals appraise their projects. Just as the elicitation module models the everyday query, "What's up?," the appraisal module poses a quotidian question, "How's it going?," with respect to the person's projects.

Prior to this, another funneling procedure needs to be considered. Although for individual assessment in clinical contexts it may be desirable to have all of the personal projects from the dump appraised, for practical purposes in most research, a smaller number is typically used. We provide the instructions shown in Table 2.3.

In the early stages of our research program respondents were to select those 10 projects from their original list that they "were most likely to be engaged in during the next weeks and months" (Little, 1983). Our intent was to make the projects carried over for appraisal ecologically representative of the actual pursuits engaged in by the individual. Later, however, we realized that this particular funneling procedure decreases the chance of getting both long-term projects and shorter term but highly salient projects.

Subsequently, we began to change the winnowing instructions in a way that was more in accordance with our theoretical stance. As indicated in Table 2.3, we now ask individuals to choose those 10 personal projects from the initial dump that provide the most important information for understanding themselves and what their life is like. Although we have not yet examined the issue systematically, there does not seem to have been a significant change in the type of results we obtain in normative investigations with this changed funneling procedure.[10] We an-

---

pursuits that they could imagine, even outrageous ones. From a counseling perspective the reasons why people feel prescribed or proscribed in their project pursuits offer considerable insight into foregone possibilities that might be revisited.

[10]We consistently recover the same factors from project matrices with the changed winnowing procedure as we did with the previous instructions; for example, stress, difficulty, and challenge have been recovered as a factor in virtually every investigation, irrespective of whether all projects, representative ones, or more meaning-based projects are rated.

TABLE 2.3

Instructions for Selecting Projects for Appraisal (Electronic Version)

Select Project List

Now, please select 10 of the projects you've listed that provide the most important information for understanding yourself and what your life is like.

Project #	Project Description	Check 10 Projects
1	Lose ten pounds	☑
2	Be a better Druid	☑
3	Maybe apologizing to my brother	☑
4	Become more extraverted	☑
⌄	⌄	⌄
10	Figure out how to pay rent	☑
11	Continue to "grow" as a person	☑
12	Organize a neighborhood watch program	☑
13	Tell my sister to get rid of her sickening boyfriend	☑
14	Help my husband get through Christmas	☑
15	Finish renovating Mom's basement	☑

ticipate that this will provide for a richer base from which to explore project appraisals in clinical and applied contexts.

Personal Project Appraisals: Standard, Ad Hoc, and Open Column Dimensions

Three different types of appraisal dimensions have been used in PPA. The first is a set of standard appraisal dimensions that have been developed and then retained for use in most studies. The second are ad hoc dimensions that have been developed to assess distinctive aspects of a particular group of respondents or the attributes of a particular behavior setting or ecosystem. The third are open columns that require the respondent to provide answers to questions such as where the project is primarily undertaken or, if the project involves others, with whom the project is being carried out. Each of these forms of appraisal provides useful information for both person-centered and variable-centered research.

The Evolution of Standard Dimensions of Personal Project Appraisal: Continuing Development.   The earliest versions of PPA only used a few dimensions relating to enjoyment, perceived control, stress, and how visible the project was to other individuals as well as two open columns (discussed later) asking where and with whom the project was carried out. By the time PPA was published (Little, 1983), it comprised 17 standard dimensions that were used in most subsequent studies. Although researchers are encouraged to take advantage of the modular nature of PPA and select relevant dimensions for their purposes, the number of dimensions that we regard as standard has increased over the years. The appraisal matrix is now divided into two components: essentially cognitive appraisals and those dealing with more affective appraisals of ongoing projects.

What guided the addition of standard appraisal dimensions in PPA? First, theoretical constructs emerging in psychology and other fields of the social sciences were added. The construct of self-identity, for example, was seen as relevant to concepts of alienation critical to political and social theory. People pursuing projects with which they are unable to identify are more likely to feel alienated and disengaged from society. Absorption was added to enable PPA to tap into issues relating to experiences of flow (Csikzentmihalyi, 1975). The stage dimension indicates where a project is situated on the continuum of inception, planning, action, and termination (Little, 1983), allowing us to assess the temporal unfolding of personal projects that was central to its early formulation. It also afforded a bridge to action psychology dealing with temporal aspects of goal pursuit (e.g., Blunt, 1998; Blunt & Pychyl, 2005). Other dimensions were added to provide for more subtle differentiations of important psychological constructs. For instance, the dimension of challenge was added as a way of differentiating negative stress from a more positive, energizing demand on individuals.

The process of flexible addition of relevant appraisal dimensions in PPA contrasts with orthodox trait assessment. In trait assessment fixed items are difficult to change without subverting the whole measurement philosophy underlying the assessment device. Consequently, revisions to traditional multi-item inventories are major ventures involving considerable labor and expense.

In early versions, all the standard appraisal dimensions were presented on a single sheet, but with the expansion of the number of affective dimensions we now present the appraisal matrix in two sections (A and B), with headings asking the respondents "what they think" about each project and "how they feel" about each project, respectively, along with a sheet explaining the meaning of each of the appraisal dimensions (see Tables 2.4 and 2.5 and Appendix B).

Through a gradual, iterative process of exploratory empirical analysis and of theoretical postulations about the major influences shaping effective project pursuit, five themes emerged: project meaning, structure, community, efficacy and stress (Little, 1989, 1998). Project meaning was anchored by the dimensions of self-identity and value congruency. Project structure was anchored by the dimensions of control and time adequacy. Project community was a consistent, although relatively small factor, comprised of only two dimensions: visibility and others' view of the importance of the project. In later years, the dimension of support has clarified and strengthened this factor. Project efficacy comprised both progress and anticipated successful outcome. It too has been more securely anchored by the addition of a dimension of competency. Finally, project stress was primarily defined by the dimension of the same name, and by challenge and difficulty. These five themes of personal projects, each of which addressed a major area of psychological research, proved to be robust predictors of a variety of outcome measures relating to quality of life and flourishing, both as measured by positive scales, such as life satisfaction and ratings of effectiveness, and by negative scales, such as measures of depression and burnout. As discussed by Little (chap. 1, this volume), the cumulative evidence indicates that human flourishing is related to having projects that are relatively high on meaning, structure, community, and efficacy and relatively low on stress (Little, 1999b).

In recent years, as affective processes have attracted considerable attention in the psychological research literature, we have added dimensions that capture the emotional experiences accompanying project pursuit. Although two of the original dimensions were clearly affective (enjoyment and stress), we have expanded both positive and negative dimensions.

With the expansion of the affective dimensions in PPA, a new five-theme model has been emerging, again a product of both empirical analysis of factor structure and theoretical changes in the ways we conceive of how personal projects are pursued. Currently we refer to the five themes as project meaning, manageability, community/support, positive affect, and negative affect. Project meaning comprises dimensions such as self-identity and absorption; manageability combines dimensions previously split between efficacy and structure (e.g., control, likelihood of successful

TABLE 2.4

Personal Projects Appraisal Matrix A (Cognitive Dimensions)

Personal Project Appraisal Matrix A: What Do You Think About What You Are Doing?

Please rate each project below from 0 to 10 on the series of dimensions listed above them.

For example, Michelle might rate her project "Get the car muffler replaced" as an 8 on Importance, 3 on Difficulty, 5 on Visibility, 7 on Control, 9 on Responsibility, 2 on Time Adequacy, and so on.

Your Projects:	Importance	Difficulty	Visibility	Control	Responsibility	Time adequacy	Outcome/ Likelihood of success	Self-identity	Others' view	Value congruency	Progress	Challenge	Absorption	Support	Competence	Autonomy	Stage
1 Lose 10 pounds																	
2 Be a better Druid																	
3 Maybe apologizing to my brother																	
4 Become more extroverted																	
5 Figure out how to pay rent																	
6 Continue to "grow" as a person																	
7 Organize a neighborhood watch program																	
8 Tell my sister to get rid of her sickening boyfriend																	
9 Help my husband get through Christmas																	
10 Finish renovating Mom's basement																	

TABLE 2.5

Personal Projects Matrix B (Affective Dimensions)

Personal Project Appraisal Matrix B: How Do You Feel About What You Are Doing?

Please rate from 0 to 10 the extent to which you feel each emotion while engaged or thinking about each project.

Use 10 if you experience the emotion very strongly, and 0 if you don't feel it at all. In the "Other emotion" column, you have the opportunity to write in any specific emotion that you feel characterizes your project, but may not have been mentioned.

	Your Projects:	*Sad*	*Fearful/Scared*	*Full of love*	*Angry*	*Happy/with enjoyment*	*Hopeful*	*Stressed*	*Uncertain*	*Depressed*	*Other emotion*
1	Lose 10 pounds										
2	Be a better Druid										
3	Maybe apologizing to my brother										
4	Become more extroverted										
5	Figure out how to pay rent										
6	Continue to "grow" as a person										
7	Organize a neighborhood watch program										
8	Tell my sister to get rid of her sickening boyfriend										
9	Help my husband get through Christmas										
10	Finish renovating Mom's basement										

Other examples of feeling words that have been provided by respondents: affectionate, aggressive, annoyed, anxious, apologetic, ashamed, bitter, blissful, bored, cautious, cheerful, confident, confused, determined, disgusted, ecstatic, enraged, exasperated, enraptured, enthusiastic, excited, exhausted, exuberant, frustrated, fun-filled, grief-stricken, horrified, hurt, indifferent, innocent, jealous, love-struck, lustful, meditative, miserable, numb, obstinate, optimistic, paranoid, playful, pleased, puzzled, regretful, relieved, resentful, satisfied, serene, shocked, smug, surly, surprised, suspicious, sympathetic, terrified, thrilled, undecided, vigilant, withdrawn, wild, or any others you prefer ...

completion); and community/support includes visibility, the importance of the project as viewed by others, and support given by others. Positive and negative affect consistently emerge as sharp and clear orthogonal factors (Chambers, 2001; Little & Chambers, 2004).

For data analytic purposes, one can conceive of the broad five themes as the equivalent of traits in five-factor theories and the dimensions as the equivalent of facets (e.g., Costa & McCrae, 1992). Thus we can sum a person's ratings across projects for each of the appraisal dimensions and use these as a person's score on each of the appraisal dimensions and as predictors of outcome measures relating to well-being and effectiveness. Alternatively, theme or factor scores can be used to provide a higher order level of analysis for the prediction of relevant outcome measures. Clearly, with a large number of participants it is possible to use a fairly large number of standard dimensions; with small numbers, we can use the theoretical themes in which the relevant dimensions are aggregated with unit weights into an overall theme score (e.g., project meaning or project negative affect). More frequently, we have used factor scores obtained from particular samples, which typically map clearly on to the five-theme framework, albeit with some idiosyncratic loadings that are reflective of such factors as the nature of the sample or the time of year. The use of such a strategy creates the need for caution in extrapolating to other samples and ideally there will be cross-validation of the empirically derived factors with different but relevant samples of other respondents.

Ad Hoc Dimensions.   One of the foundational criteria underlying PPA is the desire to provide appraisals of individuals that are sensitive to the particular contexts within which they enact their projects. More broadly still, we wish to have flexible, representative assessment that brings into focus aspects of the social ecologies of our respondents. Accordingly, we have encouraged the use of ad hoc dimensions; that is, dimensions designed specifically for a particular group or eco-setting. Typically, these do not replace, but are used in addition to the standard dimensions. This allows us to keep a cumulative record in SEAbank for comparison of groups over time on the standard dimensions.[11] The

---

[11] SEAbank's cumulative record of PPA protocols together with associated measures of individual differences, demographic, and outcome data has allowed us to do meta-analytic studies on predictors of well-being and depression (e.g., Wilson, 1990) as well as examine the stability of personal project appraisals over several decades (Seldon & Little, 2000). It also allows us to check on the extent to which the new dimensions may be redundant with the standard dimensions.

choice of ad hoc dimensions may be based on the researcher's distinctive understanding of a particular setting or may be derived from direct solicitation from respondents about dimensions relevant to appraising their projects. In the latter case we have used a variety of ways of generating new dimensions for a particular group, including grounded theory (e.g., Pychyl, 1996; Pychyl & Little, 1998) and repertory grid techniques (e.g., Cameron, 1984).

One of the most interesting trends we have observed over the years has been for the ad hoc or special dimensions to frequently emerge as among the best unique predictors of well-being for various groups. For example, in a study of Southeast Asian immigrants to Canada during the early 1980s, an excellent predictor of well-being was the extent to which people's projects did not pose language difficulties for them (Loh, 1981). Similarly, with mothers who were single parents, an ad hoc dimension tapping into the sense that the women felt "self-completion" in their projects also had substantial predictions with well-being (Doyle, 1980). A physician interested in predicting coronary risk from project dimensions compared the standard dimensions of time adequacy with time urgency associated with projects, with the latter dimension serving as a better predictor (Mickelson, 1984). Over the years, literally hundreds of such ad hoc dimensions have been used in personal projects research. Chambers (1997) prepared an exhaustive and authoritative compendium of these dimensions, the rationale for their being used, and their empirical utility.

Interlude: On the Personal Saliency of Personal Project Dimensions. It is appropriate here to raise an important issue about the criterion of personal saliency that is essential to the project analytic framework and that differentiates it from other assessment techniques such as trait measurement. Although we can make strong claims that personal projects are salient because participants generate them as idiosyncratically relevant, the dimensions on which they rate their projects have been provided to them rather than generated by them. Have we in this respect compromised the Kellian roots of our methodology?

We have explored this in some detail (Cameron, 1984; LeLacheur, 1993) by creating a measure of the extent to which each of the standard dimensions correlates with dimensions that are spontaneously generated by individuals when comparing and contrasting their personal projects. A personal projects rep grid procedure yields what we call a *mappability coefficient* for each of the standard project dimensions.

These exploratory studies indicated that each project dimension mapped onto the idiosyncratic constructs of respondents to a significant degree. For example, the scores on the standard dimension of difficulty were found to have highly significant correlations with such idiosyncratic dimensions as "pain in the neck to do." There was an interesting gradient of these mappability coefficients, such that the most abstract and theoretical dimensions showed the least mappability (although still significantly so), whereas the more everyday dimensions of stress and enjoyment showed the highest levels of match with individuals' own constructs. We conclude that, although we do supply rather than solicit rating dimensions for appraising projects, the standard dimensions appear to be personally salient to most respondents. For clinical purposes where no normative comparisons are deemed appropriate, it is possible to use both idiosyncratic projects and uniquely generated appraisal dimensions. Given findings that even inactive projects can be related to well-being (Hotson & Little, 2000), we further advise the attentive clinician to attend to what is not present as much as to what is present in the list.

It should also be noted that the modular flexibility of PPA is not restricted to the use of ad hoc dimensions in the appraisal matrices. We have also supplied projects to participants when there is a chance that such projects may not have appeared spontaneously in the project dump or selection, but are of focal theoretical concern in the research. For example, Goodine (1986) studied the personal projects of women with eating disorders compared with those who were "weight preoccupied" but not displaying clinical symptoms. She supplied the project of "control my weight" as a project for all participants who had not previously listed it. Appraisals of this supplied project indicated that it was indeed an important project, and appraisals of that project alone were successful in differentiating clinical patients from normal controls and anorexic from bulimic patients. Similarly, Gee (1992) used the common project of taking a course he was teaching and having it appear as a supplied project at different intervals throughout the term, finding that students' appraisals of the common course project predicted both dropout rates and grades in the course.

Open Column Dimensions: Tapping Into the Social Ecology of Project Pursuit. In the original version of the PPA appraisal matrix two open columns were introduced, one asking the individual to write in the initials of any other people who were involved in the project, the other asking for the location where the project is typically worked on. Both the With Whom and Where columns generate data that operationalize aspects of the social ecology in which projects are pursued. For example, some individuals list many different individuals in their matrix, others list the same person as involved in all projects, and others regard the project pursuits as solitary ventures. Indexes of the extent to which the interdependence with others is focal or diffuse (i.e., with very few or very many others involved, respectively) were used in our early research (Palys, 1980; Palys & Little, 1983). Measures of the actual distance between locations in which one is engaged in personal projects may serve as a measure of the transportation load impacting a person (Martennson, 1977).

In the Social Ecology Laboratory, the use of these two open column dimensions has waned over the years (for an important exception see James, 2001). However, several new open columns have been developed, such as the age one feels (Mavis, 1981) and the type of emotions experienced when engaged in each project (e.g., Goodine, 2000). One of the early exploratory columns we used both intrigued us and posed a dilemma. We asked individuals to write out any personal symbols that may be associated with each project. We gave as an example how "working on my thesis" might be vividly symbolized by associations with the smell of coffee, background music, and a vague sense of muscular tension. For some students this was the most interesting aspect of the whole PPA procedure, and they would effortlessly jot down the symbolic accompaniments of their projects, sometimes with a richness suggesting that their projects were vividly connected with affective and sensory experience. For others there was an uncomfortable look of incomprehension. It appears then that some dimensions, particularly those that require the generation of information rather than ratings on the PPA matrix, may prove difficult for some respondents and a delight for others. Further research on the differential evocativeness of both PPA modules and dimensions is needed. This would include examining how different categories of personal projects may be differentially evocative to certain types of open column probing (e.g., interpersonal projects may be more evocable in this respect than administrative projects). Such research should also examine how individual differences, particularly openness to experience, may be associated with the symbolic richness associated with projects irrespective of category.

Again, we emphasize that the methodology encourages the addition of relevant probes concerning projects that address the theoretical or applied concerns of the investigation. Although of decreased use in our own lab, the original With Whom and Where open columns have been explored in depth by other researchers. For example, Ruehlman and Wolchik (1988) and James (2001) performed extensive examinations of the nature of support, looking not only at the key people involved in each project but also the specific kind of support or hindrance those people played in that particular project. Wallenius (1999), similarly, has carried out detailed and informative studies of the Where column, providing a nice line of continuity with issues originally raised by applying PPA to environmental psychology (Little, 1983, 1987c).

Although we have discussed these open columns in the context of different types of columns used in the appraisal module of PPA, such open-ended questions about personal projects have been extended to encompass narrative accounts about the meaning and significance of one's projects (Goodine, 2000).

Hierarchical Analysis Module: Starting in the Middle

We have already discussed how, by looking at the phrasing level of personal projects, insights are afforded into their manageability and meaning (see also Wallenius, 2000). The hierarchical analysis module allows us to do a more detailed and systematic exploration of this aspect of personal projects. We conceive of personal projects as typically middle-level constructs. Hierarchically, they occupy a position between the molecular or subordinate level of acts and molar, superordinate attributes. The hierarchical analysis modules of PPA provide a means of locating the level of molarity of each project by adaptation of a laddering procedure originally used in repertory grid methodology (Hinkle, 1965). In this procedure, individuals are asked of each project why they are engaged in it and how they accomplish it. These questions are asked iteratively, with each answer being regarded as a rung on a ladder, the number of ladder rungs being a measure of the distance that a project is from a schedulable act ("how" laddering) or to a terminal value or overarching goal ("why" laddering; Little, 1983).

For example, for the project "lose ten pounds" a person may answer the why question by saying "to look better." When asked why he wishes to look better, he may say, "to appeal more to Felicia." If appealing to

Felicia were the ultimate concern in this person's life, then this particular project would be two ladder rungs away from a terminal value. Similarly, in response to the how question, the respondent might describe the steps as "work out more," followed by "go to the gym every Thursday." This would also comprise a distance of two rungs.

In short, laddering proceeds down until it reaches a schedulable act (Little, 1983), similar to what one would elicit in time-budget research (e.g., Harvey, Szalai, Elliott, Stone, & Clark, 1984) and up until it reaches a terminal value or core concern. We posit that the closer the distance of a given project to a terminal value, the greater the meaning of that project to the individual. The closer the distance of a project to a schedulable act, the greater the manageability of that project.

We also assume that this typically engenders a meaning–manageability trade-off, such that some people's projects, although eminently achievable because they are phrased as the level of doable acts, may lack meaning. Contrastingly, a project that may be phrased at the level of a core value may be a considerable distance from achievable acts, or even lack any plausible action steps and thus be essentially unmanageable. Part of the repertoire of skills necessary to pursue projects effectively is having the flexibility to switch to different levels of construal of a personal project or different levels of action identification (Vallacher & Wegner, 1989). A similar case was made by Apter (1989) regarding the flexibility of shifting or reversing between various experiential states during action. For example, the ability to shift between serious goal-oriented telic states and more playful paratelic states during the pursuit of a project is postulated by reversal theory as being highly adaptive.

Although there has been notable interest in this module, particularly from clinicians, it has not received as much research attention as the other modules. In part, this is because it can be time consuming and therefore, on practical grounds particularly if other PPA modules are being used, laddering can only be done on a few of the respondent's projects. Also, it is readily apparent, once one begins the laddering procedure, that a person can have multiple reasons for engaging in a project, each at the same level of molarity, as well as multiple acts through which it may be accomplished, again at the same level. In short, the hierarchical form that best characterizes projects may well be more like a lattice than a ladder (Little & Chambers, 2000, 2004). Clearly more research is needed to clarify the most efficient way in which to access the hierarchical level at which projects are phrased and the implication of different phrasing levels for successful pursuit of projects and for well-being.

The Assessment of Core Projects: Expanding the Modules

As reviewed in chapter 1, a key concept in personal projects analysis is that of *core projects*. Such core projects are postulated to serve as a stabilizing force for individuals over extended periods of time, if not an entire lifetime. We believe that such core projects typically reflect central values that the person holds dear, and both laddering and latticing procedures can be used to uncover such projects. Another approach, and one strongly recommended, has been explored in detail (MacDiarmid, 1990). This expanded module involves asking several questions about the degree of linkage a project has with other projects and the degree of resistance a person would have to giving up or relinquishing each project. Those familiar with Hinkle's (1965) research on implication grids and resistance to change grids in personal construct research will see the close links between exploring core constructs and core projects. Essentially, under this approach, a core project is one that, were it to be removed from the project system, would cause the greatest chaos in the system as a whole. Such projects are those that are most protected and most resistant to change (Little & Chambers, 2004; MacDiarmid, 1990). We accord high priority to further explorations of ways of eliciting, measuring, and examining the correlates and consequences of core projects in our continuing research agenda.

Personal Project Cross-Impact Module: Projects as Interacting Systems

In any given day a person is likely to be pursuing several different personal projects, although at any particular moment, one project may be the focus of conscious deliberative action, as the other projects are on hold. We have developed a module that systematically examines this aspect of personal projects. We do this through the use of cross-impact matrices as illustrated in Table 2.6. They are based on the assumption that projects form interacting systems with other projects both in one's own system and with the projects of others, such that any two projects in the system may have a positive effect (facilitating, assisting) or a negative effect (frustrating, impeding) on each other, and that this effect may be reciprocal or not (that Project 1 may facilitate 2, but 2 frustrates work-

TABLE 2.6
Cross Impact Matrix

Matrix 3: How do your projects impact each other?
Please rate from 0 to 10 the extent to which you feel each project affects the others.

	Your Projects:	Lose ten pounds	Be a better Druid	Maybe apologizing to my brother	Become more extraverted	Figure out how to pay rent	Continue to "grow" as a person	Organize a neighborhood watch program	Tell my sister to get rid of her sickening boyfriend	Help my husband get through Christmas	Finish renovating Mom's basement
1	Lose ten pounds	*	0	0	+ +	–	+ +	+–	0	–	–
2	Be a better Druid	0	*	+ +	+	+	+ +	+	+	+–	+ +
3	Maybe apologizing to my brother	0	+ +	*	–	0	+ +	0	+–	+ +	+
4	Become more extraverted	+	Etc.		*						
5	Figure out how to pay rent	0				*					
6	Continue to "grow" as a person	+–					*				
7	Organize a neighborhood watch program	–						*			
8	Tell my sister to get rid of her sickening boyfriend	–							*		
9	Help my husband get through Christmas	–								*	
10	Finish renovating Mom's basement	+ +									*

ing on Project 1). Our original assumption was that project systems characterized by a high degree of mutual facilitation will be more adaptive for the individuals than those filled with a similar degree of mutual frustration, although the research yield on this is complex (see Riediger, chap. 4, this volume).

The instructions are for the respondents to examine each project, starting with the first row (Project 1) and to scan across the list of other projects on the top, indicating the impact of Project 1 on each of the others by placing + if it has a positive impact, + + if it strongly facilitates it, – if it has a negative impact, – – if it has a strong negative impact, and 0 if it has no impact. Any combination of these can be used; thus + +– would indicate that one project strongly facilitates (in one respect) another, but also has a smaller negative impact. Note that this notational system assumes that positive and negative impact are separate, not bipolar dimensions (see Riediger, chap. 4, this volume, for an extensive discussion of this issue). This module yields a number of indexes. For normative research one can look at the overall degree of coherence or conflict in the cross-impact matrix. One can also examine if certain categories of projects (e.g., work projects) have a disproportionate degree of negative impact on other projects.

In single-case studies, one can see which project in the overall system has the highest degree of negative (or positive) effect on the rest of the system. As discussed earlier, a project that has a high degree of positive facilitation of others in the system may well be a core project; they serve to ground the system as a whole, prove resistant to change, and provide a source of strength during periods of turbulence in the person's life. However, it is entirely possible that core projects, to be sustainable, may exact costs on other projects. Instead of a highly balanced system, we may find that during periods of sustained core project pursuit some strategic imbalance may be required. Clearly, a high priority for future research is the longitudinal examination of sustainable core projects and how they impact on a person's overall project system.

As highlighted throughout this book, personal projects are intimately impacted by the projects of others, and the logic of the cross-impact matrix can easily be generalized to assess such relations. A joint cross-impact matrix involves listing the projects of one person down the side of the matrix and the projects of another person (e.g., a spouse or coworker) across the top. Scores of mutual positive and negative impact can be calculated and again, it seems plausible to suggest that the greater the degree of conflict in the project systems, the more problems there may be between the two individuals. As explored in more detail by Salmela-Aro and Little (chap. 7, this volume), there are now several studies that have examined the relational issues between couples using variations on the joint cross-impact matrix.

Extensions to the PPA Suite

To sum up our discussion so far, the four major modules of PPA provide ways of looking at the content, appraisal, systemic features, and impact of one's personal projects. We have also developed other assessment techniques for looking at the characteristics of personal projects that are not part of the standard PPA suite and, as they are not given prominence in this volume, two of these are simply noted here.

For individuals wishing to examine personal project ratings at a global level, the Personal Project System Rating Scale (Little, 1988) asks individuals to rate from 0 to 10 their overall set of projects and pursuits on the five factors of meaningful versus meaningless, manageable versus chaotic, supported by others versus not supported, highly likely to succeed versus highly unlikely to succeed, and highly stressful versus not at all stressful. These simple, direct magnitude scales have been used in several studies in the Social Ecology Laboratory and show substantial predictive validity and moderate levels of convergent and discriminant validity with the corresponding dimensions of PPA.[12] A Q-deck procedure for PPA has also been developed, comprising items that describe how individuals manage their overall set of personal projects and capturing many of the dimensional themes of the original PPA (e.g., "My projects are generally very stressful"). This includes a computer-based version that allows individuals (or other judges such as peers, work partners, or spouses) to describe their personal project management style. The strength of this measure is that it can be used with archival data, opening up a vast territory of possible explorations into, for example, the ways in which various historical figures carried out their personal projects.

Personal Projects Analysis in Retrospect and Prospect: Concluding Thoughts

This chapter has provided a guide to how to do PPA, together with some technical commentary explaining the purpose or justification for some of its features. The methodology, as the title denotes, comprises essentially a set of four modules for eliciting, appraising, determining the hierarchical placement, and estimating the impact of a person's projects. PPA also employs a set of winnowing devices that make the potentially unmanageable project of studying projects more doable. It is helpful for us, first, to cast a retrospective glance at these components of PPA and to

---

[12]We have been influenced by Burisch's (1984) research on the validity of single scales item for certain aspects of our research and have been able, independently, to show that the considerable utility of such scales does not compromise validity and is consistent with the orientation toward respondents discussed in chapter 1. Despite their psychometric unorthodoxy, there is mounting evidence of the use and value of single items in personality research (see John & Benet-Martinez, 2000).

underscore their significance. Then we look at the prospects for future developments.

Retrospect and Review: Why Use Personal Projects Analysis?

Elicitation Module: What's Up?   In the elicitation module we ask individuals to generate examples of their ongoing or planned personal projects. Why do it this way? Why not get a set of prespecified common activities or projects and ask individuals whether they are engaged in them? It would certainly make issues of commensurability and comparability across respondents a lot easier and, depending on one's purposes, can be an entirely worthwhile task. However, we are concerned with the singular and idiosyncratic aspects of human conduct as well as the common and conventional. We do not want to sacrifice the possibility of discovering special facts about unique people—such as someone in southeastern Ontario wanting to be a better Druid. We suspect that clinicians, in particular, would find the self-generation of projects to be helpful to the therapeutic enterprise.

However, there are other ways of preserving a focus on individual activity without forcing it into precast categories. We could simply engage in naturalistic observation and follow individuals around to discern what their projects are. However, the outward and visible aspects of action do not always align with the inwardly formulated reasons as viewed by the project pursuer. We may get high interrater reliability on the behavior settings entered and time spent in them by an individual, yet miss the personal project that makes those comings and goings part of a larger concern. Behavior setting analysis and time-budget research are entirely compatible with PPA but they ask and answer different questions.

The Appraisal Matrix: How's It Going?   The appraisal module asks individuals to rate each of their personal projects on a set of dimensions, some of which are theory driven and others that are more applied in nature. Does this approach make sense? Do people actually appraise their projects along the kind of dimensions that we specify? Isn't it possible, even likely, that people will distort or at least be unreliable in their appraisals?

Our answer here is both theoretical and empirical. Theoretically, there are variables such as perceived control, stress, and social support that need to be operationalized to advance our conceptual agenda. By using such dimensions as commensurable within a single case, but also allowing them to be treated as normative dimensions for comparison across individuals, we suggest that PPA contributes to the theoretical exploration of variables of significance in the fields of personality and developmental science and ancillary fields. Moreover, through its modular and modifiable nature, it can keep apace and even drive theoretical explorations in a way that is more difficult with methodologies that are fixed, such as traditional trait inventories.

Empirically, as briefly summarized in this chapter, there is no evidence that we have compromised our Kellian roots by providing dimensions instead of having them elicited. There is an encouraging degree of mappability between the standard dimensions and those generated idiosyncratically by respondents. For clinical purposes, there is no reason not to make both projects and appraisal dimensions fully idiosyncratic. The final justification for the use of appraisal dimensions is their predictive utility in domains that matter, such as measures of well-being or rated effectiveness in a work context.

Hierarchical Analysis Module: Getting There From Here   In the hierarchical analysis module we place personal projects within a hierarchical structure ranging from schedulable acts at the most molecular level to core values or overarching concerns at the most molar level. By starting with the personal project as the elicitation unit we allow access to each of the other levels through the laddering or latticing procedures. This is important because if we were to start at either of the other levels of analysis (superordinate goals or the kind of acts that might be generated from beeper methods), we might miss the opportunity of tracing through the linkages between all three levels. Because both extremes of the action hierarchy are important, it is critical that we are able to get to one from the other.

We suggest that the more subordinated acts of daily lives are linked to the more superordinate concerns of human affairs through the everyday projects that constitute the middle-level gateway. Thus higher level aspirations or possible selves may be provisionally tried out by engaging in a project that is new and challenging. This, in turn, leads to the small acts of daily life that, on direct inquiry, may not be thought to represent much of anything at all. However, by providing a method for detecting linkages, however fragile or fragmentary they may be, we are encouraging a view of human activity that spans the full spectrum of human concerns. Thus, for example, we can get from the ethereal "being a better person" to the earthly "using a pooper scooper" by eliciting the middle-level project "take Cujo for a walk."

Cross-Impact Matrices: Conflict and Core Projects

The cross-impact matrix, both in its individual and group version, allows us to chart conflict among and between individuals. Conversely, it affords us the opportunity to look at a person's projects as a system, albeit a personal system (Little, 1972), in which we can discern which projects are playing a supporting role in the system and even forming synergistic relations with other undertakings.

When we look at the impact of personal projects on others and on the social ecology more generally, we are able to spot areas where conflict may play a corrosive role in a partnership (be it domestic or business). One of the most intriguing questions, and one that is amenable to study by PPA impact research is whether core projects—those most central to one's self-definition—might actually impact in a negative way the rest of one's projects. In many respects, the laying out of a person's cross-impact matrix, particularly if done alongside that of a partner in the joint cross-impact matrix, may reveal both conflicts and supports that had not been noticed before. Again, PPA is meant to be a microcosm of the life spaces of individuals and when explicated may provide insights and sudden recognitions that redound to the benefit of those engaged in the exercise. Indeed, one of the most encouraging aspects of working with the methodology has been the observation that engaging in PPA can provide personal insights that are intriguing to the participants who may not need to be bribed with monetary inducements to participate in further research (e.g., Omodei & Wearing, 1990).

PROSPECTS FOR PPA: SMALL STEPS, GIANT LEAPS

Small Steps: Consolidating and Expanding the Psychometric and Empirical Base of PPA

One of the exciting aspects of working with PPA over the years has been its rapid adoption, particularly in thesis and dissertation research; in the mainstream literatures of personality, social, and developmental psychology; and in fields as diverse as optometry and town planning. However, there has been a downside: Until this volume, there has been little in the way of easily accessible information on the methodological and psychometric aspects of PPA. One of the most important needs for future research is making this work, which has been extensively documented in internal reports from the Social Ecology Laboratory, more available to researchers and practitioners interested in adopting or adapting the methodology. Although much of this is available on the Web (http://www.brianrlittle.com/ppa/index.htm), we intend to continue confirming and consolidating the psychometric and empirical base of personal projects analysis.

For example, there is good evidence for the internal coherence and temporal stability of indexes derived from PPA and it will be helpful to draw on SEAbank to efficiently summarize that evidence using multiple samples. Also, there is clear evidence that the original five factors of project dimensions are robust predictors of various measures of well-being, even after controlling for the effects of stable traits of behavior. However, that research remains largely confined to dissertations and unpublished technical reports. With the addition of project affect factors, it is readily apparent that we can, not surprisingly, boost even further those already notable correlations with important outcome measures. A final example of a small but important future research project that would help consolidate the past is that the original publication (Little, 1983) contained a large number of predictions regarding individual differences (e.g., in extraversion, self-monitoring, locus of control, Machiavellianism) in how people would handle different stages of personal project pursuit. Although data are available in SEAbank for testing those predictions, a systematic review of them has yet to be undertaken. These projects are all on our agenda as small-scale but important undertakings to consolidate and strengthen the evidentiary base of PPA, and we encourage other researchers to join in on the enterprise.

Giant Leaps: Harnessing Technology and Expanding the Human Reach of PPA

We have already alluded to the fact that PPA readily lends itself to computerization and the case has been made that we need to be far more audacious in using multimedia and other technological tools to make human assessment an exciting venture (Little, 2005). Traditional testing and assessment can sometimes be extremely tedious and we have found even with the intrinsically engaging assessment provided by PPA that, with the addition of more dimensions and modules, the procedure risks overloading the participants. Beyond using graphically pleasing computer and Web versions of PPA we have seen highly imaginative adaptations of the methodology, which we would further encourage. For example, occupational therapists have been particularly drawn to PPA because it speaks virtually the same language as they do (the content of daily action and occupation; Christiansen, Little, & Backman, 1998; Christiansen, Little, Backman, & Nguyen, 1999). Occupational therapists and occupational scientists have used unconventional ways of presenting PPA, including the low-tech but highly engaging process of having patients write out their projects on large sheets on a wall and sitting back and engaging in conversations about them. We anticipate major leaps in both high- and low-tech developments of PPA methodology in the coming years. Unlike conventional fixed tests, PPA's modular structure lends itself to interactive assessment and to incorporation of interviews into the process, some of which can be done by nonhuman "embodied conversational agents" (Bickmore & Cassell, 2004). Our hope is for the assessment of personal projects to be an engaging and even exciting aesthetic experience.

There is also considerable current interest in applying the project analytic perspective to issues in both cross-cultural psychology and cultural psychology. PPA modules have been translated into approximately two dozen languages and research on cross-national comparisons is growing (e.g., Richardson, 2002). We are hoping to carry out some major cross-national comparisons in the near future. It is important here to underline one crucial aspect of the methodology: Its unit of analysis is tractable. That is, in contrast with most philosophical and psychometric views on traits, personal projects can be changed. If, for example, a project is found to be stressful and meaningless and it interferes with your and others' core projects, it might be a candidate for termination. There must be 50 ways to leave your project. Sometimes projects cannot be dropped, however, because they are essentially the conative glue that holds one's whole system together. Rather, the means through which one enacts the project might be reconsidered, or its stress might be reduced by breaking the project down into more accomplishable small tasks.

Whereas some individuals suffer from a surfeit of projects under which they are straining, others suffer from a dearth of anything meaningful into which they can invest themselves. We have been exploring the use of an orally administered variant of PPA for use in developing countries, where many projects are politically proscribed or too dangerous to undertake. As a way of capturing the concerns and possible projects of those who have been precluded from meaningful project pursuit, PPA might aid those who see human assessment and the amelioration of human misery as potential partners. We are hopeful that PPA and related approaches, unconventional as they might be, can play a role in extending the human reach of assessment. A methodology that might yield both aesthetic delight and the hope of promoting human flourishing is a giant aspiration, but one we hold dear.

REFERENCES

Apter, M. J. (1989). *Reversal theory: Motivation, emotion and personality.* London: Routledge.

Bickmore, T., & Cassell, J. (2004). Social dialogue with embodied conversational agents. In J. Van Kuppevelt, L. Dybkjaer, & N. Bernsen (Eds.), *Natural, intelligent and effective interaction with multimodal dialogue systems.* New York: Kluwer.

Blunt, A. K. (1998). Task aversiveness and procrastination: A multi-dimensional approach to task aversiveness across stages of personal projects (Master's dissertation, Carleton University). *Masters Abstracts International, 36,* 1409.

Blunt, A. K., & Pychyl, T. A. (2005). Project systems of procrastinators: A personal project-analytic and action control perspective. *Personality and Individual Differences, 38,* 1771–1780.

Burisch, M. (1984). Approaches to personality inventory construction: A comparison of merits. *American Psychologist, 39,* 214–227.

Cameron, L. (1984). *A personal projects rep grid.* Unpublished bachelor's thesis, Carleton University, Ottawa, ON, Canada.

Cantor, N. (1994). Life task problem solving: Situational affordances and personal needs. *Personality and Social Psychology Bulletin, 20,* 235–243.

Chambers, N. C. (1997). *Personal projects analysis: The maturation of a multi-dimensional methodology.* Retrieved May 1, 2005, from http://www.brianrlittle.com/research/index.htm

Chambers, N. C. (2001). Time and personal action: Tenses and aspects of project pursuit (Doctoral dissertation, Carleton University, 2000). *Dissertation Abstracts International, 62*(2B), 1130.

Christiansen, C. H. (1996). Three perspectives on balance in occupation. In R. Zemke & F. Clark (Eds.), *Occupational science: The evolving discipline* (pp. 431–451). Philadelphia: Davis.

Christiansen, C. H., Little, B. R., & Backman, C. (1998). Personal projects: A useful approach to the study of occupation. *American Journal of Occupational Therapy, 52,* 439–446.

Christiansen, C. H., Little, B. R., Backman, C., & Nguyen, A. (1999). Occupations and well-being: A study of personal projects. *American Journal of Occupational Therapy, 53,* 91–100.

Chulef, A. S., Read, S. J., & Walsh, D. A. (2001). A hierarchical taxonomy of human goals. *Motivation and Emotion, 25,* 191–232.

Costa, P. T., & McCrae, R. R. (1992). *NEO PI–R professional manual.* Odessa, FL: Psychological Assessment Resources.

Csikszentmihalyi, M. (1975). *Beyond boredom and anxiety.* San Francisco: Jossey-Bass.

Dowden, C. E. (2004). *Managing to be "free": Personality, personal projects and well-being in entrepreneurs.* Unpublished doctoral dissertation, Carleton University, Ottawa, ON, Canada.

Doyle, R. E. (1980). *Personal projects and the social ecology of single motherhood.* Unpublished bachelor's thesis, Carleton University, Ottawa, ON, Canada.

Emmons, R. A. (1986). Personal strivings: An approach to personality and subjective well-being. *Journal of Personality and Social Psychology, 51,* 1058–1068.

Gee, T. L. (1992). *Personal project dimensions—Of course!* Unpublished manuscript, Carleton University, Social Ecology Laboratory, Ottawa, ON, Canada.

Gee, T. L. (1997). *On redefining reliability for the single case.* Unpublished manuscript, Carleton University, Ottawa, ON, Canada.

Gee, T. L. (1999). Individual and joint-level properties of personal project matrices: An exploration of the nature of project spaces (Doctoral dissertation, Carleton University, 1998). *Dissertation Abstracts International, 59*(10B), 5609.

Goodine, L. A. (1986). *Anorexics, bulimics and highly weight preoccupied women: A comparison of personal project systems and personality factors.* Unpublished master's thesis, Carleton University, Ottawa, ON, Canada.

Goodine, L. A. (2000). An analysis of personal project commitment. (Doctoral dissertation, Carleton University, 1999). *Dissertation Abstracts International, 61*(4-B), 2260.

Harvey, A. S., Szalai, A., Elliott, D. H., Stone, P. J., & Clark, S. M. (1984). *Time budget research: An ISSC workbook in comparative analysis.* Frankfurt, Germany: Campus Verlag.

Hinkle, D. (1965). *The change of personal constructs from the viewpoint of a theory of construct implications.* Unpublished doctoral dissertation, Ohio State University Columbus.

Hotson, A. H., & Little, B. R. (2000, June). *Inactive personal projects: The impacts of unfinished tasks.* Paper presented at the 61st annual conference of the Canadian Psychological Association, Ottawa, ON.

James, D. (2001). The nature of the self and well-being: A relational analysis using personal projects (Doctoral dissertation, Carleton University, 2000). *Dissertation Abstracts International, 61,* 4475.

John, O. P., & Benet-Martinez, V. (2000). Measurement: Reliability, construct validation, and scale construction. In H. Reis & C. M. Judd (Eds.), *Handbook of research methods in social and personality psychology* (pp. 339–369). Cambridge, UK: Cambridge University Press.

LeLacheur, P. (1993). *The personal construing of personal projects: An omnigrid analysis.* Unpublished bachelor's thesis, Carleton University, Ottawa, ON, Canada.

Little, B. R. (1968). Psychospecializaton: Functions of differential orientation toward persons and things [Abstract]. *Bulletin of the British Psychological Society, 21*(70), 113.

Little, B. R. (1972). Psychological man as scientist, humanist and specialist. *Journal of Experimental Research in Personality, 6,* 95–118.

Little, B. R. (1976). Specialization and the varieties of environmental experience: Empirical studies within the personality paradigm. In S. Wapner, S. B. Cohen, & B. Kaplan (Eds.), *Experiencing the environment* (pp. 81–116). New York: Plenum.

Little, B. R. (1983). Personal projects: A rationale and method for investigation. *Environment and Behavior, 15,* 273–309.

Little, B. R. (1987a). Personal projects analysis: A new methodology for counselling psychology. *NATCON, 13,* 591–614.

Little, B. R. (1987b). Personal projects and fuzzy selves: Aspects of self-identity in adolescence. In T. Honess & K. Yardley (Eds.), *Self and identity: Perspectives across the life span* (pp. 230–245). London: Routledge & Kegan Paul.

Little, B. R. (1987c). Personality and the environment. In D. Stokols & I. Altman (Eds.), *Handbook of environmental psychology* (pp. 205–244). New York: Wiley.

Little, B. R. (1988). *Personal projects analysis: Theory, method and research.* Ottawa, ON, Canada: Social Sciences and Humanities Research Council of Canada.

Little, B. R. (1989). Personal projects analysis: Trivial pursuits, magnificent obsessions, and the search for coherence. In D. M. Buss & N. Cantor (Eds.), *Personality psychology: Recent trends and emerging directions* (pp. 15–31). New York: Springer-Verlag.

Little, B. R. (1993). Personal projects and the distributed self: Aspects of a conative psychology. In J. Suls (Ed.), *Psychological perspectives on the self* (Vol. 4, pp. 157–181). Hillsdale, NJ: Lawrence Erlbaum Associates.

Little, B. R. (1998). Personal project pursuit: Dimensions and dynamics of personal meaning. In P. T. P. Wong & P. S. Fry (Eds.), *The human quest for meaning: A handbook of psychological research and clinical applications* (pp. 193–212). Mahwah, NJ: Lawrence Erlbaum Associates.

Little, B. R. (1999a). Personal projects and social ecology: Themes and variation across the life span. In J. Brandtstädter & R. M. Lerner (Eds.), *Action and self-development: Theory and research through the life span* (pp. 197–221). Thousand Oaks, CA: Sage.

Little, B. R. (1999b). Personality and motivation: Personal action and the conative evolution. In L. A. Pervin & O. P. John (Eds.), *Handbook of personality theory and research* (2nd ed., pp. 501–524). New York: Guilford.

Little, B. R. (2000a). Free traits and personal contexts: Expanding a social ecological model of well-being. In W. B. Walsh, K. H. Craik, & R. Price (Eds.), *Person environment psychology* (2nd ed., pp. 87–116). New York: Guilford.

Little, B. R. (2000b). Persons, contexts and personal projects: Assumptive themes of a methodological transactionalism. In S. Wapner, J. Demick, T. Yamamoto, & H. Minami (Eds.), *Theoretical perspectives in environment–behavior research* (pp. 79–88). New York: Plenum.

Little, B. R. (2005). Personality science and personal projects: Six impossible things before breakfast. *Journal of Research in Personality, 39,* 4–21.

Little, B. R., & Chambers, N. C. (2000). Analyse des projets personnels: Un cadre intégratif pour la psychologie clinique et le counselling [Personal projects analysis: An integrative framework for clinical and counseling psychology]. *Revue Québécoise de Psychologie, 21,* 153–190.

Little, B. R., & Chambers, N. C. (2004). Personal project pursuit: On human doings and well beings. In M. Cox & E. Klinger (Eds.), *Handbook of motivational counseling: Concepts, approaches and assessment* (pp. 65–82). Chichester, UK: Wiley.

Little, B. R., & Gee, T. L. (in press). Personal projects analysis. In N. Salkind (Ed.), *Encyclopedia of measurement and statistics.* Thousand Oaks, CA: Sage.

Little, B. R., Lecci, L., & Watkinson, B. (1992). Personality and personal projects: Linking Big Five and PAC units of analysis. *Journal of Personality, 60,* 501–525.

Little, B. R., & Ryan, T. J. (1979). A social ecological model of development. In K. Ishwaran (Ed.), *Childhood and adolescence in Canada* (pp. 273–301). Toronto: McGraw-Hill Ryerson.

Little, T. D., Schnabel, K. U., & Baumert, J. (Eds.). (2000). *Modeling longitudinal and multilevel data: Practical issues, applied approaches and specific examples.* Mahwah, NJ: Lawrence Erlbaum Associates.

Loh, P. F. (1981). *Personal projects, social networks, and the adaptation of Indochinese refugees.* Unpublished bachelor's thesis, Carleton University, Ottawa, ON, Canada.

MacDiarmid, E. W. (1990). *Level of molarity, project cross impact and resistance to change in personal project systems.* Unpublished master's thesis, Carleton University, Ottawa, ON, Canada.

Martennson, S. (1977). Childhood interaction and temporal organization. *Econ Geography, 53,* 99–115.

Mavis, B. (1981). *Personal projects as indicators of change in men at mid-life.* Unpublished master's thesis, Carleton University, Ottawa, ON, Canada.

Mickelson, W. P. (1984). *Personal project systems and health status.* Unpublished master's thesis, Carleton University, Ottawa, ON, Canada.

Ogilvie, D. M., & Rose, K. M. (1995). Self-with-other representations and a taxonomy of motives: Two approaches to studying persons. *Journal of Personality, 63,* 643–679.

Ogilvie, D. M., Rose, K. M., & Heppen, J. B. (2001). A comparison of personal project motives in three age groups. *Basic and Applied Social Psychology, 23,* 207–215.

Omodei, M. M., & Wearing, A. J. (1990). Need satisfaction and involvement in personal projects: Toward an integrative model of subjective well-being. *Journal of Personality and Social Psychology, 59,* 762–769.

Palys, T. S. (1980). Personal projects systems and perceived life satisfaction (Doctoral dissertation, Carleton University, 1979). *Dissertation Abstracts International, 41*(5B), 1894.

Phillips, S. D., Little, B. R., & Goodine, L. A. (1996). *Organizational climate and personal projects: Gender differences in the public service* (Canadian Centre for Management Development Research Paper No. 20). Ottawa, ON, Canada: Minister of Supply and Services.

Phillips, S. D., Little, B. R., & Goodine, L. A. (1997). Reconsidering gender and public administration: Five steps beyond conventional research. *Canadian Journal of Public Administration, 40,* 563–581.

Palys, T. S., & Little, B. R. (1983). Perceived life satisfaction and the organization of personal project systems. *Journal of Personality and Social Psychology, 44,* 1221–1230.

Pychyl, T. A. (1996). Personal projects, subjective well-being and the lives of doctoral students (Doctoral dissertation, Carleton University, 1995). *Dissertation Abstracts International, 56*(12B), 7080.

Pychyl, T. A., & Little, B. R. (1998). Dimensional specificity in the prediction of subjective well-being: Personal projects in pursuit of the PhD. *Social Indicators Research, 45,* 423–473.

Rankin, N. (1967). *The measurement of traits: A new approach emphasizing the measurement of the individual case.* Unpublished manuscript, University of California, Berkeley, CA.

Richardson, K. (2002). Personal projects analysis and well-being: Cultural explorations. (Master's thesis, Carleton University, 2001). *Masters Abstracts International, 40,* 1630.

Ruehlman, L. S., & Wolchik, S. A. (1988). Personal goals and interpersonal support and hindrance as factors in psychological distress and well-being. *Journal of Personality and Social Psychology, 55,* 293–301.

Seldon, K., & Little, B. R. (2000, June). *Personal projects: Generational effects in project systems.* Presentation at the 61st annual conference of the Canadian Psychological Association, Ottawa, Canada.

Simpson, E. H. (1951). The interpretation of interaction in contingency tables. *Journal of the Royal Statistical Society, 13,* 238–241.

Vallacher, R. R., & Wegner, D. M. (1989). Levels of personal agency: Individual variation in action identification. *Journal of Personality and Social Psychology, 57*, 660–671.

Wallenius, M. A. (1999). Personal projects in everyday places: Perceived supportiveness of the environment and psychological well-being. *Journal of Environmental Psychology, 19*, 131–143.

Wallenius, M. A. (2000). Personal project level of abstraction and project conflict: Relations to psychological well-being. *European Journal of Personality, 14*, 171–184.

Wilson, D. A. (1990). *Personal project dimensions and perceived life satisfaction: A quantitative synthesis.* Unpublished master's thesis, Carleton University, Ottawa, ON, Canada.

Zimmerman, D., & Little, B. R. (1972). *Mathematical and applied characteristics of ipsative measurement.* Unpublished manuscript, Carleton University, Ottawa, ON, Canada.

APPENDIX A
PSYCHOMETRIC ISSUES
IN PERSONAL PROJECTS ANALYSIS

From the outset, PPA was designed to measure features of individual cases and the internal structure of a person's projects as well as to provide data in vector form that, like orthodox traits, could serve as predictor variables regarding measures of well-being and flourishing. Some of these assumptions were similar to Kelly's repertory grid technique, but PPA posed its own distinctive psychometric challenges, which we briefly and selectively discuss in this appendix.

Data in personal projects analysis can be treated at the individual level of analysis, can be aggregated to form normative scales or vectors, and can be treated at the project level (e.g., all health projects listed from a set of studies can be examined and compared with interpersonal projects on the project dimensions). It is important to underscore several assumptions about this approach to measurement (Little & Gee, in press).

First, like a repertory grid technique, we assume that the basic level of measurement is that of the individual's personal project system. We further assume that the sample of projects elicited represents the current state of that system. This is somewhat problematic for classical approaches to reliability, which have involved either correlations between scores over time or internal consistency measures such as Cronbach's alpha. These methods have invariably been developed assuming that $N > 1$, and mathematically suffer from the deficiency that they are not defined when $N = 1$ (and perform rather poorly when N is not much more than 1). Rankin (1967) devised an ipsative reliability coefficient by invoking the notion of maximum possible variance, which we denote as $V_{max,}$ which was the maximum amount of change that could possibly be observed in an individual's score, given the structure of the test. This was originally devised for binary items and extended to multi-item scales by Zimmerman and Little (1982). Gee (1997) extended their work to multi-item polytomous Likert scales and showed through simulation that Cronbach's alpha is heavily dependent on the distribution of what by then we referred to as Rankin's Rho in the sample. Using a formula where we denote the minimum value on the scale as Min and the maximum value on the scale as Max, we see that for n items, the expected value for the mean score on the scale (when maximum variance is attained) is (Min + Max)/2 (for an even number of items). Thus, for an even number n of items, the maximum possible variance can be arbitrarily written as either

$$V_{max,} = n[Max - ((Min + Max) / 2)^2] / (n - 1)$$

or

$$V_{max,} = n[Min - ((Min + Max) / 2)^2] / (n - 1).$$

For an odd number of items, the mean may reflect an imbalance in extreme scores at either end of the distribution. As a result, for any odd number of items greater than or equal to 3, the theoretical midpoint for an extreme pattern is not so simple. The bias introduced by having an odd number of items is small for a large number of items, but should be factored in, particularly for a small number of items. When N is odd, the midpoint will be either [MID = ((n/2 – 0.5) * MIN + ((n/2 + 0.5) * MAX) / n] or [MID = ((n2 – 0.5) * MAX + ((n/2 + 0.5) * MIN / n], depending on the imbalance of extremes induced by the odd number of items. If we assume either and proceed consistently, both methods give the same value of V_{max}. If for example we assume the midpoint [((3/2 + 0.5 * MAX + (3/2 – 0.5) * MIN) / 3] form, we need to specify a preponderance of MAX values over MIN values in competing V_{max}, in a quantity that mirrors the assumed split in extreme responses. For any odd number n items that reflect the most extreme response pattern, there will be $(n / 2 – 0.5)$ deviations of the MIN value from the bias-adjusted midpoint, and $(n / 2 + 0.5)$ deviations of the MAX value. Thus, we may write

$$V_{max} = [(n / 2 – 0.5)(MIN – MID)^2 + (n / 2 + 0.5)(MAX – MID)^2]/(n - 1)$$

If we consider, for example, the stress factor (stress/difficulty/challenge) commonly identified in PPA research (Little, 1988), and imagine someone rating a project with the S/D/C scores (9, 10, 8) we see immediately how this works. First, we consider that the worst possible (i.e., most inconsistent) pattern of responding on a 3-item, 0-to-10 Likert scale would be (10, 0, 10) or (0, 10, 0). The observed variance of the items (9, 10, 8) is 1, whereas the maximum possible variance would be that of the scores (0, 10, 0) or 33.33. Here we can check the formula by inserting the values:

$$V_{max} = [(3/2 - .5)(0 - (0 + 2(10))/3)^2 + (3/2 + .5)(10 - (0 + 2(10))/3)^2]/(3 - 1)$$

$$= [1(0 - 20/3)^2 + (2(10 - 20/3)^2]/2$$

$$= (-6.66^2 + 2(3.33^2))/2$$

$$= (44.44 + 22.22)/2$$

$$= 66.66/2$$

$$= 33.33$$

Therefore for this case, the ipsative reliability of the scale would be $1 - 1/33.33$ or .97. Equally, for the pattern (7, 7, 7) it would be 1, as observed variance goes to zero. With such numbers, we can examine the distribution of this statistic across projects for that case, and estimate both a mean and a standard deviation for the ipsative reliability for that case. Once we have estimated the internal consistency for each case, then in the sample we can make the usual statistical inferences about the population with equal validity. It would seem that mean ipsative reliability is a better indicator than classical indexes for these reasons:

- It is defined for the single case.
- It gives a direct measure of the average ipsative reliability in a sample.
- It does not assume that reliability is the same for all individuals.
- It provides a direct measure of dispersion of the reliability across the sample.
- It also allows identification of outliers, for whom the scale may not be valid.

Factor analysis and single-case matrices: In adopting an idiographic view, we limit immediately the volume of data that we can process to what can be collected comfortably at a given time, in a given place. Obtaining data on 12 projects, but having them rated on 17 dimensions, for instance, creates a problem for factor analysis when looking at a single case. The fact that intraclass correlations exist when project-level data are pooled over many cases further violates the assumption of independence of observations that factor-analytic techniques requires to be satisfied.

Fortunately, there are other methods that do not collapse when the n-to-variable ratio is below critical thresholds, or other assumptions are violated. Gee (1999) demonstrated the multidimensional scaling of correlation matrices computed from individual PPA matrices could be used to reveal essentially the same underlying structure as did overall factor analysis, both of means and of raw project-level data taken across many participants. Mixed model analysis is now available that permits modeling of covariance structures that we expect will, in future research, demonstrate the viability of data collected at multiple levels, and elaborate extant findings (Little, Schnabel, & Baumert, 2000).

APPENDIX B
PROJECT APPRAISAL DIMENSION DESCRIPTIONS

Cognitive Project Dimension	Dimension Description
Importance	How important is this project to you? Use 10 if you consider it to be very important, and 0 if it is not at all important.
Difficulty	How difficult do you find it to carry out this project? Use 10 for a project that is extremely difficult to carry out, and 0 for one that is not difficult at all.
Visibility	How visible is this project to others that are close to you? Use 10 for a project that is very visible to those around you, and 0 for a project, which is not at all visible to those around you.
Control	How much do you feel you are in control of this project? Use 10 if you feel completely in control of the project, and 0 if you feel you have absolutely no control over the project.
Responsibility	How responsible are you for carrying out this project? Use 0 is you do not feel any responsibility for making progress in this project, and 10 if you feel entirely responsible for the project.
Time Adequacy	How adequate is the amount of time you spend working on this project? Use 10 if you feel the amount of time is perfectly adequate, and 0 if you feel that the amount of time you spend working on the project is not at all adequate.
Outcome/ Likelihood of Success	How successful do you believe this project will be? Use 10 if you expect the project to be entirely successful, and 0 if you think the project will turn out to be a total failure.

(continued)

Cognitive Project Dimension	Dimension Description
Self Identity	All of us have things we do that we feel are typical or truly expressive of us. These things can be thought of as our "trade marks." For example, some people engage in sports every chance they get, others prefer to read, and others prefer to socialize. Think of what your own personal "trade marks" are, and then rate this project on the extent to which it is typical of you. Use 10 if a project is very typical of you, and 0 if it is not typical at all.
Others' View	How important is this project seen to be by those people who are close to you? Use 10 if others see a project as very important, and 0 if it is seen as not important at all.
Value Congruency	To what extent is each project consistent with the values that guide your life? Use 10 if a project is totally consistent with your values, and 0 if a project is totally at odds with them.
Progress	How successful have you been in this project so far? Use 10 to indicate that you have been very successful and 0 to indicate that you have had no success at all.
Challenge	How challenging do you find this project? Use 10 if it is very challenging, perhaps more than you can handle, and 0 if it is not at all challenging, indeed you find it almost boring.
Absorption	To what extent do you become engrossed or deeply involved in a project? Use 10 if you generally get absorbed in an activity, and 0 if you tend to be uninvolved when doing it.
Support	To what extent do you feel other people support each project? Support may come in different forms, e.g., emotional (encouragement, approval), financial (money, material possessions) or practical (active assistance). Use 10 if you feel other people support the project a lot, and 0 if there is no support at all.
Competence	To what extent do you feel competent to carry out this project? Use 10 if you feel completely competent to carry out the project, and 0 if you do not feel competent to carry it out.
Autonomy	How much is this project one which you feel you are pursuing autonomously? (That is, you are engaged of your own free will in the project, not because anyone else wants you to do it.) Use 10 if you are engaged in this project entirely of your own free will, and 0 if this project is one that you feel totally obliged to complete because of or for someone else.

Cognitive Project Dimension	*Dimension Description*
Stage	Projects often go through several stages, which can be visualized along a time-line. Think of each project as moving through stages on such a time-line. Using the scale on this page, rate each project's stage: 0—1 Awareness: The idea for the project has just come to you. 2 Transition: You have decided to proceed with the project. 3—4 Planning: You are planning it and obtaining whatever personal and material support it may require. 5 Transition: You have the project planned out and you are beginning to (or trying to) actively start the project. 6—7 Action: You are actively working on the project and trying to balance it with your other projects, resources and time commitments. 8 Transition: You are evaluating the project and your motivation to continue with it, or bring it to completion/disengage from it. 9—10 Completion: The project is coming to a close or has actually been completed or terminated.

II

Basic Processes of Project Pursuit:
Internal Regulatory Functions

3

Approach–Avoidance: A Central Characteristic of Personal Goals

Andrew J. Elliot and Ron Friedman

Motivated behavior may be energized or directed by a positive or negative event or possibility. For example, a person may desire to attain success or seek to deepen a friendship or, alternatively, a person may desire to avoid failure or seek to avoid the dissolution of a friendship. The former examples represent *approach* motivation, whereas the latter represent *avoidance* motivation. This distinction between approach and avoidance motivation has a long history in intellectual thought in general, dating back to the writings of the ancient Greek philosophers, and in scientific psychology more specifically, dating back at least as far as the work of William James (1890). This distinction also has a broad history, as it has been shown to have conceptual and empirical utility within a diversity of psychological literatures (for reviews see Elliot, 1999; Elliot & Covington, 2001).

Given the long and richly documented utility of the approach–avoidance distinction, it is surprising that it is ignored or overlooked in many contemporary analyses of motivation and personality. Approach–avoidance concepts have certainly garnered substantial attention in the past decade (see Cacioppo & Berntson, 1994; Carver & Scheier, 1998;

Davidson, 1992; Elliot, 1997; Gray, 1987; Higgins, 1997; Lang, 1995), yet theories, models, constructs, and hypotheses are still often espoused with little consideration of this distinction (see Elliot & Mapes, 2005, for a discussion of possible reasons for this oversight).

In our hierarchical model of approach–avoidance motivation (Elliot, 1997, 1999; Elliot & Thrash, 2002), we proposed that the approach–avoidance distinction is fundamental and basic to any analysis of affect, cognition, and action. Indeed, we view this distinction as a unifying conceptual thread that may be used to organize and integrate various levels of investigation. Thus, the approach–avoidance distinction is applicable at the dispositional, domain-specific, and situation-specific levels of analysis, and is integral to the study of temperaments, motives, strategies, goals, and reflexes. In this chapter, we focus on the approach–avoidance distinction as it applies to goal constructs, specifically, to idiographic personal goals.

APPROACH AND AVOIDANCE PERSONAL GOALS: DEFINED, ASSESSED, AND CODED

A goal is a cognitive representation of a possible state or outcome that an individual seeks to attain (Austin & Vancouver, 1996; Elliot & Thrash, 2001; Tolman, 1923). All goals focus on either a positive or a negative possibility, and goals serve a directional function in motivation by guiding the individual toward potential positive outcomes or away from potential negative ones (Elliot & Church, 1997).[1] For instance, one may jog every morning with the aim of attaining a slender and attractive physique, or one may jog every morning with the aim of not embarrassing oneself (or one's significant other) at the beach. The approach–avoidance distinction is an inherent, structural feature of goal constructs, and any given goal may be identified as an approach goal or an avoidance goal. This separates approach–avoidance from most other features of goals such as expectancy, difficulty, importance, and so on. These latter features are viewed as indicative of goal appraisal and commitment, whereas approach–avoidance refers to a structural aspect of the goal itself.

---

[1]We conceptualize approach and avoidance goals in terms of what are commonly considered normal, health-inducing aims to approach positive possibilities and avoid negative possibilities. We acknowledge that there are instances in which individuals seek to avoid positive possibilities (e.g., the anorexic who seeks to avoid food) or approach negative possibilities (e.g., the masochist who seeks to approach pain), but consider these abnormal or aberrant motivational tendencies that commonly have ill consequences for health and well-being.

The goal construct has many different manifestations, one of which is the consciously embraced, personally meaningful objectives that individuals pursue in their daily lives (Emmons, 1986; Little, 1983). This type of goal has been operationalized in several different ways, most notably as personal projects (Little, 1983), personal strivings (Emmons, 1986), possible selves (Markus & Nurius, 1986), and current concerns (Klinger, 1977; see Little, 1999, for a discussion of similarities and differences among these operationalizations). In our research, we use the term *personal goal* for this type of goal, which is meant to serve as a generic, inclusive equivalent of the aforementioned operationalizations.

Personal goals are assessed with an *idiographic* procedure (the personal goals elicitation procedure [PGEP]) in which individuals write short statements indicating what they are trying to do in their daily behavior. The manner in which individuals present their goals lexically is presumed to correspond to the way that the goal is represented in memory and, accordingly, the way the goal is utilized in daily regulation. That is, we believe that the precise wording that individuals use in listing their personal goals is neither random nor accidental, but carries important information as to the structure and psychological meaning of the goal.

As with any type of goal, a personal goal may be approach or avoidant in nature. Indeed, nearly any possibility that an individual may focus on in daily life may be framed in terms of a positive possibility that he or she is trying to move toward or maintain, or a negative possibility that he or she is trying to move away or stay away from. For example, a person may articulate his or her goals in terms of "trying to do well in school" and "trying to be respectful toward my mother" or, alternatively, in terms of "trying to avoid doing poorly in school" and "trying not to be disrespectful toward my mother." Given our belief that the way in which a goal is worded corresponds to the way in which the goal is represented in memory, we have devised an objective coding system to categorize personal goal statements for approach–avoidance. In our research, we ask participants to list eight personal goals using the PGEP (see Appendix A and Appendix B), which was devised on the basis of similar procedures used by Little (1983) and Emmons (1986). We have found that essentially all of our participants can readily list eight goals in a relatively short amount of time (i.e., 10 minutes) using this procedure, and that this number of goals is sufficient for the purposes of deriving an approach–avoidance measure with adequate variability. In this procedure, the personal goals concept is defined, and examples of personal goals are provided. The examples presented feature actual goals generated by participants in pilot research, cover several different life domains (e.g., achievement, affiliation), and vary in terms of approach–avoidance. Following the examples, the personal goals concept is further defined with several additional notes indicating that personal goals may involve trying to approach or avoid something, may represent what a person is trying to do regardless of whether the person is actually able to do it, may be broad or specific, and may last for varying lengths of time. The time focus of the elicitation procedure may be varied depending on the research question at hand; participants may be asked to list their goals for a specific time period (e.g., 3 months or an upcoming semester) or they may be asked to list their goals in general without designating a specific time period. Confidentiality and the importance of openness and honesty are emphasized in an attempt to maximize the truly personal nature of the goals elicited.

Participants list their eight personal goals on a separate page. They are provided with scratch paper for brainstorming so that they may be sure to list the eight goals that best describe what they are trying to do in their daily lives. A single, relatively short line is provided for each goal to encourage participants to list a single goal in a concise fashion. We have learned from experience that providing a longer line or multiple lines increases the likelihood that participants will list statements that contain multiple goals or both a goal and a reason for pursuing the goal (see Elliot & Thrash, 2001; Thrash & Elliot, 2001, for a discussion of the distinction between goal and reason; see Ogilvie & Rose, 1995, for a procedure that focuses on reasons rather than goals per se).

Once participants' goal lists have been obtained, a minimum of two independent coders categorize each goal as an approach or avoidance goal. The conceptual core of approach–avoidance is the *valence* of the end state that is the focus of the goal, and it is assumed that individuals construe positive end states as appetitive things to approach and negative end states as aversive things to avoid. Thus, our coding system (see Appendix C) uses information regarding both the positive or negative focus of the goal statement, and the appetitive or aversive tendency with respect to that focus in ascertaining the approach or avoidance nature of a goal.

In most instances, the focus of the goal statement, whether that focus is positive or negative, and whether the tendency with regard to that focus is appetitive or aversive are all clearly discerned, and coding for approach–avoidance is extremely easy. However, some goals are worded in an ambiguous way, contain multiple goals or goal–reason combinations, or are difficult to interpret given translation issues. The rules for coding these relatively infrequent instances are detailed in the coding system. The general strategy underlying the system is to use approach as the default category, because the clear majority of goals in any given sample are approach (thus using approach as the default is the conservative option). Independent coders always reach greater than 99% agreement in their coding. Indeed, in one published study (Elliot & Thrash, 2002) this was the case for a research assistant and the first author's 10-year-old son, a fact testifying to the clarity with which approach and avoidance is manifest in most goal statements.

Once all goals in a sample are coded for approach–avoidance, the number of approach and avoidance goals is summed for each participant, and an avoidance (relative to approach) goals index is created for each participant for use as an independent or dependent variable. It is this index that is the primary measure used in the studies discussed in this chapter. Use of our goal elicitation and coding procedures with U.S. participants tends to yield samples with approximately 10% avoidance goals (of course, this percentage varies somewhat across samples).

Our goal elicitation and coding procedures may be contrasted with those of other researchers who have focused on approach–avoidance or conceptually equivalent distinctions. First, our elicitation of personal goals is fundamentally idiographic in that participants are not requested to provide a particular content or valence of goals, but are completely free to list any type of goals they would like to list. Even in instances where we use a special version of our elicitation procedure focused on the achievement domain, participants are provided with many different examples of achievement-based goals to guide them toward the domain of interest, but remain free to list whatever content and valance of goals they would like within that domain (Elliot & Sheldon, 1997). Others have used procedures that are fully idiographic with regard to goal content, but not with regard to the approach–avoidance nature of the goals. For example, Roberson (1990) provided participants with separate pages on which to write their positively focused and negatively focused goals. Likewise, Coats, Janoff-Bulman, and Alpert (1996) had participants begin each of their goals with an explicitly approach-based or avoidance-based stem (e.g., "It is important for me to obtain ..." or "It is important for me to avoid ...").

Second, our coding system for approach–avoidance relies on individuals other than participants themselves to determine the approach–avoidance nature of the goals. As such, our coding system relies exclusively on the objective, manifest content of the goal statement itself to determine the approach or avoidance designation. Others have had participants code their own goals for approach–avoidance (or conceptually equivalent distinction). However, this opens the coding process to numerous response biases as there are as many coders as participants and, as their own coders, participants may use quite different implicit criteria or assumptions. In addition, in coding their own goals, individuals undoubtedly use information beyond the manifest content of the goal itself (e.g., the reason behind the goal) to determine its approach or avoidance designation (see, e.g., Klinger, Barta, & Maxeiner, 1980; Moffitt & Singer, 1994). In short, although these other elicitation and coding procedures certainly generate interesting and useful goal data, it is important to acknowledge that these data are not really idiographic with regard to the approach–avoidance distinction, and likely represent something other than information about the approach–avoidance nature of the goal per se.

Research on Avoidance (Relative to Approach) Personal Goals

In the hierarchical model, the approach–avoidance nature of motivation at different levels of analysis, including the goal level of analysis, is posited to have important implications for psychological functioning and well-being. Accordingly, it is important to conduct research that examines the consequences of the ratio of avoidance to approach personal goals, the processes responsible for such consequences, and the antecedents of avoidance personal goal adoption. Over the past decade we have carried out a research program guided by this aim, and we overview this work in the following. Our overview also includes the two other empirical studies conducted by other investigators who used a goal elicitation and coding procedure that, like our own, yields a truly idiographic assessment of approach–avoidance goals (or conceptual equivalent). We also make brief note of other research that has focused on approach–avoidance goals or their conceptual equivalents, but in a less fully idiographic fashion.

Consequences and Mediational Processes. Our research in this area is grounded in the proposition that the pursuit of avoidance (relative to approach) goals typically has negative consequences. The focus on negative possibilities inherent in avoidance goal regulation is presumed to evoke and sustain a host of processes (see Table 3.1) that are deleterious to the individual's goal attainment, psychological adjustment, and physical health. Such processes are broad in scope, and include perceptual processes (e.g., appraising information as a threat), attentional processes (e.g., heightened sensitivity to and vigilance for negative information), mental control processes (e.g., difficulty concentrating and sustaining focus), memorial processes (e.g., biased search for and recall of negative information), emotional processes (e.g., anxiety and worry), volitional processes (e.g., feeling internally forced or obligated to expend effort), and behavioral processes (e.g., escaping or selecting oneself out of goal-relevant situations). Using negative possibilities as the hub of goal regulation is also presumed to be inefficient and ineffective because it provides the individual with something to move away from but not something to move toward, and does not afford the person a clear sense of goal progress. Indeed, even if one succeeds at an avoidance goal, one simply acquires the absence of a negative outcome, not the presence of a positive outcome that is needed to satisfy the individual's psychological and physical needs (see Elliot & Sheldon, 1998; Elliot, Sheldon, & Church, 1997, for overviews of the problems associated with avoidance goal regulation). Avoidance personal goals are not necessarily always expected to have inimical consequences, but in the main they are expected to produce negative processes that eventuate in negative outcomes.

In our brief overview, we focus primarily on the empirical findings of the research, rather than the specific theoretical explanations for the findings. Space considerations preclude the presentation of such information, and readers interested in the theoretical underpinnings are en-

TABLE 3.1
Processes Evoked by Avoidance (Relative to Approach) Personal Goals

Process	Example
Perceptual	Appraising information as a threat
Attentional	Heightened sensitivity to and vigilance for negative information
Mental control	Difficulty concentrating and sustaining focus
Memorial	Biased search for and recall of negative information
Emotional	Anxiety and worry
Volitional	Feeling internally forced or obligated to expend effort
Behavioral	Escaping or selecting oneself out of goal-relevant situations

couraged to proceed to the original articles themselves. The studies discussed in this chapter were conducted with undergraduate participants unless otherwise indicated.

We began our research by focusing on personal goals in the achievement domain (Elliot & Sheldon, 1997). At the beginning of a 4-month study, participants completed both implicit and explicit measures of fear of failure. A week later, participants listed their personal achievement goals, and rated each of their goals in terms of importance, expected competence, and intended effort. Participants also reported their subjective well-being (SWB; life satisfaction, positive affectivity, and [absence of] negative affectivity) during the past few weeks. Three times over the course of the 4-month period, participants reported their current perceptions of competence for each of their goals. At the end of the 4-month period, participants again reported their SWB during the past few weeks (thereby affording a longitudinal analysis of SWB), and completed a retrospective report of their SWB during the entire 4-month period. They also completed retrospective, goal-specific measures regarding adjustment (e.g., the extent to which their goal pursuit influenced their self-esteem) and the experience of goal regulation (e.g., the extent to which they perceived goal pursuit to have been an enjoyable experience).

Following data collection, participants' goals were coded for level of specificity, and the order in which participants' goals were listed provided an indicator of goal representativeness (i.e., salience). The results from this study indicated that the avoidance–approach index of personal goals was a negative predictor of all indicators of SWB, adjustment, and experience. All of these findings held when possible alternative predictor variables (implicit and explicit fear of failure, goal importance, goal expectancy, goal importance × goal expectancy, intended effort, goal specificity, and goal representativeness) were controlled. Perceived competence was shown to mediate the direct relations observed, such that the ratio of avoidance to approach goals undermined perceptions of competence, which in turn undermined SWB, adjustment, and experience. Ancillary within-subjects analyses conducted with the goal-specific measures yielded essentially identical results to those obtained in the between-subject analyses.

In a subsequent study (Elliot et al., 1997, Study 2), we used the same short-term longitudinal procedure used in Elliot and Sheldon (1997) to extend the work beyond the achievement domain to personal goals in general. The results conceptually replicated the core findings of the

Elliot and Sheldon study. Avoidance (relative to approach) personal goals were a negative predictor of both retrospective and longitudinal SWB, and these relations proved robust across low and high scores on self-regulatory skills, social skills, goal importance, goal expected progress, and goal importance × goal expected progress. Participants' perceived progress was documented as a mediator of the direct relation between avoidance goal pursuit and SWB. Again, ancillary within-subjects analyses with the goal-specific perceived progress measure replicated the between-subject analyses.

Next, we used our short-term longitudinal procedure to examine the link between approach–avoidance personal goals and physical symptomatology, as well as possible mediators of this link. In an initial study (Elliot & Sheldon, 1998, Study 1), the avoidance ratio was shown to be a positive predictor of both retrospective and longitudinal physical symptoms (e.g., headaches, chest or heart pain, stomachache), and these findings held when controlling for neuroticism, Type A personality, and optimism. The study was distinctive in that it was conducted over a month-long period, participants listed five personal goals, and the goal elicitation procedure simply instructed participants to list the "individual, specific goals" that they would be pursuing during the next month (no other information regarding personal goals was provided). In a 4-month follow-up study (Elliot & Sheldon, 1998, Study 3), avoidance personal goals were again shown to positively predict both retrospective and longitudinal physical symptoms, and these findings were robust across neuroticism, extraversion, neuroticism × extraversion, and behavioral inhibition system (BIS) sensitivity. Avoidance goals negatively predicted participants' goal-specific perceptions of competence and autonomy, and positively predicted goal-specific perceptions of control. Further, participants' perceived competence and perceived control were documented as joint mediators of the direct relation between avoidance goal pursuit and physical symptomotology. Ancillary within-subjects analyses with the goal-specific perceived competence, perceived autonomy, and perceived control measures replicated the between-subject analyses. A unique feature of this study is the use of "past few days" as the temporal referent in the longitudinal assessment of physical symptoms over the study period.

After documenting the inimical influence of avoidance (relative to approach) goals on SWB and physical symptomatology, we turned to an examination of the generalizability of these findings across cultures. Specifically, we conducted two studies designed to examine the concurrent relation between the ratio of avoidance to approach goals and SWB in an individualistic country—the United States (where all of our prior work had been conducted)—and two collectivistic countries—South Korea (which is typically characterized as highly collectivistic) and Russia (which is typically characterized as moderately collectivistic). In the comparative U.S.–South Korea study (Elliot, Chirkov, Kim, & Sheldon, 2001, Study 3), avoidance (relative to approach) goals were negatively related to SWB in the U.S. sample, but were unrelated to SWB in the South Korean sample. Likewise, in the U.S.–Russia study (Study 4), avoidance goals were negatively related to SWB in the U.S. sample, but were unrelated to SWB in the Russian sample. In each of these studies, participants' goals were coded for achievement and affiliation content, and the preceding findings held when these variables and several demographic variables (e.g., parental education, family income) were controlled.

We then proceeded to examine whether our longitudinal SWB findings extended to the psychotherapy context. The participants in our study (Elliot & Church, 2002) were individuals seeking short-term (12-session) psychotherapy in a university counseling center. Prior to their first therapy session, participants listed five therapy goals and completed goal-specific measures of importance and expected progress. They also reported their SWB with regard to the past few days. After their final therapy session, participants reported their satisfaction with their therapist, perceived problem improvement, and perceived goal progress, as well as their SWB with regard to the past few days. Results indicated that a higher ratio of avoidance therapy goals led to a smaller increase in SWB during therapy; this finding was observed across goal importance, goal expected progress, and goal importance × goal expected progress. Sequential mediation of the direct relation was documented: More avoidance goals led to less therapist satisfaction, which led to low perceptions of problem improvement and goal progress, which led to less of an increase in SWB during the course of therapy.

In a recent study, Elliot and Friedman (2004) examined a characteristic of personal goals that is independent of, but clearly relevant to, the approach–avoidance distinction: the presence–absence distinction. Like approach–avoidance, the presence–absence distinction is an inherent, structural feature of goals; any goal can be characterized in terms of whether it focuses on something that is currently present or currently absent. This presence–absence distinction carries information regarding whether the goal is focused on maintenance or change. Approach/presence and avoidance/absence goals focus on maintaining a current situation, and approach/absence and avoidance/presence goals focus on changing a current situation. In the study, participants' personal goals were coded for both approach–avoidance and presence–absence, and SWB reports (over a period of "the past few days") were acquired at the beginning and end of the 4-month study. Results indicated that avoidance (relative to approach) goals undermined SWB, and an approach–avoidance × presence–absence interaction was also observed. Avoidance goals were found to be most deleterious for SWB when they focused on getting away from something negative that was already present.

Finally, other studies have been conducted using less idiographic assessments of approach–avoidance goals (or conceptual equivalent), and the results of these studies are briefly noted.[2] Klinger et al. (1980) linked the ratio of positively focused to negatively focused goals to concurrent negative expectations of positive affect. Roberson (1990) found that a higher ratio of positively focused goals was negatively related to concurrent low job satisfaction. Coats et al. (1996, Study 1) reported a negative correlation between avoidance goals and reports of optimism and self-esteem, and a positive correlation between avoidance goals and depression. Updegraff, Gable, and Taylor (2004) demonstrated that approach social goals were a positive predictor of positive social outcomes and that avoidance social goals were a positive predictor of negative social outcomes. Furthermore, the number of social events encountered and the reactivity to social events were shown to mediate the approach and avoidance goal relations, respectively.

Antecedents. What determines whether people tend to avoid or approach their goals? Given the negative influence of a high proportion of avoidance personal goals on a variety of different processes and outcomes, it is clearly important to determine what leads people to adopt and pursue these maladaptive forms of regulation. Several studies have examined antecedents of avoidance personal goals, and we overview

---

[2]In this paragraph, and the corresponding paragraph in the antecedents section, we exclude some studies that nevertheless focused on approach or avoidance goals (or conceptual equivalent) component. These include studies that (a) only assessed approach goals or only assessed avoidance goals (e.g., Ogilvie, 1987), (b) assessed expected rather than desired outcomes (e.g., Oyserman & Markus, 1990), (c) assessed approach and avoidance goals via a fully nomothetic procedure (e.g., Dunkel, 2000), and (d) assessed approach and avoidance goals but did not report results on the consequences or antecedents of these goals (e.g., Robinson, Davis, & Meara, 2003).

this research here. Our research in this area is grounded in a basic premise of the hierarchical model—that goals, including personal goals, signify concrete, cognitive representations of possible outcomes that help channel and guide general motivational tendencies toward specific aims (Elliot, 1999; Elliot & Thrash, 2002). Thus, our work focuses on general, motivationally relevant constructs that are likely to prompt avoidance goals in the process of self-regulation. As in our earlier review of consequences and mediational processes, we primarily detail the empirical results of the research, and encourage readers interested in additional conceptually based information to read the original articles themselves.

One potential explanation is that the tendency to frame goals as avoidance is related to age or gender. Heckhausen (1997) tested age as a predictor of gain- and loss-framed personal goals and found that older adults did adopt more loss-framed (and less gain-framed) goals than younger adults. In all extant studies in which gender has been examined as a predictor variable, however, it has failed to produce significant results. Indeed, gender seems clearly unrelated to avoidance goal adoption.

Other research has looked to a variety of personal predispositions or enduring temperaments. Emmons and McAdams (1991) hypothesized that individuals who are highly inhibited in their behavior (as indicated by use of the word *not* in projective protocols) are preoccupied with avoiding negative outcomes and are thus likely to adopt more negatively focused goals. Their data supported this proposition, as activity inhibition was a positive predictor of negatively focused (relative to positively focused) goals. Elliot and Sheldon (1997) posited that emotion-based motive dispositions, such as implicit and explicit fear of failure, prompt the adoption of more cognitively based avoidance goals that function to channel the general motive-based tendencies toward specific aims. As expected, both implicit and explicit fear of failure were shown to positively predict the ratio of avoidance to approach achievement goals. Elliot et al. (1997) examined the hypothesis that individuals with poor self-regulatory skills would be more likely to adopt ineffective forms of regulation such as avoidance personal goals. The data conformed to predictions as self-regulatory skills were found to be a negative predictor of avoidance goal adoption.

Other explanations look to external or cultural factors as antecedents. Elliot and Church (2002), for example, reasoned that relational loss or disruption would produce a self-protective tendency in individuals, and prompt them to focus on avoiding negative possibilities in their goal pursuits. The data supported this contention in that parental loss due to separation, divorce, or death was a positive predictor of avoidance (relative to approach) goals in a psychotherapy context. Elliot et al. (2001) posited that collectivism, with its emphasis on fitting in and eliminating negative characteristics that could create relational disruption, would lead to more avoidance goal adoption than individualism, with its emphasis on standing out and acquiring positive characteristics that establish one's distinctiveness. This hypothesis was supported across the three most common representations of the individualism–collectivism construct: psychological construal, ethnic category, and cultural attribute (i.e., country). In Study 1, interdependent self-construals were positive and independent self-construals were negative predictors of avoidance (relative to approach) goals. In Study 2, Asian Americans were shown to adopt relatively more avoidance goals than White Americans. In Studies 3 and 4, South Koreans and Russians were found to adopt more avoidance (relative to approach) goals than those from the United States.

Elliot and Thrash (2002) examined approach and avoidance temperaments, operationalized in terms of behavioral activation system (BAS) and BIS sensitivity, respectively, as predictors of the adoption of avoidance achievement goals. Approach and avoidance temperaments were portrayed as general, biologically grounded orientations that prompt like-valenced goals in the process of self-regulation. As anticipated, approach temperament was shown to be a positive predictor and avoidance temperament was shown to be a negative predictor of avoidance (relative to approach) achievement goals. In focusing more specifically on social goals, Gable (2006) showed that BAS sensitivity and hope for affiliation were positive predictors of social-approach goals, whereas BIS sensitivity and fear of rejection were positive predictors of social-avoidance goals.

The security of attachment may also shape inherent preferences for avoidance or approach goal in important ways. Elliot and Reis (2003) posited that secure attachment reflects unconditional support and acceptance that allows individuals to freely engage in approach-oriented exploration, whereas insecure attachment reflects conditional support and acceptance that reorients individuals toward the avoidance of mistakes and failures. As such, insecurely attached individuals (both anxious/ambivalent and avoidant) were expected to list relatively more avoidance personal achievement goals than securely attached individuals. The data were in accord with these predictions. Similarly, individuals with low self-esteem, argued Heimpel, Wood, and Elliot (2005), are motivated by self-protection (i.e., concealing their faults and preventing further self-worth decrements). They therefore use avoidance goals in their daily self-regulation. Furthermore, self-esteem was conceptualized by Elliot and Thrash (2002) as a mediator of the link between avoidance temperament and avoidance goal adoption. The results of three studies supported these hypotheses. In Study 1, self-esteem was shown to negatively predict avoidance goal adoption. Study 2 replicated this finding, and additionally documented self-esteem as a mediator of the relation between avoidance temperament (neuroticism) and the avoidance–approach index. Study 3 replicated Study 2 with achievement personal goals and a different indicator of avoidance temperament (BIS sensitivity).[3]

CONCLUSIONS

The research reviewed here attests to the fact that the investigation of approach and avoidance personal goals has yielded many insights into the nature of motivation and self-regulation. The ratio of avoidance to approach personal goals has been shown to exert a deleterious influence on many different outcomes in many different contexts. Avoidance goals have been shown to exert their negative impact through a variety of different processes, and they have been shown to emerge from a host of different factors. Clearly, approach–avoidance is an important conceptual distinction at the personal goal level of analysis.

---

[3]The pattern of results of Elliot and colleagues has been supported by other studies that have used less explicitly idiographic assessments of approach–avoidance goals (or equivalent units), notably in the study of possible selves. Cross and Markus (1991) demonstrated that the number of both hoped-for and feared possible selves decreases from late adolescence to late adulthood. Carver, Reynolds, and Scheier (1994) reported that optimism was inversely related to the diversity of hoped-for possible selves, but was unrelated to the diversity of feared possible selves. Hooker and Kaus (1994) showed that young and middle-aged adults had more feared than hoped-for possible selves in the health domain. Hooker, Fiese, Jenkins, Morfei, and Schwagler (1996) found that parents of infants were more likely to have hoped-for parenting selves than parents of preschoolers, and mothers were more likely to have feared parenting selves than fathers. Morfei, Hooker, Fiese, and Cordeiro (2001) found substantial continuity in hoped-for and feared parenting selves over time, and showed that mothers had more feared parenting selves than fathers. Dunkel and Anthis (2001) showed that individuals who decreased in identity commitment over time (relative to those who increased) had a greater decrease in both hoped-for and feared possible selves. Dickson and MacLeod (2004a, 2004b) found that depression was a negative predictor of approach goals, and that anxiety was a negative predictor of avoidance goals.

From our perspective, research on approach–avoidance personal goals is at only a nascent stage of development. Although many antecedents, processes, and consequences have been documented, much remains unknown about the adoption and pursuit of approach and avoidance personal goals. For example, research to date has clearly documented that avoidance personal goals have negative consequences for many different outcomes, but research has barely begun to explore the degree to which these findings generalize across cultures, contexts, personality characteristics, types of avoidance goals, and so on. It is possible that for for some tasks (e.g., air-traffic controlling) or in some situations (e.g., immediately responding to a dangerous event), avoidance goals may actually be beneficial forms of regulation. Likewise, it is possible that avoidance goals focused on a negative outcome that is currently present are most deleterious for well-being when the goals are personal goals pursued over a lengthy time period (see Elliot & Friedman, 2004), whereas avoidance goals focused on a negative outcome that is currently absent may be most inimical for performance in specific achievement situations (Elliot, 1999).

One seriously underexplored issue concerns the processes that mediate the link between avoidance goal pursuit and goal progress. We have posited that avoidance goals possess a number of features that are detrimental in the process of regulation (see Elliot & Sheldon, 1998), but research has yet to be conducted on this issue. Furthermore, given the negative implications of avoidance goal pursuit, a pressing question is whether interventions may be developed to shift an individual toward the pursuit of approach goals and away from the pursuit of avoidance goals. We suspect that relatively straightforward intervention procedures may be effective for some individuals. For those who have adopted avoidance goals out of deeply engrained avoidance tendencies, such as neuroticism or BIS sensitivity, however, more elaborate procedures would likely be necessary.

In sum, approach and avoidance personal goals are easily assessed, easily coded, and easy to investigate using a diversity of research methodologies. Approach–avoidance goals may be examined in studies designed a priori with this focus in mind, but, importantly, approach– avoidance goals may also be examined in nearly any extant data set containing idiographic goal lists. Given the clear predictive utility of the approach–avoidance distinction and the conceptual importance and centrality of approach–avoidance motivation, we are hopeful that other researchers will join the effort to contribute to empirical work in this area.

ACKNOWLEDGMENTS

Preparation of this chapter was facilitated by support from the William T. Grant Foundation (Grant No. 2565) and a Friedrich Wilhelm Bessel Research Award from the Alexander von Humboldt Foundation. We thank Bettina Wiese and the editors of this book for their helpful comments on an earlier draft of this chapter.

REFERENCES

Austin, J. T., & Vancouver, J. B. (1996). Goal constructs in psychology: Structure, process, and content. *Psychological Bulletin, 120,* 338–375.

Cacioppo, J., & Berntson, G. (1994). Relationship between attitudes and evaluative space: A critical review with emphasis on the separability of positive and negative substrates. *Psychological Bulletin, 115,* 401–423.

Carver, C. S., Reynolds, S. L., & Scheier, M. F. (1994). The possible selves of optimists and pessimists. *Journal of Research in Personality, 28,* 133–141.

Carver, C. S., & Scheier, M. F. (1998). *On the self-regulation of behavior.* New York: Cambridge University Press.

Coats, E. J., Janoff-Bulman, R., & Alpert, N. (1996). Approach versus avoidance goals: Differences in self-evaluation and well-being. *Personality and Social Psychology Bulletin, 22,* 1057–1067.

Cross, S., & Markus, H. (1991). Possible selves across the life span. *Human Development, 34,* 230–255.

Davidson, R. J. (1992). Emotion and affective style: Hemispheric substrates. *Psychological Science, 3,* 39–43.

Dickson, J. M., & MacLeod, A. K. (2004a). Approach and avoidance goals and plans: Their relationship to anxiety and depression. *Cognitive Therapy and Research, 28,* 415–432.

Dickson, J. M., & MacLeod, A. K. (2004b). Brief report: Anxiety, depression and approach and avoidance goals. *Cognition and Emotion, 18,* 423–430.

Dunkel, C. S. (2000). Possible selves as a mechanism for identity exploration. *Journal of Adolescence, 23,* 519–529.

Dunkel, C. S., & Anthis, K. S. (2001). The role of possible selves in identity formation: A short-term longitudinal study. *Journal of Adolescence, 24,* 765–776.

Elliot, A. J. (1997). Integrating "classic" and "contemporary" approaches to achievement motivation: A hierarchical model of approach and avoidance achievement motivation. In P. Pintrich & M. Maehr (Eds.), *Advances in motivation and achievement* (Vol. 10, pp. 143–179). Greenwich, CT: JAI.

Elliot, A. J. (1999). Approach and avoidance motivation and achievement goals. *Educational Psychologist, 34,* 149–169.

Elliot, A. J., Chirkov, V. I., Kim, Y., & Sheldon, K. M. (2001). A cross-cultural analysis of avoidance (relative to approach) personal goals. *Psychological Science, 12,* 505–510.

Elliot, A. J., & Church, M. A. (1997). A hierarchical model of approach and avoidance achievement motivation. *Journal of Personality and Social Psychology, 72,* 218–232.

Elliot, A. J., & Church, M. A. (2002). Client articulated avoidance goals in the therapy context. *Journal of Counseling Psychology, 49,* 243–254.

Elliot, A. J., & Covington, M. V. (2001). Approach and avoidance motivation. *Educational Psychology Review, 12,* 73–92.

Elliot, A. J., & Friedman, R. (2004). *Maintenance-change as a characteristic of goals independent of the approach–avoidance distinction.* Unpublished data, University of Rochester, Rochester, NY.

Elliot, A. J., & Mapes, R. R. (2005). Approach–avoidance motivation and self-concept evaluation. In A. Tesser, J. Wood, & D. Stapel (Eds.), *On building, defending, and regulating the self: A psychological perspective* (pp. 171–196). Washington, DC: Psychological Press.

Elliot, A. J., & Reis, H. (2003). Attachment and exploration in adulthood. *Journal of Personality and Social Psychology, 85,* 317–331.

Elliot, A. J., & Sheldon, K. M. (1997). Avoidance achievement motivation: A personal goals analysis. *Journal of Personality and Social Psychology, 73,* 171–185.

Elliot, A. J., & Sheldon, K. M. (1998). Avoidance personal goals and the personality–illness relationship. *Journal of Personality and Social Psychology, 75,* 1282–1299.

Elliot, A. J., Sheldon, K. M., & Church, M. A. (1997). Avoidance personal goals and subjective well-being. *Personality and Social Psychology Bulletin, 23,* 915–927.

Elliot, A. J., & Thrash, T. M. (2001). Achievement goals and the hierarchical model of achievement motivation. *Educational Psychology Review, 12,* 139–156.

Elliot, A. J., & Thrash, T. M. (2002). Approach–avoidance motivation in personality: Approach and avoidance temperaments and goals. *Journal of Personality and Social Psychology, 82,* 804–818.

Emmons, R. A. (1986). Personal strivings: An approach to personality and subjective well-being. *Journal of Personality and Social Psychology, 51,* 1058–1068.

Emmons, R. A., & McAdams, D. P. (1991). Personal strivings and motive dispositions: Exploring the links. *Personality and Social Psychology Bulletin, 17,* 648–654.

Gable, S. L. (2006). Approach and avoidance social motives and goals. *Journal of Personality, 74,* 175–222.

Gray, J. A. (1987). *The psychology of fear and stress* (2nd ed.). Cambridge, UK: Cambridge University Press.

Heckhausen, J. (1997). Developmental regulation across adulthood: Primary and secondary control of age-related challenges. *Developmental Psychology, 33,* 176–187.

Heimpel, S., Wood, J., & Elliot, A. J. (2005). *Self-esteem and avoidance (relative to approach) personal goals.* Unpublished data, University of Rochester, Rochester, NY.

Higgins, E. T. (1997). Beyond pleasure and pain. *American Psychologist, 52,* 1280–1300.

Hooker, K., Fiese, B. H., Jenkins, L., Morfei, M. Z., & Schwagler, J. (1996). Possible selves among parents of infants and preschoolers. *Developmental Psychology, 32,* 542–550.

Hooker, K., & Kaus, C. R. (1994). Health-related possible selves in young and middle adulthood. *Psychology and Aging, 9,* 126–133.

James, W. (1890). *The principles of psychology.* New York: Holt.

Klinger, E. (1977). *Meaning and void: Inner experience and the incentives in people's lives.* Minneapolis: University of Minnesota Press.

Klinger, E., Barta, S. G., & Maxeiner, M. E. (1980). Motivational correlates of thought content frequency and commitment. *Journal of Personality and Social Psychology, 39,* 1222–1237.

Lang, P. J. (1995). The emotion probe: Studies in motivation and attention. *American Psychologist, 50,* 372–385.

Little, B. R. (1983). Personal projects: A rationale and method for investigation. *Environment and Behavior, 15,* 273–309.

Little, B. R. (1999). Personality and motivation: Personal action and the conative evolution. In L. A. Pervin & O. P. John (Eds.), *Handbook of personality: Theory and research* (2nd ed., pp. 501–524). New York: Guilford.

Markus, H., & Nurius, P. (1986). Possible selves. *American Psychologist, 41,* 954–969.

Moffit, K. H., & Singer, J. A. (1994). Continuity in the life study: Self-defining memories, affect, and approach/avoidnace personal strivings. *Journal of Personality, 62,* 21–43.

Morfei, M. Z., Hooker, K., Fiese, B. H., & Cordeiro, A. M. (2001). Continuity and change in parenting possible selves: Longitudinal follow-up. *Basic and Applied Social Psychology, 23,* 217–223.

Ogilvie, D. M. (1987). The undesired self: A neglected variable in personality research. *Journal of Personality and Social Psychology, 52,* 379–385.

Ogilvie, D. M., & Rose, K. M. (1995). Self-with-other representations and a taxonomy of motives: Two approaches to studying persons. *Journal of Personality, 63,* 643–679.

Oyserman, D., & Markus, H. (1990). Possible selves in balance: Implications for delinquency. *Journal of Social Issues, 46,* 141–157.

Roberson, L. (1990). Prediction of job satisfaction from characteristics of personal work goals. *Journal of Organizational Behavior, 11,* 29–41.

Robinson, B. S., Davis, K. L., & Meara, N. M. (2003). Motivational attributes of occupational possible selves for low-income rural women. *Journal of Counseling Psychology, 50,* 156–164.

Thrash, T. M., & Elliot, A. J. (2001). Delimiting and integrating achievement motive and goal constructs. In A. Efklides, J. Kuhl, & R. Sorrentino (Eds.), *Trends and prospects in motivational research* (p. 1–19). Dordrecht, Netherlands: Kluwer Academic.

Tolman, E. C. (1923). A behavioristic account of emotions. *Psychological Review, 30,* 217–227.

Updegraff, J. A., Gable, S. L., & Taylor, S. E. (2004). What makes experiences satisfying? The interaction of approach–avoidance motivations and emotions in well-being. *Journal of Personality and Social Psychology, 86,* 496–504.

APPENDIX A
PERSONAL GOALS ELICITATION PROCEDURE
(PGEP)

Personal Goals

In this study, we are interested in the things that you typically or characteristically are trying to do in your daily life—your "personal goals." Here are some examples of personal goals that others have provided in our previous studies (this can help you understand what we mean by "personal goal"):

"be physically attractive to others"
"persuade others that I am right"
"avoid being lonely"
"do well in my place of employment"
"avoid procrastination"
"not feel inferior to others"

Here are some things to note about personal goals:

1. Personal goals may involve trying to *approach* something or trying to *avoid* something. For example, you may typically try to "get attention from others" or you may typically try to "avoid calling attention to yourself."

2. Personal goals are phrased in terms of what a person is *trying* to do, regardless of whether the person is actually successful. For example, a person might try to "be on time for all of my appointments" without necessarily being successful.

3. Personal goals may be fairly *broad* such as "avoid making other people angry" or more *specific* such as "avoid making my roommate angry in the morning." Also, personal goals can last for varying lengths of time, but in this study, we would like you to identify a set of goals that you expect to last at least through the end of the semester.

On the next page, we would like you to list the *8 personal goals* that you think *best* describe what you will typically be trying to do in your daily life during this semester.

Before you write down your final set of 8 personal goals, you may want to take a few minutes to "brainstorm" by jotting down various possibilities on the "scratch paper" that we have provided. When considering your personal goals, please be as honest and open as possible. Remember, your name will not be on this list, and all of your responses will be kept completely *confidential*.

Now, please turn the page and begin by listing possibilities on the "scratch paper." When you have selected your final set of personal goals for the semester, please write them down in the spaces provided on the "Your Personal Goals" page.

APPENDIX B
PERSONAL GOALS LIST

Your Personal Goals

In the spaces below, please list the *8 personal goals* that *best* describe what you will typically be trying to do in your daily life during this semester.

Personal Goal #1: _____

Personal Goal #2: _____

Personal Goal #3: _____

Personal Goal #4: _____

Personal Goal #5: _____

Personal Goal #6: _____

Personal Goal #7: _____

Personal Goal #8: _____

APPENDIX C
APPROACH–AVOIDANCE PERSONAL GOALS
CODING SYSTEM

Approach–Avoidance Personal Goals Coding System

Codes

1 = approach
2 = avoidance
3 = approach, then avoidance
4 = avoidance, then approach

Guidelines

1. Structurally, approach goals focus on a positive possibility that a person is trying to move toward or maintain, whereas avoidance goals focus on a negative possibility that a person is trying to move away from or stay away from.

2. The foci of goals vary tremendously across participants; the tendencies with regard to the foci also vary, but to a lesser extent. Thus, it is possible to identify a set of words or phrases that commonly appear in avoidance goals: not, no more, get away from, keep away from, stay away from, stop, omit, reduce, get out of, get rid of, prevent, turn away from, lose, diet, avoid, escape, quit, be free from, refrain from, eliminate, squash, lessen, forget, do away with, _____ less. This set of words and phrases is meant to be illustrative, not exhaustive.

3. Most goals should be easy to code for approach–avoidance. However, some goals are worded in an ambiguous way, seem to possess a mismatch between the focus of the goal and the tendency regarding that focus, or contain multiple goals or goal–reason combinations. Each of these issues is discussed in the following points.

a. For some goals such as "be nonjudgmental" it is difficult to know whether the focus is positive (i.e., nonjudgmental, which is a desirable characteristic the person wants to approach) or negative (i.e., judgmental, which is an undesirable characteristic the person wants to avoid). If this goal was phrased "not be judgmental" it would clearly be coded avoidance, but when phrased "be nonjudgmental" it is best to assume that nonjudgmental is a positive characteristic that the person wants to approach, and to code it as an approach goal.

b. Some goals such as "get a handle on my temper" seem, on first glance, to contain a negative focus coupled with an approach tendency. However, this apparent mismatch is resolved if one considers the focus of the goal to be "a handle on my temper," as opposed to "my temper." Thus "get a handle on my temper" clearly represents an approach goal in which the focus is positive and the tendency is approach.

c. Some goal statements contain multiple goals such as "take life as it comes and be less uptight" or contain both an aim (i.e., goal) and a reason for pursuing the aim, such as "avoid chocolate so that I can get in better shape." The first example should be coded approach, then avoidance, whereas the second should be coded avoidance, then approach. For goals written in English, it is assumed that the most important goal or the aim comes first or at the beginning of the statement, and that the less important goal or the reason for pursuing the aim comes second or at the latter part of the statement (see Elliot & Thrash, 2001, for details on the aim vs. reason distinction and its importance). As such, approach, then avoidance should be collapsed into the approach category, and avoidance, then approach should be collapsed into the avoidance category. For goals written in a language in which the most important goal or the aim would not systematically come at the beginning of the statement (e.g., Chinese, Japanese, Korean), both approach, then avoidance and avoidance, then approach should be collapsed into the avoidance category. In other words, in this instance, goal statements containing any avoidance content are coded as avoidance goals. Furthermore, for the sake of comparability, this latter approach should be used for all samples in cross-cultural work in which this issue applies to any sample in the study.

4. In general, use approach as the default code, because the majority of goals in any given sample will be approach goals. So, a goal must clearly fit the avoidance category to be coded avoidance.

4

Interference and Facilitation Among Personal Goals: Age Differences and Associations With Well-Being and Behavior

Michaela Riediger

Some years ago, I went to a New Year's party with my friend Barbara. It was midnight. Glasses were clinking, people were hugging, but Barbara was not there. Minutes later I found her, alone in some corner, writing. She told me that she had written down her New Year's resolutions. "Just to make sure that I don't forget. You know, I realized that there are quite a few things that I want to do next year," she said, and showed me her pocket diary. She had scribbled a long list of goals all over the front cover: Lose 10 pounds! Write a really good dissertation! Become fluent in Spanish! Travel to South America! Exercise three times a week! More time with friends! Call home once a week! Enjoy life! "Well," she sighed, "I will have to give it more thought. Some of this goes really well together. But then again, I wonder if I will have enough time for everything." She looked at her watch. "Oh no! It's past midnight already," she exclaimed startled, "Let's get back to the party! Happy New Year!"

When people think about what they want to attain or avoid in their future, they typically realize that they have multiple goals, perhaps pertaining to different domains of their lives. Such multiple goals are not always independent of each other. As probably everybody knows from their own experiences, goals may interfere with each other. Examples are Barbara's goals to write a really good dissertation and to become fluent in Spanish. Pursuing one goal may take away time and energy from pursuing the other goal. Goals, however, may also mutually facilitate each other. Pursuing the goal to travel to South America, for example, may offer Barbara many good opportunities for pursuing her goal to become fluent in Spanish.

The purpose of this chapter is to review empirical evidence on *intraindividual* relations among different goals of an individual.[1] It starts with definitions of intergoal facilitation and interference and a brief clarification of a basic conceptual question: Are intergoal facilitation and interference opposites on a single dimension, or are they distinct characteristics? Following that, three topics of empirical research on intergoal relations are reviewed. This review begins with the most prominent theme thus far, namely, potential associations between intergoal relations and people's psychological well-being. I summarize the partly inconsistent findings and propose an explanation that may reconcile the differences. The second topic addresses associations between intergoal relations and people's actual behavior or action, a theme that is receiving increasing attention. This section presents research that has investigated implications of intergoal relations for people's active involvement in goal pursuit. The third topic has only recently been investigated in research on intergoal relations. Joining a developmental and a motivational perspective, it addresses adulthood changes in intergoal relations and their potential developmental-regulatory functions. Following a discussion of this recently emerging line of research, I conclude the chapter by integrating the re-

---

[1]Related topics that are not within the scope of this chapter are (a) ambivalence toward single goals; that is, an approach–avoidance conflict a person might have about a goal (i.e., wanting and at the same time not wanting to attain it; Emmons & King, 1988; Emmons, King, & Sheldon, 1993); (b) relations between goals and broader motivational themes, such as possible selves, needs, or motives (e.g., Brunstein, Schultheiss, & Grässman, 1998; Kehr, 2004; McGregor & Little, 1998; Omodei & Wearing, 1990; Schultheiss & Brunstein, 1999; Sheldon & Emmons, 1995); and (c) relations between goals of different persons (e.g., Argyle, Furnham, & Graham, 1981; Lewis, Reitsma, Wilson, & Zigurs, 2001) or between individual and team or organizational goals (e.g., DeShon, Kozlowski, Schmidt, Milner, & Wiechmann, 2004; Kristof-Brown & Stevens, 2001).

search reviewed and outlining future research perspectives. Figure 4.1 depicts the central topics that are discussed in this chapter.

As is typically the case in goal research, the studies reviewed in this chapter partly employed different theoretical goal concepts, such as personal projects (Little, 1983) or personal strivings (Emmons, 1986). For the sake of the flow and clarity of argumentation, and because several authors have proposed that the various theoretical goal concepts are largely comparable on an empirical level (e.g., Brunstein, 1993; Kehr, 2003; Omodei & Wearing, 1990), this chapter treats the goal concepts in the reviewed studies as more or less equivalent.

THE CONCEPT AND MEASUREMENT OF INTERGOAL RELATIONS

Theoretically, three different qualities of relations among an individual's goals (or, more precisely, the impact of pursuing one goal on the pursuit of another goal) are possible: (a) independence, (b) facilitation, and (c) interference (Argyle, Furnham, & Graham, 1981; Little, 1983).

Goal independence refers to a constellation of goals in which the pursuit of one has no impact, either positive or negative, on the pursuit of any other goal of the individual.

Intergoal facilitation occurs when the pursuit of one goal simultaneously increases the likelihood of success in reaching another goal. It may result, for example, from instrumental relations among goals (Riediger & Freund, 2004; Wilensky, 1983). These exist when progress toward one goal also represents a step toward another goal (e.g., when

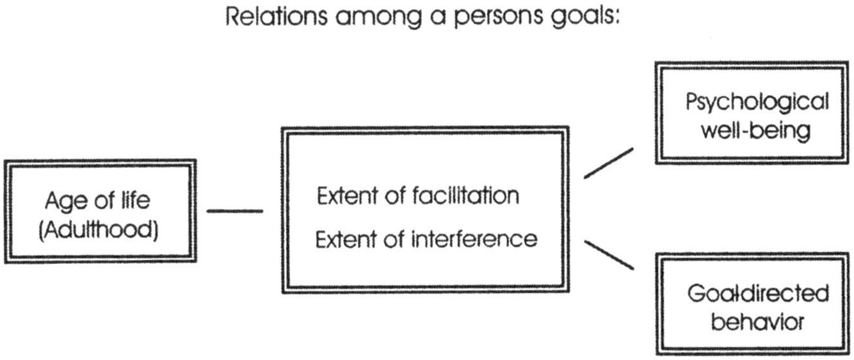

Figure 4.1. Overview of topics reviewed in this chapter.

being successful in establishing a professional career generates resources for financially supporting one's partner). Intergoal facilitation may also result from overlapping goal attainment strategies (Riediger & Freund, 2004; Wilensky, 1983). These exist if strategies for pursuing one goal represent a subset of strategies for pursuing another goal (e.g., when exercising regularly is effective for both improving one's cardiovascular fitness and improving one's appearance).

Intergoal interference occurs when the pursuit of one goal impairs the likelihood of success in reaching another goal. This phenomenon has also been referred to as *goal conflict*. To stay within the terminology used by the various authors, the terms *interference* and *conflict* are used interchangeably throughout this chapter. Interference among goals may result, for example, when the pursuits of different goals of an individual require the same limited resource, such as time or money, of which an insufficient quantity is available. Intergoal interference may also occur when the strategies for attaining different goals are incompatible (Greenhaus & Beutell, 1985; Riediger & Freund, 2004; Wilensky, 1983). "To keep my relationships on a 50–50 basis" and "to dominate, control, and manipulate people and situations" are examples of two conflicting goals cited by Emmons and King (1988, p. 1042) that imply such an inherent logical incompatibility.

The research reviewed in this chapter employed different methods for assessing interrelations among personal goals. Two general approaches can be distinguished: a bipolar assessment strategy, which anchors both negative or interference and positive or facilitation impacts as opposite ends of the same scale, and a unipolar approach, which measures the degree of interference or facilitation on the scale and requires two separate scales if both interference and facilitation are to be assessed. As I elaborate later, both strategies partly yield different empirical results. To provide the basis for an adequate reflection of these findings, a brief illustration of the history of both assessment strategies and a discussion of the central conceptual question that distinguishes them follows: Are intergoal conflict and facilitation mutually exclusive opposites, or are they distinct characteristics of the interrelations among a person's goals?

INTERFERENCE AND FACILITATION AMONG GOALS DO NOT EXCLUDE EACH OTHER

To date, the majority of research on intergoal relations has been based on the assumption that interference and facilitation among goals are mutually exclusive opposites. This assumption may be intuitively appealing at first glance. Empirical evidence, however, suggests that facilitation and interference among goals are more adequately conceptualized as two independent dimensions: Goals might interfere with each other in some aspects, but facilitate each other in others. For example, a person might perceive the goal of exercising regularly to facilitate her other goal of professional success because exercising might help with relieving stress and thus enhance efficacy at work. At the same time, she might also experience exercising to interfere with the work goal because it takes time that cannot be spent working. This part of the chapter briefly discusses this issue and its implications for the assessment of intergoal relations and the interpretation of research results.

To my knowledge, the first attempt at assessing interrelations among a person's goal was published by Little (1983) and accounted for the possibility that two goals might be both interfering and facilitative. Using this approach, participants first report a certain number of current goals (or personal projects, in this case). They then complete a cross-impact matrix, the rows and columns of which are labeled with short summary phrases of the reported projects. Each cell of this matrix represents a pair of two projects. Participants decide whether carrying out the project indicated by the column has a positive, negative, neutral, or ambivalent (i.e., both positive and negative) impact on the project indicated by the row, and they write their responses into the respective cell (see Figure 4.2).

The assumption that a goal may have both a positive and a negative impact on another goal was later dropped by researchers introducing bipolar assessment procedures, which presuppose intergoal facilitation and interference to be mutually exclusive opposites. An example is the striving instrumentality matrix (SIM) by Emmons and King (1988), which has been frequently adapted (e.g., Kehr, 2003; King, Richards, & Stemmerich, 1998; Michalak & Schulte, 2002; Sheldon & Kasser, 1995). Again, participants first report a certain number of goals, pair each of these goals with each of the remaining goals, and rate the pairwise goal relations. This time, however, participants rate the impact that being successful in one goal has on the other goal using a scale ranging from –2 (*very harmful*), to 0 (*no effect*), to +2 (*very helpful;* see Figure 4.2). This scale has been interpreted in different ways. Most researchers recoded responses so that higher scores indicate more unfavorable intergoal relations, and interpreted the average of these ratings as indicating the extent of conflict among the participant's goals (e.g.,

Step 1: Free reports of personal goals (strivings, projects)
Step 2: Pairwise combination of all reported goals

Example (3 goals):

	Goal A	Goal B	Goal C
Goal A	-	BA	CA
Goal B	AB	-	CB
Goal C	AC	BC	-

Step 3: For each pairwise goal combination, assessment of intergoal relation:

Example 1: Cross-Impact Matrix (Little, 1983)

What impact does carrying out the first project have on the second project?

: :	:	+	+ +	0	+/
(very negative)	(negative)	(positive)	(very positive)	(neutral)	(ambivalent)

Example 2: Striving Instrumentality Matrix (Emmons & King, 1988)

What effect does being successful in the first striving have on the second striving?

: 2	: 1	0	+ 1	+ 2
(very harmful)		(no effect)		(very helpful)

Example 3: Intergoal Relations Questionnaire (Riediger & Freund, 2004)

(a) Interference:

How often can it happen that , because of the pursuit of Goal A, you do not invest as much time/money/energy into Goal B as you would like to?

How often can it happen that you do something in the pursuit of Goal A that is incompatible with Goal B?

(b) Facilitation:

How often can it happen that you do something in the pursuit of Goal A that is simultaneously beneficial for Goal B?

The pursuit of Goal A sets the stage for the realization of Goal B.

1	2	3	4	5
(very rarely/ not at all true)				(very often/ very true)

Figure 4.2.   Assessment of intergoal relations: Comparison of different approaches at the example of three instruments.

Emmons & King, 1988; Kehr, 2003; King et al., 1998). Michalak, Heidenreich, and Hoyer (2004), however, pointed out that the scale means reported in various studies are too low to warrant an interpretation as indicator of goal conflict. They argued that, "the SIM seems to be a method of assessing a greater or lesser degree of integration between a person's goals rather than a measure of intrapsychic conflict" (p. 91). In line with this, Sheldon and Kasser (1995) recoded responses such that higher scores indicate more favorable intergoal relations and interpreted this SIM composite as an indicator of coherence among goals.

To date, bipolar assessment methods have been very prominent in research on intergoal relations. Some studies, however, employed unipolar measures, typically of intergoal interference only (e.g., McKeeman & Karoly, 1991; Pomaki, Maes, & ter Doest, 2004). An example of a unipolar instrument that assesses both interference and facilitation among goals is the Intergoal Relations Questionnaire (IRQ; Riediger & Freund, 2004). Participants respond, for each possible pair of their self-reported personal goals, to six unipolar items (see Figure 4.2, Example 3). Interference among goals is assessed in terms of resource constraints (time, financial, and energy constraints) and in terms of incompatible goal attainment strategies. Mutual facilitation among goals is assessed in terms of instrumental goal relations and overlapping goal attainment strategies.

Whereas some measures leave it to the participants to decide on which criteria to base their judgment of interference or facilitation, the IRQ specifies explicit reference standards (i.e., specific forms of intergoal interference and facilitation), which presumably enhances the interindividual comparability of responses. Furthermore, the unipolar assessment approach of the IRQ allows empirical testing of the association between intergoal interference and facilitation. In fact, in two independent adult samples ($N_1 = 111$, $N_2 = 145$), Riediger and Freund (2004) found a clear two-factor structure of intergoal facilitation and interference. Correlations between the respective facilitation and interference composite scores were small ($| r | \leq .19$). Interestingly, the cross-impact matrix (Little, 1983) shows a similar two-dimensional structure: The positive impact score (facilitation) and the negative impact score (interference) are independent of each other (B. R. Little, personal communication, December 2, 2004).

These findings indicate that it is possible (although not necessarily the case) that two or more of an individual's goals can interfere with each other, while also being mutually facilitative. A bipolar instrument cannot unambiguously reflect such a constellation. Its midpoint, for example, could signify either that two goals are neither interfering nor facilitative or that they are about equally interfering and facilitative.

In short, intergoal conflict and facilitation appear to be most adequately conceptualized as distinct characteristics. The reviews of empirical results in the following two parts of this chapter further support this conclusion. These findings show that intergoal interference and facilitation are differentially related to subjective well-being and persistent goal pursuit.

INTERGOAL RELATIONS
AND PSYCHOLOGICAL WELL-BEING

Throughout the history of psychology, it has been repeatedly theorized that intraindividual conflict is linked to negative experiences both in the pathological and in the nonpathological range, and that psychological health and well-being require that different aspects of the person are harmoniously integrated (for reviews, see Epstein, 1982; Hoyer, 1992; McReynolds, 1991). Applied to interrelations among personal goals, these propositions suggest that interference among goals should impair, and mutual facilitation among goals should enhance, psychological well-being. The available empirical evidence, however, is not as clear as one might expect (and as it is sometimes described to be; e.g., Emmons, Cheung, & Tehrani, 1998; Kehr, 2003). Next, I briefly summarize the available findings and propose an explanation for the inconsistent pattern of results. This review first addresses research using bipolar assessment scales of intergoal relations and then turns to research using unipolar scales. For the sake of brevity, it is restricted to studies that assessed interrelations among personal goals specifically and directly. It does not include studies that investigated interrelations among other psychological concepts (e.g., Hoyer, 1992; Lauterbach, 1996), nor does it include studies that inferred intergoal relations indirectly without assessing the participants' goals (e.g., Perring, Oatley, & Smith, 1988).

Research Using Bipolar Assessment Strategies

Overall, the empirical picture provided by studies using bipolar assessment instruments is not very clear. Emmons and King (1988) reported a series of studies that did not yield consistent results concerning the association between the bipolar SIM, described earlier, and various indicators of mental health. In a first study ($N = 40$ undergraduates), the SIM composite (interpreted by the authors as an indicator of goal conflict) was unrelated to measures of positive affect, but was positively related to negative affect ($r = .28$), anxiety ($r = .29$), and depression ($r = .34$). In a second study ($N = 48$ undergraduates), the authors did not replicate the associations with negative affect, anxiety, and depression.

A number of other authors also found no associations of the SIM with indicators of psychological well-being. Sheldon and Kasser (1995), in a sample of 161 psychology students, found no association between the SIM composite (interpreted as an indicator of goal coherence) and self-esteem, positive, and negative affect or vitality. Similarly, King et al. (1998), in a sample of 80 undergraduate students, found no concurrent associations between the SIM composite and life satisfaction, self-esteem, or depression. Furthermore, Michalak et al. (2004) reported that the SIM composite was unrelated to psychological symptoms in two recent studies with undergraduate participants and outpatients with anxiety and affective disorders.

Kehr (2003) reported ambiguous results regarding concurrent associations between the SIM composite and measures of positive and negative affect in a longitudinal study of 99 German managers. Participants completed the SIM at two time points about 5 months apart. At Time 1, the SIM composite (interpreted as an indicator of goal conflict) was unrelated to concurrent reports of positive and negative affect. At Time 2, the SIM composite was unrelated to concurrent reports of positive affect, but showed a significant although small positive association with concurrent negative affect ($r = .21$). Longitudinally, an interesting interaction emerged in the prediction of change in positive (but not negative) affect. During the course of 5 months, an increase in the SIM composite (interpreted by Kehr as emerging conflict) was associated with a decrease in positive affect, whereas stability of the SIM composite at high levels (interpreted by Kehr as enduring conflict) was associated with a slight increase in positive affect. Without speculating about the underlying mechanisms, Kehr concluded that, "goal conflicts offer the benefit of buffering against fluctuations in well-being" (p. 205).

In sum, this empirical picture is relatively inconsistent. It is clarified, however, by research using unipolar assessment methods, which yield a consistent pattern of results.

Research Using Unipolar Assessment Strategies

Palys and Little (1983) reported two studies (N_1 = 178 university students, N_2 = 72 community residents) in which participants indicated for each pair of their self-reported personal projects whether pursuing Project A facilitated, conflicted with, both facilitated and conflicted with, or was irrelevant for the pursuit of Project B (see the cross-impact matrix, described earlier). The authors restricted their reported analyses, however, to unipolar information pertaining to the extent of goal conflict only. In both studies, project conflict was among the characteristics that discriminated significantly between participants with low versus high life satisfaction. Participants with low life satisfaction reported more conflict (M = 15.03, theoretical range 0–90) among their goals than did participants who were highly satisfied with their lives (M = 11.46).

In line with this are recent findings by Pomaki et al. (2004). In a large-scale study of 3,088 health care employees, participants reported their most important work goal for the coming 12 months, and responded to four items assessing facets of conflict associated with this goal (e.g., "Pursuing this goal conflicts with other goals I find important"). This goal conflict measure was significantly associated with various facets of psychological well-being at the workplace, such as job satisfaction (r = $-.24$) and emotional exhaustion (r = .32). Employees were less satisfied with their jobs and more emotionally exhausted the more conflictful they perceived their most important work goals to be. These associations remained robust when controlling for a host of demographic and workplace characteristics.

Riediger and Freund (2004), in three studies with younger and older adult participants (N_1 = 111, N_2 = 145, N_3 = 81), found strong evidence for differential associations of intergoal interference and facilitation as assessed with the IRQ, described earlier, with various facets of both state and trait subjective well-being. In all three studies and independent of the participants' age, intergoal interference was associated with impairments in various facets of psychological well-being (i.e., positive psychological functioning, life satisfaction, state and trait measure of emotional well-being; $.19 \leq \mid r \mid \leq .44$), whereas intergoal facilitation did not contribute significantly to these various predictions. Only in 1 of 10 analyses did intergoal facilitation show a significant positive association with participants' diary reports of positive affect in everyday life (r = .27). There were no significant interference × facilitation interactions in any of these analyses.

In Study 3, Riediger and Freund (2004) demonstrated similar differential associations in people's day-to-day experiences. Here, participants kept nine detailed activity diaries that were distributed throughout 3 weeks. Each diary consisted of three diary entries to be completed at noon, at 6 p.m., and immediately before going to bed. In each diary entry, participants first rated their positive and negative affect during the preceding hours. They then chronologically listed all activities they had been engaged in during that time. For each reported activity, they indicated if and how much it had furthered each of a number of goals they had reported prior to the diary phase. We considered it an expression of the everyday experience of intergoal facilitation if the same activity was rated as simultaneously furthering more than one goal. Participants further indicated whether they would have liked to do or should have done something else instead of the reported activities. Affirmative responses were regarded as indicators of the everyday experience of interference between motivational tendencies. Consistent with the differential association pattern obtained in the other studies, everyday experiences of intergoal facilitation—that is, the experience that one's activities further several goals at once—were unrelated to within-person fluctuations in emotional well-being. In contrast, everyday experiences of motivational conflict—that is, the feeling that one wants to or should do something else instead of what one is doing—accounted for fluctuations of people's emotional well-being below their personal average. Experiencing motivational conflict was associated with less-than-average positive and more-than-average negative affect (about 8% modeled variance in multilevel regressions).

In short, recent evidence indicates that interference among goals is associated with impairments in subjective well-being, whereas mutual goal facilitation appears to be unrelated. This differential pattern is in line with research demonstrating that people react stronger to losses than to gains (Hobfoll, 1998; Kahneman & Tversky, 1984). Interference among goals may imply that the attainment of one's goals is threatened. Associated impairments in psychological well-being may serve the function of directing people's attention to the problem, and of motivating them to solve it (cf. Bagozzi, Baumgartner, & Pieters, 1998; Carver & Scheier, 1990).

The differential association pattern of intergoal facilitation and interference with psychological well-being offers an explanation for the inconsistency of results obtained with bipolar measures of intergoal relations. It seems likely that these are a consequence of not separating the assessment of intergoal interference (which is negatively related to well-being) and of intergoal facilitation (which is not related to well-being).

INTERGOAL RELATIONS AND GOAL-DIRECTED BEHAVIOR

Setting personal goals is only a first step toward accomplishing them, which also requires the investment of effort and other resources into the initiation and pursuit of goal-directed actions (Freund & Baltes, 2000). Yet, motivation (i.e., setting goals) does not necessarily lead to volition (i.e., pursuing goals). Many goals remain exactly that: goals. A highly relevant research topic in motivational psychology, therefore, is the identification of factors that contribute to the initiation and maintenance of goal-directed behavior. This part of the chapter briefly reviews available research addressing the question of whether interrelations among personal goals influence people's engagement in persistent goal pursuit. I again first summarize research using bipolar assessment scales of intergoal relations, and then turn to research using a unipolar assessment strategy. As before, this review is restricted, as it only refers to studies that investigated the association between intergoal relations and goal-directed behaviors directly and explicitly.

Research Using Bipolar Assessment Strategies

Overall, research using bipolar assessment strategies found that intergoal relations tend to be related to people's engagement in goal-directed behaviors. The researchers' interpretations of these associations vary, however. For example, using an experience sampling approach, Emmons and King (1988, Study 3) randomly collected momentary thoughts and activities over a 3-week period in a sample of 40 undergraduates. At the end of the 3 weeks, participants judged whether the reported thoughts and activities were related to their previously reported goals. Participants with higher scores on the bipolar SIM (interpreted by the authors as an indicator of goal conflict) tended to act less, but to think more about their goals. The size of these associations, however, was small ($r = -.17$ and $r = .14$, respectively).

Michalak and Schulte (2002) investigated the association between intergoal relations and goal-related behavior in a clinical setting. In a sample of 24 outpatients with anxiety disorders, goal-related behaviors were assessed with respect to the goal "get relief from symptoms." At the end of each therapy session, psychotherapists rated the participants' goal-pursuit behaviors in terms of five categories: seeking treatment, cooperation, self-disclosure (vs. refusal), willingness to test new patterns of behavior, and (lack of) resistance. Intergoal relations were assessed among the participants' goals to get relief from symptoms and their other self-reported goals using the bipolar SIM. In contrast to Emmons and King (1988), these authors interpreted the SIM composite as an indicator of coherence rather than of conflict among goals, because participants rarely rated their goals as conflictful on this scale. The study yielded marked positive associations between the bipolar SIM composite and the various goal-pursuit behaviors ($.44 \leq |r| \leq .62$). The assessed behaviors, in turn, were positively related to retrospective evaluations of therapeutic success (not, however, to pre–post changes in symptoms). The authors concluded that, "coherence ... of client's goal systems seems to facilitate motivational support of goal enactment in psychotherapy" (p. 92).

In short, research using bipolar assessment strategies showed that intergoal relations tend to be related to people's engagement in goal-directed behaviors. As a consequence of the ambiguity in interpreting bipolar scale scores, however, the researchers' interpretations of these associations vary, a problem that can be circumvented by using unipolar assessment methods. Recent research with unipolar scales suggests that it is particularly the extent of intergoal facilitation (rather than of interference) that contributes to a high involvement in behaviors directed at the pursuit of personal goals. The next section briefly summarizes the available studies.

Research Using Unipolar Assessment Strategies

McKeeman and Karoly (1991) retrospectively assessed goal conflict associated with attempts to quit smoking in a sample of college students. The sample consisted of three groups: participants who smoked at least 15 cigarettes a day and had not recently attempted to quit (smokers, $n = 38$), participants who currently smoked at least 15 cigarettes a day and had recently made an unsuccessful attempt to quit (relapsers, $n = 40$), and participants who had recently stopped smoking and who had smoked at least 15 cigarettes a day prior to quitting (self-quitters, $n = 36$). All participants reported their five most important current goals. They then rated the extent to which each goal might have interfered with their attempt to quit smoking on unipolar response scales. Potential facilitative intergoal relations were not assessed in this study. Self-quitters retrospectively reported significantly lower conflict (M = 8.28; theoretical range = 3–27) than did both current smokers (M = 11.54) and relapsers (M = 10.75). Smokers and relapsers did not differ from each other with respect to reported goal conflict. The authors concluded that people tend to pursue the goal to quit smoking less if it interferes with their other goals. The retrospective assessment procedure, however, is a major methodological shortcoming in this study. The authors acknowledged that a "sour grapes" (i.e., excuse-making) explanation of the observed association is possible because smoking and particularly one's apparent inability to quit are commonly viewed as relatively undesirable.

One of the aims of the studies reported by Riediger and Freund (2004) was to overcome this limitation. Apart from investigating associations with subjective well-being (see earlier), we also investigated associations between intergoal interference and intergoal facilitation on the one hand and multiple (including objective) indicators of goal pursuit on the other, using cross-sectional and prospective study designs. The samples included younger and older adult participants. In all three studies, a consistent differential association pattern that was independent of the participants' age emerged. There were no interference × facilitation interactions in any of the analyses.

In Study 1, intergoal interference (as assessed with the IRQ) was not predictive of the participants' self-reported goal involvement. The higher the extent of intergoal facilitation, however, the more involved participants reported being in activities directed at the realization of their goals (r = .29).

These findings were replicated in a prospective diary study (Study 3). Here, everyday goal-directed behaviors were assessed using a diary method throughout a period of 3 weeks following the assessment of intergoal relations. As in Study 1, intergoal interference was unrelated to the participants' everyday goal involvement. Intergoal facilitation, however, was associated with an enhanced involvement in goal pursuit (r = .42).

To obtain objective (rather than self-reported) information on goal-related behaviors, we investigated exercise beginners in another study; that is, people who shared the goal to start regular physical exercise. Using the IRQ, participants evaluated how much their exercise goal interfered with, and was facilitative for, other important goals in their lives. Objective information on the participants' involvement in goal pursuit (i.e., exercise adherence) was obtained from the participants' sports facilities throughout 5 months following the assessment of inter-goal relations. In the first 3 months, exercise-specific intergoal facilitation and interference did not contribute significantly to the predictions of the participants' monthly exercise adherence. In months 4 and 5, however, a differential prediction pattern consistent with that observed in the other two studies emerged. Participants exercised more frequently the more exercise-specific intergoal facilitation they had initially reported ($r = .25$), whereas the degree of exercise-specific intergoal interference did not contribute to these predictions.

These results do not contradict the findings obtained with bipolar response scales. Rather, they may contribute to a clarification of the diverse interpretations proposed for these results. It seems that the observed negative association between the SIM composite and goal involvement does not reflect an inhibition of goal-directed activities by intergoal conflict (as Emmons & King, 1988, proposed), but a lack of enhancement of goal-directed activities by low levels of intergoal facilitation (as Michalak & Schulte, 2002, argued).

Consequently, theoretical approaches to the implementation of goal-directed activities would benefit from incorporating the notion of facilitative intergoal relations. So far, theoretical attempts at explaining differences in goal-related activities in terms of intergoal relations have exclusively focused on the role of conflictual relationship qualities (e.g., Maes & Gebhardt, 2000).

It seems likely that mutual facilitation among goals enhances goal-directed activities by allowing an efficient utilization of one's limited resources (e.g., time). Facilitative goals can be pursued simultaneously with little or no additional effort and without exhausting one's resources. For example, Riediger and Freund (2004, Study 3) observed a high positive association between the IRQ facilitation composite and participants' tendency to evaluate their everyday activities as simultaneously furthering two or more of their goals ($r = .67$). This appears to be particularly important for the long-term maintenance of goal-pursuit behaviors even in the context of new situations, demands, or interests.

Interference among goals may play a less important role in the prediction of goal-directed behaviors because it is possible (although not necessarily the case) that people mobilize efforts and other resources to compensate for interference among their goals. For example, they may extend their waking day to have more time to engage in the accomplishments of their goals. Intergoal interference might thus not be reflected in fewer goal-pursuit activities (but could well have long-term health implications; Emmons & King, 1988). In situations of very severe resource limitations or when people perceive a goal not to be worth the effort, however, they might not engage in such compensatory efforts. In such situations, interference among goals may lead to a selective inhibition of goal-directed activities, very likely at the cost of the comparatively least important goals (for an empirical demonstration of selective goal pursuit associated with goal conflict in situations with clear resource limitations, see Locke, Smith, Erez, Chah, & Schaffer, 1994). Apart from the methodological problem of retrospective evaluation of goal conflict, this reasoning offers another interpretation of why McKeeman and Karoly (1991) observed that people with higher smoking-related goal conflict were less likely to be successful in attempts at quitting. To "quit smoking" may have been comparatively less important to the participants than their other goals. Consequently, they may have been more likely to disengage from attempts to quit in the interest of pursuing their other goals than to mobilize resources to realize all goals despite their interference.

In sum, the findings reviewed so far underscore that intergoal facilitation and interference are functionally distinct properties of intergoal relations. Whereas intergoal interference is associated with impairments in psychological well-being, intergoal facilitation is associated with enhanced involvement in goal-directed activities. The direction and size of these associations do not differ between younger and older adults (Riediger & Freund, 2004). There is, however, evidence that there are age-group mean differences in the nature of intergoal relations. The following section reviews this evidence.

A DEVELOPMENTAL PERSPECTIVE ON INTERGOAL RELATIONS

Current developmental theories increasingly acknowledge the importance of motivational and volitional processes for understanding human development in general, and successful aging in particular (for an overview, see Freund & Riediger, 2003). Examples are the theories of selection, optimization, and compensation (Baltes & Baltes, 1990; Freund & Baltes, 2000), of assimilative and accommodative coping (Brandtstädter & Renner, 1990), of primary and secondary control (Heckhausen & Schulz, 1995), or of socioemotional selectivity (Carstensen, 1993). One of the common assumptions of these various theories is that people, within the limits given by social, cultural, historical, and biological constraints, actively shape their own environment and life course (Baltes, Lindenberger, & Staudinger, 1998; Brandtstädter, 1998; Lerner & Busch-Rossnagel, 1981). Setting and pursuing personal goals play an important role in this respect, particularly in adolescence and adulthood (e.g., Freund & Riediger, 2006; Lerner & Busch-Rossnagel, 1981; Nurmi, 1991; Salmela-Aro, Nurmi, Saisto, & Halmesmäki, 2000).

Life-span developmental psychologists further propose that adult development is characterized by decline and loss as well as a potential for continuing developmental gains (e.g., Baltes, 1987, 1997; Labouvie-Vief, 1981; Ryff, 1985). Empirical evidence of the fact that losses occur in later adulthood, and are particularly prevalent in very old age (i.e., 80+ years of age), is overwhelming (e.g., decreasing cognitive processing speed, increasing vulnerability to disease and disability, increasing risk of losing close social partners; for an overview see Freund & Riediger, 2003). The empirical evidence of developmental gain throughout adulthood, however, is relatively scarce. To date, it stems primarily from studies on some potential age-related gains in knowledge-associated aspects of cognitive functioning (Baltes, Staudinger, & Lindenberger, 1999; Krampe & Baltes, 2003) as well as from research in personality-associated domains of functioning, such as coping (e.g., Aldwin, 1994; Diehl, Coyle, & Labouvie-Vief, 1996; Folkman, Lazarus, Pimley, & Novacek, 1987), or emotion regulation (e.g., Carstensen & Charles, 1998; Gross et al., 1997).

In light of the increasing interest in the active role that adults of all ages play in shaping their development, it is surprising to note how little we know about age-related changes in motivational and volitional processes (for an overview, see Freund & Riediger, 2006). Only recently has research slowly begun to accumulate empirical evidence indicating that motivation and volition may be among the functional domains that show positive developmental trajectories throughout adulthood (Bauer & McAdams, 2004; Sheldon & Kasser, 2001). Among this research are a few studies showing adulthood advances in intergoal relations, which appear to have positive implications for people's persistent goal pursuit (Kehr, 2003; Locke et al., 1994; Riediger, Freund, & Baltes, 2005).

Kehr (2003) investigated German managers aged 21 to 62 years ($M = 39.8$). Intergoal relations were assessed with the bipolar SIM at two time points 5 months apart. Age was negatively associated with the SIM composite (interpreted as an indicator of goal conflict) at the second measurement occasion ($r = -.27$). Furthermore, the older the participants, the more they tended to report progress on previously self-selected goals ($r = .23$).

Locke et al. (1994) asked 274 university professors ($M = 46.58$ years, $SD = 10.36$) to indicate the degree of conflict they felt about "the desire to be a good teacher ... and the desire to be a good researcher/scholar" (p. 83). The older the participants, the less they tended to report experiencing conflict between research and teaching. The size of this association was small, however ($r = -.14$).

My colleagues and I (Riediger et al., 2005) investigated potential behavioral functions of age-related differences in intergoal relations. Our hypothesis was that more mutually facilitative relations among personal goals in older adulthood might serve the behavioral function of ensuring high levels of goal pursuit despite decreasing external and internal resources. In developmental terms, we expected that older adults, in part through having mutually facilitative goals, stay highly involved in actively influencing their life course according to their own priorities.

We investigated this prediction with the data set described earlier. Older participants ($n = 58$, range $= 60$–78 years, $M = 65.2$) in a first cross-sectional study reported more mutual facilitation among their goals (as assessed with the IRQ; partial $\eta^2 = .08$) and a higher involvement in goal pursuit (partial $\eta^2 = .07$) than did younger participants ($n = 53$, range $= 20$–30 years, $M = 24.3$). Younger and older participants did not differ in the extent of intergoal interference. Mediational analyses revealed that the older adults' higher behavioral involvement in the pursuit of their goals was partly mediated by the higher degree of mutual facilitation among their goals.

Another short-term longitudinal study investigated 99 younger and 46 older exercise beginners. Recruiting younger and older adults who had one goal in common (i.e., the goal to start regular physical exercise) had two advantages. It increased the overlap between younger and older participants' goals, thus partially controlling for age-group differences in goal content, and it allowed prospective investigations of objective indicators of goal pursuit (exercise adherence). Interrelations between the participants' exercise goal and their other important goals were assessed with the IRQ. Consistent with the other study, older participants ($M = 64$ years) reported higher degrees of exercise-specific intergoal facilitation than did younger participants ($M = 25$ years, partial $\eta^2 = .13$). Older participants also reported less interference between exercising and their other goals (partial $\eta^2 = .04$). Furthermore, older adults maintained their exercise adherence throughout a longer period of time. In the later part of the study interval (beginning with the fourth month following the assessment of intergoal relations), older adults tended to exercise more frequently than younger adults (partial $\eta^2 = .15$). Mediational analyses again confirmed that the older adults' higher levels of exercise-specific intergoal facilitation partly mediated this age-group difference in pursuing the exercise goal.

This finding was replicated in a diary phase with a subsample of participants ($n = 52$ younger, $n = 29$ older adults). In-depth activity diaries throughout a period of 9 days indicated that older adults tend to be more involved in the everyday pursuit of their goals than younger adults (partial $\eta^2 = .22$). Control analyses revealed that this age-group difference could not be accounted for by the fact that older adults typically have available more free time and are less involved in study or work activities than younger adults. Again, this higher goal-pursuit involvement of the older adults was partially mediated by the higher extent of intergoal facilitation in that age group.

In effect, this provides the first empirical evidence to suggest that establishing a system of mutually facilitative personal goals is among the competencies that show positive adult developmental trajectories, at least into "young" old adulthood (i.e., up to about 80 years of age; Baltes, 1997; Baltes & Smith, 2003). This finding is in line with the general argument that higher levels of structural integration of different aspects of life and personality characterize developmental growth in adulthood (e.g., Erikson, 1959; Jung, 1933; Werner, 1967). These results further indicate that having more mutually facilitative goals serves an important developmental-regulatory function in older adulthood, namely, the maintenance of very high levels of active involvement in life management (goal pursuit) despite age-associated declines in available resources.

SUMMARY

The empirical evidence reviewed in this chapter shows that a person's goals are not necessarily independent of each other. They may influence each other in positive (facilitative) and negative (interfering) ways. Although it may seem intuitively appealing to assume that facilitation and interference among goals are mutually exclusive opposites on one dimension, they appear to be more adequately conceptualized as distinct characteristics. Goals may interfere with one another in some aspects, and mutually facilitate each other in other aspects.

This chapter reviewed empirical evidence on three central issues in research on intergoal relations: (a) associations with psychological well-being, (b) associations with persistent goal pursuit, and (c) implications of adult developmental changes in intergoal relations on goal involvement in a social ecology of increasingly limited resources.

In sum, the reviewed studies show that the nature of interrelations among a person's goals is associated with his or her experiences and behaviors. Recent findings emphasize that it is particularly the extent of intergoal interference (rather than facilitation) that is associated with impairments in subjective well-being. Conversely, it is particularly the extent of intergoal facilitation (rather than interference) that is associated with an enhanced behavioral involvement in goal pursuit. Age-comparative research demonstrates that these associations hold in younger and older adults. There are, however, age-associated differences in the nature of interrelations among younger and older adults' goals. Older adults tend to report more mutually facilitative goals than younger adults. This, in turn, appears to ensure high levels of engagement in goal pursuit in older adulthood (or, in developmental terms, of active involvement in shaping one's life and environment according to one's own priorities), even despite age-associated declines in external and internal resources. These findings contribute to a recently evolving line of research suggesting that motivational and volitional processes are among the domains of functioning that have the potential for positive developmental trajectories in adulthood.

Outlook

The understanding of motivational and developmental mechanisms relevant to this field of research would considerably benefit from future research that refines and integrates the various findings reviewed in this chapter. I consider four approaches to be particularly fruitful in this respect.

First, the field would be advanced by studies that focus on potential moderators of the extent, development, and functions of intergoal relations (e.g., gender, goal characteristics).

Second, another promising route for expanding our knowledge would be to investigate potential mediators; that is, to identify the mechanisms underlying the findings reviewed in this chapter. Relevant research questions pertain, for example, to the psychological processes underlying the associations between intergoal interference and psychological well-being, and between intergoal facilitation and persistent goal pursuit. Another important line of fruitful future investigation involves the identification of life circumstances or strategies that contribute to systems of more mutually facilitative goals in older as compared to younger adulthood.

Third, equally important is the investigation of the intraindividual development of goal selection and pursuit competencies (Baltes, Reese, & Nesselroade, 1977; Nesselroade & Baltes, 1979). So far, the available evidence on age-related differences in intergoal relations is cross-sectional. It thus potentially confounds age and cohort effects. Longitudinal research would yield a more precise picture of within-person developments (for one of the first attempts in this direction, see Kehr, 2003).

Fourth, future research might further differentiate the currently available empirical picture by providing more adequate insights into potential causal sequences with the help of experimental and longitudinal study designs. It is possible, for example, that associations between intergoal facilitation and subjective well-being evolve over time. The higher involvement in behaviors directed at the pursuit of mutually more facilitative goals could ultimately result in comparably more successful realization of these goals (King et al., 1998), which over time could result in higher levels of satisfaction and well-being (Brunstein, 1993). Longitudinal research might also lead to the identification of potential positive aspects of intergoal interference. It has been repeatedly argued that the acknowledgment, confrontation, and eventual solution of intraindividual conflict might play an important role in stimulating developmental growth (e.g., Brim & Kagan, 1980; Riegel, 1975; Turiel, 1974). Empirical evidence on this proposed positive role of conflict in developmental regulation is rare. The study of ontogenetic change in intergoal interference and its solution might be a suitable way to investigate this question. Impairments in psychological well-being associated with intergoal interference might initiate attempts to resolve the interference, and thus, in the long run, promote the attainment of more integrated goal systems.

REFERENCES

Aldwin, C. M. (1994). *Stress, coping, and development: An integrative perspective.* New York: Guilford.

140 ☙ RIEDIGER

Argyle, M., Furnham, A., & Graham, J. A. (1981). *Social situations*. New York: Cambridge University Press.
Bagozzi, R. P., Baumgartner, H., & Pieters, R. (1998). Goal-directed emotions. *Cognition and Emotion, 12,* 1–26.
Baltes, P. B. (1987). Theoretical propositions of life-span developmental psychology: On the dynamics between growth and decline. *Developmental Psychology, 23,* 611–626.
Baltes, P. B. (1997). On the incomplete architecture of human ontogeny: Selection, optimization, and compensation as foundation of developmental theory. *American Psychologist, 52,* 366–380.
Baltes, P. B., & Baltes, M. M. (1990). Psychological perspectives on successful aging: The model of selective optimization with compensation. In P. B. Baltes & M. M. Baltes (Eds.), *Successful aging: Perspectives from the behavioral sciences* (pp. 1–34). New York: Cambridge University Press.
Baltes, P. B., Lindenberger, U., & Staudinger, U. M. (1998). Life-span theory in developmental psychology. In R. M. Lerner (Ed.), *Handbook of child psychology: Vol. 1. Theoretical models of human development* (5th ed., pp. 1029–1143). New York: Wiley.
Baltes, P. B., Reese, H. W., & Nesselroade, J. R. (1977). *Life-span developmental psychology: Introduction to research methods*. Monterey, CA: Brooks/Cole.
Baltes, P. B., & Smith, J. (2003). New frontiers in the future of aging: From successful aging of the young old to the dilemmas of the fourth age. *Gerontology, 49,* 123–135.
Baltes, P. B., Staudinger, U. M., & Lindenberger, U. (1999). Lifespan psychology: Theory and application to intellectual functioning. *Annual Review of Psychology, 50,* 471–507.
Bauer, J. J., & McAdams, D. P. (2004). Growth goals, maturity, and well-being. *Developmental Psychology, 40,* 114–127.
Brandtstädter, J. (1998). Action perspective on human development. In W. Damon (Series Ed.) & R. Lerner (Vol. Ed.), *Handbook of child psychology: Vol. 1. Theoretical models of human development* (5th ed., pp. 807–863). New York: Wiley.
Brandtstädter, J., & Renner, G. (1990). Tenacious goal pursuit and flexible goal adjustment: Explication and age-related analysis of assimilative and accommodative strategies of coping. *Psychology and Aging, 5,* 58–67.
Brim, O. G., & Kagan, J. (1980). Constancy and change: A view of the issues. In O. G. Brim & J. Kagan (Eds.), *Constancy and change in human development* (pp. 1–25). Cambridge, MA: Harvard University Press.
Brunstein, J. C. (1993). Personal goals and subjective well-being: A longitudinal study. *Journal of Personality and Social Psychology, 65,* 1061–1070.
Brunstein, J. C., Schultheiss, O. C., & Grässman, R. (1998). Personal goals and emotional well-being: The moderating role of motive dispositions. *Journal of Personality and Social Psychology, 75,* 494–508.
Carstensen, L. L. (1993). Motivation for social contact across the life span: A theory of socioemotional selectivity. In J. E. Jacobs (Ed.), *Nebraska Symposium on Motivation, 1992: Developmental perspectives on motivation. Current theory and research in motivation* (Vol. 40, pp. 209-254). Lincoln, NE: University of Nebraska Press.
Carstensen, L. L., & Charles, S. T. (1998). Emotion in the second half of life. *Current Directions in Psychological Science, 7,* 144–149.
Carver, C. S., & Scheier, M. F. (1990). Origins and functions of positive and negative affect: A control-process view. *Psychological Review, 97,* 19–35.

DeShon, R. P., Kozlowski, W. J., Schmidt, A. M., Milner, K. R., & Wiechmann, D. (2004). A multiple-goal, multilevel model of feedback effects on the regulation of individual and team performance. *Journal of Applied Psychology, 89,* 1035–1056.

Diehl, M., Coyle, N., & Labouvie-Vief, G. (1996). Age and sex differences in strategies of coping and defense across the life span. *Psychology and Aging, 11,* 127–139.

Emmons, R. A. (1986). Personal strivings: An approach to personality and subjective well-being. *Journal of Personality and Social Psychology, 51,* 1058–1068.

Emmons, R. A., Cheung, C., & Tehrani, K. (1998). Assessing spirituality through personal goals: Implications for research on religion and subjective well-being. *Social Indicators Research, 45,* 391–422.

Emmons, R. A., & King, L. A. (1988). Conflict among personal strivings: Immediate and long-term implications for psychological and physical well-being. *Journal of Personality and Social Psychology, 54,* 1040–1048.

Emmons, R. A., King, L. A., & Sheldon, K. M. (1993). Goal conflict and the self-regulation of action. In D. M. Wegner & J. W. Pennebaker (Eds.), *Handbook of mental control: Century psychology series* (pp. 528–551). Englewood Cliffs, NJ: Prentice-Hall.

Epstein, S. (1982). Conflict and stress. In L. Goldberger & S. Breznitz (Eds.), *Handbook of stress* (pp. 49–68). New York: The Free Press.

Erikson, E. H. (1959). Identity and the life cycle. *Psychological Issues, 1,* 1–171.

Folkman, S., Lazarus, R. S., Pimley, S., & Novacek, J. (1987). Age differences in stress and coping processes. *Psychology and Aging, 2,* 171–184.

Freund, A. M., & Baltes, P. B. (2000). The orchestration of selection, optimization and compensation: An action-theoretical conceptualization of a theory of developmental regulation. In W. J. Perrig & A. Grob (Eds.), *Control of human behavior, mental processes, and consciousness: Essays in honor of the 60th birthday of August Flammer* (pp. 35–58). Mahwah, NJ: Lawrence Erlbaum Associates.

Freund, A. M., & Riediger, M. (2003). Successful aging. In R. M. Lerner, M. A. Easterbrooks, & J. Mistry (Eds.), *Handbook of psychology: Vol. 6. Developmental psychology* (pp. 601–628). New York: Wiley.

Freund, A. M., & Riediger, M. (2006). Goals as building blocks of personality and development in adulthood. In D. K. Mroszek & T. D. Little (Eds.), *Handbook of personality development.* Lawrence Erlbaum Associates.

Greenhaus, J. H., & Beutell, N. J. (1985). Sources of conflict between work and family roles. *Academy of Management Roles, 10,* 76–88.

Gross, J. J., Carstensen, L. L., Pasupathi, M., Tsai, J., Goetestam Skorpen, C., & Hsu, A. Y. C. (1997). Emotion and aging: Experience, expression, and control. *Psychology and Aging, 12,* 590–599.

Heckhausen, J., & Schulz, R. (1995). A life-span theory of control. *Psychological Review, 102,* 284–304.

Hobfoll, S. E. (1998). *Stress, culture, and community: The psychology and philosophy of stress.* New York: Plenum.

Hoyer, J. (1992). *Intrapsychischer Konflikt und psychopathologische Symptombelastung [Intrapsychic conflict and psychopathological symptom severity].* Regensburg, Germany: S. Roderer.

Jung, C. (1933). *Modern man in search of a soul.* New York: Harcourt.

Kahneman, D., & Tversky, A. (1984). Choices, values, and frames. *American Psychologist, 39,* 341–350.

Kehr, H. M. (2003). Goal conflicts, attainment of new goals, and well-being among managers. *Journal of Occupational Health Psychology, 8,* 195–208.

Kehr, H. M. (2004). Implicit/explicit motive discrepancies and volitional depletion among managers. *Personality and Social Psychology Bulletin, 30,* 315–327.

King, L. A., Richards, J. H., & Stemmerich, E. (1998). Daily goals, life goals, and worst fears: Means, ends, and subjective well-being. *Journal of Personality, 66,* 713–744.

Krampe, R. T., & Baltes, P. B. (2003). Intelligence as adaptive resource development and resource allocation: A new look through the lenses of SOC and expertise. In R. J. Sternberg & E. L. Grigorenko (Eds.), *Perspectives on the psychology of abilities, competencies, and expertise* (pp. 31–69). New York: Cambridge University Press.

Kristof-Brown, A. L., & Stevens, C. K. (2001). Goal congruence in project teams: Does the fit between members' personal mastery and performance goals matter? *Journal of Applied Psychology, 86,* 1083–1095.

Labouvie-Vief, G. (1981). Proactive and reactive aspects of constructivism: Growth and aging in life-span perspective. In R. M. Lerner & N. A. Busch-Rossnagel (Eds.), *Individuals as producers of their development: A life-span perspective* (pp. 197–230). New York: Academic.

Lauterbach, W. (1996). The measurement of personal conflict. *Psychotherapy Research, 6,* 213–225.

Lerner, R. M., & Busch-Rossnagel, N. A. (Eds.). (1981). *Individuals as producers of their development: A life-span perspective.* New York: Academic.

Lewis, C., Reitsma, R., Wilson, E. V., & Zigurs, I. (2001). Extending coordination theory to deal with goal conflicts. In G. M. Olson, T. W. Malone, & J. B. Smith (Eds.), *Coordination theory and collaboration technology* (pp. 651–672). Mahwah, NJ: Lawrence Erlbaum Associates.

Little, B. R. (1983). Personal projects: A rationale and method for investigation. *Environment and Behavior, 15,* 273–309.

Locke, E. A., Smith, K. G., Erez, M., Chah, D. O., & Schaffer, A. (1994). The effects of intra-individual goal conflict on performance. *Journal of Management, 20,* 67–91.

Maes, S., & Gebhardt, W. (2000). Self-regulation and health behavior: The health behavior goal model. In M. Boekaerts, P. R. Pintrich & M. Zeidner (Eds.), *Handbook of self-regulation* (pp. 343–368). San Diego, CA: Academic.

McGregor, I., & Little, B. R. (1998). Personal projects, happiness, and meaning: On doing well and being yourself. *Journal of Personality and Social Psychology, 74,* 494–512.

McKeeman, D., & Karoly, P. (1991). Interpersonal and intrapsychic goal-related conflict reported by cigarette smokers, unaided quitters, and relapsers. *Addictive Behaviors, 16,* 543–548.

McReynolds, P. (1991). The nature and logic of intrapsychic conflicts. In C. D. Spielberger, I. G. Sarason, J. Strelau, & J. M. T. Brebner (Eds.), *Stress and anxiety* (Vol. 13, pp. 73–83). New York: Hemisphere.

Michalak, J., Heidenreich, T., & Hoyer, J. (2004). Goal conflicts: Concepts, findings, and consequences for psychotherapy. In W. M. Cox & E. Klinger (Eds.), *Handbook of motivational counseling: Concepts, approaches, and assessment* (pp. 83–98). Chichester, UK: Wiley.

Michalak, J., & Schulte, D. (2002). Zielkonflikte und Therapiemotivation [Goal conflicts and therapy motivation]. *Zeitschrift für Klinische Psychologie und Psychotherapie, 31,* 213–219.

Nesselroade, J. R., & Baltes, P. B. (Eds.). (1979). *Longitudinal research in the study of behavior and development.* New York: Academic.

Nurmi, J.-E. (1991). How do adolescents see their future? A review of the development of future orientation and planning. *Developmental Review, 11,* 1–59.

Omodei, M. M., & Wearing, A. J. (1990). Need satisfaction and involvement in personal projects: Toward an integrative model of subjective well-being. *Journal of Personality and Social Psychology, 59,* 762–769.

Palys, T. S., & Little, B. R. (1983). Perceived life satisfaction and the organization of personal project systems. *Journal of Personality and Social Psychology, 44,* 1221–1230.

Perring, C., Oatley, K., & Smith, J. (1988). Psychiatric symptoms and conflict among personal plans. *British Journal of Medical Psychology, 61,* 167–177.

Pomaki, G., Maes, S., & ter Doest, L. (2004). Work conditions and employees' self-set goals: Goal processes enhance prediction of psychological distress and well-being. *Personality and Social Psychology Bulletin, 30,* 685–694.

Riediger, M., & Freund, A. M. (2004). Interference and facilitation among personal goals: Differential associations with subjective well-being and persistent goal pursuit. *Personality and Social Psychology Bulletin, 30,* 1511–1523.

Riediger, M., Freund, A. M., & Baltes, P. B. (2003). Managing life through personal goals: Intergoal facilitation and intensity of goal pursuit in younger and older adulthood. *Journal of Gerontology: Psychological Sciences, 60,* P84–F91.

Riegel, K. F. (1975). Adult life crises: A dialectic interpretation of development. In N. Datan & L. H. Ginsberg (Eds.), *Life-span developmental psychology: Normative life crises* (pp. 99–128). New York: Academic.

Ryff, C. D. (1985). Adult personality and the motivation for personal growth. In D. A. Kleiber & M. L. Maehr (Eds.), *Motivation and adulthood* (Vol. 4, pp. 55–92). Greenwich, CT: JAI.

Salmela-Aro, K., Nurmi, J. –E., Saisto, T., & Halmesmäki, E. (2000). Women's and men's goals during the transition to parenthood. *Journal of Family Psychology, 14,* 171–186.

Schultheiss, O. C., & Brunstein, J. C. (1999). Goal imagery: Bridging the gap between implicit motives and explicit goals. *Journal of Personality, 67,* 1–38.

Sheldon, K. M., & Emmons, R. A. (1995). Comparing differentiation and integration within personal goal systems. *Personality and Individual Differences, 18,* 39–46.

Sheldon, K. M., & Kasser, T. (1995). Coherence and congruence: Two aspects of personality integration. *Journal of Personality and Social Psychology, 68,* 531–543.

Sheldon, K. M., & Kasser, T. (2001). Getting older, getting better? Personal strivings and psychological maturity across the life span. *Developmental Psychology, 37,* 491–501.

Turiel, E. (1974). Conflict and transition in adolescent moral development. *Child Development, 45,* 14–29.

Werner, H. (1967). The concept of development from a comparative and organismic point of view. In D. B. Harris (Ed.), *The concept of development* (pp. 125–148). Minneapolis: University of Minnesota Press.

Wilensky, R. (1983). *Planning and understanding.* Reading, MA: Addison-Wesley.

5

Just Doing It: Affective Implications of Project Phrasing

Neil C. Chambers

They've a temper, some of them—particularly verbs: they're the proudest—adjectives you can do anything with, but not verbs ...
—Carroll, *Through the Looking Glass*

Most linguists agree that language encodes important distinctions that we as humans make in the world around us (Lakoff, 1987; Sapir, 1921; Wierzbicka, 1996), but to date explorations in consistent differences in the patterns of usage within a single language have focused primarily on differences among social groups in the sociolinguistic tradition of Bernstein (1971). Only very recently have psychologists begun to explore the personality correlates of consistent individual differences in phrasing (Chambers, 2001; Pennebaker, 2001).

In the tradition of George Kelly (1955), I suggest that from the myriad of lexical and grammatical permutations available to any single speaker of a language, individuals will tend to chose some rather than others and this choice reflects their unique construct system, the way in which they parse the world around them into meaningful units. A systematic study of the words and grammatical turns of phrase that individuals use is therefore postulated to reflect consistent individual differences in personality.

Little (1996), responding to McAdams (1996), conceptualized three tiers in a comprehensive edifice of personality: the havings (traits), doings (conative psychology), and beings (narrative psychology) of the individual. I would like to propose that each level suggests a preferred linguistic unit of analysis. Trait psychology focused from the outset almost exclusively on the adjective (Allport & Odbert, 1936) and current trait measures ultimately place people on adjectival dimensions: neurotic, extraverted, conscientious, and so on (Costa & McCrae, 1992). Conative or action psychology emphasizes the verbs of personality, how the individual characterizes his or her own actions, as projects (Little, 1983), strivings (Emmons, 1986), or concerns[1] (Klinger, Barta, & Maxeiner, 1981), among others. Each of these related units of analysis is basically a verbal phrase that indicates intended or ongoing action, the idiosyncratic appraisals of which are assumed to be, in aggregate, a key index of personality and motivation (Little, 1999b). Finally, narrative psychology emphasizes integration in language, as it does in personality, by focusing on integrated discourse (McAdams, 1996), myth and metaphor (Sarbin, 1994), and linguistic or literary mechanisms for understanding the person as a whole. Individual differences in language can be fruitfully studied at each of these levels.

The research outlined in this chapter explores differences in phrasing at the second level of personality, that of personal action. English verbs or action words are, more than any other part of speech, highly complex grammatical entities that are inflected to convey nuanced interactions of time and action. They also reflect subtle differences in the way in which the action itself is perceived by the individual, for instance, by using the passive versus active voice or through combining principal verbs with modal (or "helping") verbs.

During my tenure as a student of personal projects, I noted over several years of data analysis a tendency among some respondents to use certain phrases ("try to," "keep on," "start ...," etc.) when listing their projects. Among the many possible phrasing options, this chapter looks at actions involving the following:

---

[1]Elsewhere (Chambers, 1997) I have made the case that concerns often focus more on the resultant state rather than the action itself; however because in English states are also conveyed by verbs (stative verbs) they are still primarily verbal phrases.

* Trying to do, rather than simply doing (explicitly conative).
* Doing more of something (augmentative).
* Doing so as not to ... (avoidant).
* Doing less of something (reductive).
* Continuing or keeping on doing (continuative).[2]

These phrasing tendencies can be contrasted with "just doing it," that is with straightforward expressions of action in progress that are not modified by prefatory phrasing.

Based on an archival data set of 2,499 personal projects, an initial exploration was made of whether English-speaking university students phrased their volitional action in ways that systematically reflected their appraisals of those actions. This research falls into what Buss (1999) characterized as "the study of human nature," that is, "the common characteristics of humans—the shared motives, goals, and psychological mechanisms that are either universal or nearly universal" (p. 31). To this we might add the constraint that it is human nature within a specific cultural context, that of North American English speakers.

Separately collected data are also explored at the level of the individual. Do people who "try to" all the time run the risk of seeing their projects as less likely to succeed than those who just do them? Are those who are always "doing more of something" happier with their projects than those who are constantly undertaking new and different endeavors? This research falls under the other major branch of personality psychology, that of individual differences (Buss, 1999), although I support Buss's contention that both themes should be regarded as inextricably linked.

Measures and Coding

The same measures were used in both studies discussed in this chapter to allow for comparability. Personal projects analysis (PPA; Little, 1983) elicits currently salient projects of the respondent, who is then asked to reflect on these projects and rate them from 0 to 10 on a series of dimensions that have been shown to be relevant to how people view their planned and ongoing actions. In both studies, key project efficacy dimensions—control, competence, likelihood of success, stage and,

---

[2]Inceptive (start X) and terminative (finish X or stop X) phrasing were also explored with interesting results at the project level. Space limitations preclude a discussion here.

where ratings were available, success to date (progress)—were used based on research that has shown efficacy to be consistently the strongest predictor of well-being in "second-level" research in personality (Little, 1989; Salmela-Aro, 1992). Commitment to the project and the perceived difficulty of the action were also included in the analyses as potential discriminating variables, and standardized enjoyment and stress scores provided a measure of project-level affect.[3]

At the individual level, subjective well-being (SWB) was measured by aggregating standardized scores from the Diener and Emmons (1985) affect scale (positive affect [PA] and negative affect [NA]) with a global measure of life satisfaction (Palys & Little, 1983) to reflect current conceptualizations of SWB as PA + Life satisfaction – NA (Diener, Suh, Lucas, & Smith, 1999). The Center for Epidemiological Studies Depression Scale (CES–D; Radloff, 1977) was used to measure depression, whereas the Personal Project System Rating Scale (PPSRS) developed by Little and Lecci (Little, 1988) was used to elicit global perceptions of efficacy and meaning in individual project systems. Trait domains were measured either using the NEO–PI–R (Costa & McCrae, 1992) or a rationally derived self-report direct magnitude scale (Little, 1988), both of which classified individuals on the Big Five personality factors: neuroticism, extraversion, openness to experience, agreeableness, and conscientiousness.

Blind to the appraisal dimension ratings, I coded 10,604 projects according to the categories already outlined. All projects in the database were compared to the original (handwritten) project elicitation to ensure that the participants' phrasing had not been modified either in transferring the project from the elicitation module to the rating matrix or in entering the project into the database. The original (elicitation) phrasing was taken as that most reflective of the idiosyncratic construal of the project, as there were virtually no constraints on the length of project phrasing, as there were in the latter two instances.

After a brief overview of the coding system, a second judge coded a random 10% of the total projects in Study 1. Interrater agreement on all categories was over 95% in all cases, sometimes reaching 100%. The high level of coding reliability is not surprising given the very clear linguistic guidelines established (e.g., to be classed as continuative, the

---

[3]Because PPA is a highly modular personality assessment methodology not all dimensions are used in every study and not all respondents rate every project on each dimension, hence sample size varies widely, particularly in the case of listwise deletion for discriminant function analysis.

phrase must include "continue," "keep on," "do more," etc.; with regard to strong interrater reliability of similar project coding see also Elliot & Friedman, chap. 3, this volume).

At the level of individual action phrasing, projects were examined as separate cases based on previous findings that the assumption of independent observations is robust in PPA. In particular, the manner of rating used does not limit degrees of freedom and the project space associated with both PPA data from complete matrices and from randomly sampled projects is effectively the same (Gee, 1999). At the individual level, frequency of phrasing tendencies were calculated for the individual and then converted to z scores. A consistent phrasing tendency was operationalized as any frequency reflected by a z score of over $+1$. Mean project appraisals were used to reflect individual levels of efficacy, enjoyment, stress, and so on associated with project systems.

PROJECT-LEVEL ACTION PHRASING

Affective project appraisal data (project enjoyment, stress) were converted to T scores for each individual; that is, the individual mean score on each dimension was specified as 50 and their project ratings defined in standard deviations ($\pm$ 10). Given the inherent difficulty in comparing affective ratings, it was deemed more useful to compare project ratings to individual-level norms than to an artificial group norm (see Omodei & Wearing, 1990, for an example of the procedure). In short, we are more interested whether "do more of" projects, for instance, are associated with greater relative enjoyment for the individual than greater absolute enjoyment across participants. The cognitive dimensions were not converted, given the underlying assumption that appraisals of success, difficulty, and so on are much more heavily influenced by common norms, particularly within a common context (university) and with peers (students). Statistical analyses were conducted using univariate and multivariate techniques.

The personal projects of 222 English-speaking undergraduate students were selected from Carleton University's Social Ecological Assessment Databank (SEAbank) based on (a) recency of the sample, and (b) native fluency in English. The former was to provide as much comparability in project appraisal as possible, given that earlier samples in SEAbank generally include fewer appraisal dimensions and hence less comprehensive data on how personal action is viewed by the respondent. English speakers were required because of the linguistic-based nature of this study, which assumes a native "feel" for language usage. Forty-five percent of the sample were male ($n = 100$) and the remainder female ($n = 122$), with an overall mean age of 23 years.

Examining first phrasing tendencies at the project level ($n = 4,339$, 2,499 of which were rated[4]), usage among the categories varied considerably as Table 5.1 shows. Of greatest interest is the relative consistency between the two samples in the overall prevalence of these verbal phrases.

Explicitly Conative Action: Try As You Might ...

Folk wisdom would suggest that it is better to do something rather than to try to do something; indeed clinicians are sensitive to the hedging that is implicit in their patients' commitments to try to change a given behavior, frequently countering "Don't try, just do it!" A project phrased with an explicit try is therefore hypothesized to be an "out" for the individual. For instance if someone says "I will quit smoking," that person can only truthfully state that he or she carried through on the action if he or she does indeed stop for good, whereas if someone says "I'll try and quit smoking," that person can claim successful engagement in the at-

TABLE 5.1
Frequency of Phrasing Use: Project Level

Phrasing type	Number of Projects ($n = 4339$)	Percent of Total	Number of Rated Projects ($n = 2499$)	Percent of Total
Explicitly conative (try)	159	3.7	93	3.7
Augmentative (more/better)	741	17.1	447	17.9
Avoidant (not)	178	4.1	93	3.7
Reductive (less)	150	3.5	85	3.4
Continuative (maintain)	165	3.8	96	3.8

[4]Personal projects are first elicited in an initial module and then a sample transferred by the respondent to a rating matrix for further rating (because it would be too onerous to rate all the projects listed, which can number as many as 50, and on average would be 15–20; Little & Chambers, 2000).

tempt even if the outcome was not as desired: "Well, I *tried* ... ." To try, in effect, redirects the focus of the action from the outcome to the process. If this is the case, intended actions that are phrased in an explicitly conative manner will be perceived as less likely to succeed and more difficult than actions expressed without the modal. It follows that the individual may have doubts about his or her self-efficacy to successfully carry the action through to termination, so we would expect to see lower levels of perceived competency and control for the given project. Trying projects, then, are expected to be appraised, on average, as less likely to succeed and more difficult and as engendering lower levels of perceived competence and control. Given the associations between low efficacy and negative affect, we would expect this to translate into lower project enjoyment and higher project stress.

Two separate random selections each of 100 unmodified (as originally phrased by respondents) projects (from 1,566 such projects in the sample) were compared to the 93 projects that were coded as explicitly conative using discriminant function analysis. The goal was to explore whether appraisals of efficacy and affect consistently discriminated explicitly conative projects along the lines hypothesized. In both samples, discriminant functions: CANCORR = .49, $\chi^2(8) = 31.89, p <$ .001; and .50, $\chi^2(8) = 34.92, p < .001$, distinguished the explicitly conative projects from the unmodified comparison group along three of the hypothesized dimensions, including difficulty, likelihood of success, and control. Competence was distinguished only in the first analysis and a lack of enjoyment only in the second. Project stress did not differ significantly in either sample.[5] It would seem that choosing to phrase one's project as an attempt generally equates to the perception that it is difficult and unlikely to succeed, and that it tests both one's sense of competence and control. The fact that such projects were no more stressful, albeit sometimes less enjoyable than the comparison group does provide some support for the interpretation that "trying to" is an out, providing a disjuncture between the negative valence usually associated with such a poor prognostication and an appraisal of just that sort of probable outcome. As long as I try, I need not feel too stressed about whether this all works out or not. Clearly, it is an impaired sense of efficacy that is the hallmark of trying projects.

---

[5]Specific statistical results for each analysis across both samples are not included given space limitations, but are available from the author at neilchambers@sympatico.ca

Augmentative Action: Give Me More ...

In listing one's personal goals or projects, an individual is providing an overview of the content and direction of daily life that, although circumscribed somewhat by social and cultural requirements, still allows him or her considerable latitude in terms of which actions to choose from all those available. If among those actions are several that are phrased as "doing more of," we might surmise that the individual is satisfied with many of his or her current projects. Why do more if it is not agreeable, beneficial, or self-enhancing in some way? It would seem logical that projects phrased as "do more of X" will, on average, be more enjoyable and less stressful than other action constructs. Similarly we would expect such projects to reflect increased perceptions of efficacy, in that it is unlikely one will consider doing more of X unless one is already doing X reasonably well. Projects that involve doing more are therefore likely to be appraised as less stressful, more enjoyable, more likely to succeed, and pursued with a greater sense of competency and control than other (unmodified) projects.

"Do more of" was the most common phrasing tendency ($n = 477$) and was compared to two random samples of 500 (unmodified) projects from a total of 1,566 such projects. Again both analyses yielded significant discriminant functions: CANCORR = .30, $\chi^2(8) = 61.10$, $p < .001$; and .32, $\chi^2(8) = 70.06$, $p < .001$, that distinguished doing more from the comparison group and provided support for the view that "doing more of X" type projects are consummately unstressful. It would appear, however, that this may not result in nor stem from perceptions of efficacy in project pursuit. Although perceived as somewhat more manageable, such projects were, at least sometimes, viewed as less likely to come to fruition. A brief perusal of the nature of augmentative projects does show that a large number of "do more of" projects were in fact desires that may well be perceived as unlikely to be realized given the daily impingements of other required tasks: "do more yoga," "read more," "practice piano more," and so on. This was supported by chi-square analyses in both samples that showed such "do more" projects were significantly more likely to be in the health and body, intrapersonal, or leisure domains and less likely to be academic or maintenance—the everyday projects of most students, $\chi^2(5) = 141.76$, $p < .001$, and $\chi^2(5) = 154.74$, $p < .001$. Thus these projects are generally less stressful than daily activities (when one actually can engage in them), but not particularly likely to happen given the exigencies of daily life.

Avoidant and Reductive Action: Doing (Less) So as Not to Be

Avoidance goals have been clearly distinguished in the literature and evidence is strong that a surfeit of such goals is associated with lower well-being (see Elliot & Freidman, chap. 3, this volume, for a thorough review). Within the context of control theory, avoidance goals are thought to lead to lower well-being because of the diffuse goal–action relation inherent in avoiding a negatively valenced state (Carver, 1996). There are usually a limited number of plausible action alternatives that will lead to a desired state, but an almost unlimited number of actions that can be taken to avoid such a state, especially if broadly construed. Furthermore it may not always be that clear whether a negative state has been successfully avoided, hence the positive affect associated with goal attainment is attenuated when the goal is a negative state (Elliot, Sheldon, & Church, 1997).

In the context of project phrasing we can distinguish two types of avoidant action: action that is planned or undertaken to ensure the avoidance of the end state (pure avoidant action), and action that is undertaken to reduce or diminish an undesired end state (reductive action). Whereas doing more of something presupposes the action is enjoyable, doing less of something suggests the opposite. Thus projects that are phrased avoidantly or reductively are likely to be perceived as more stressful, less enjoyable, and associated with lower efficacy than unmodified action constructs. No specific hypothesis is adduced regarding which of the two avoidant phrases is more pernicious: smoke less versus quit smoking.

Reductive and avoidant phrasing were initially compared to ascertain whether there are significant differences between doing something less and avoiding doing something along the five project dimensions of stress, enjoyment, likelihood of success, control, and competence. No significant differences emerged. Collapsing these into a single group ($n = 168$), avoidant projects were compared to two samples of 200 randomly selected projects. Significant discriminant functions, CANCORR = .52, $\chi^2(8) = 78.65$, $p < .001$; and .48, $\chi^2(8) = 68.34$, $p < .001$, distinguished avoidant projects from the unmodified comparison group as more difficult, less enjoyable, and associated with lower perceived competence. Avoidant projects were also seen as less likely to succeed and marginally more stressful in the first but not the second analysis.

The analyses support the view that avoidant goal phrasing is problematic, both in terms of perceived efficacy and the associated negative valence (or at least here, the absence of positive valence). This is congruent with Carver's (1996) contention noted earlier that the inability to actually achieve a positive goal (rather than avoid a negative one) lowers considerably the potential positive affect associated with action.

Among the efficacy dimensions, it is a lack of competence that stands out as particularly characteristic of avoidant projects (Elliot & Sheldon, 1997). Competence is a more clearly self-focused efficacy dimension, as opposed to low likelihood of success or difficulty, which may more easily be attributed to environmental factors. Examining avoidant projects by domain in both samples, we find a significant lack of independence, $\chi^2(5) = 393.48, p < .0001, \chi^2(5) = 194.74, p < .001$, with the overwhelming majority of avoidant projects (almost 87%) falling into two categories: health or body and intrapersonal. Both these categories are closely related to perceptions of self (Little, 1993) with many students concerned about body image and health (Goodine, 1986; Melia-Gordon, 1992) and with specifically self-changing projects such as being less aggressive or less shy (Zomer, 2000). Indeed, in comparing perceptions of project self-identity between avoidantly phrased and unmodified projects, we find the former to be consistently significantly less identified with the self: $t(360) = 3.50, p < .001$, and $t(360) = 4.77, p < .001$, respectively. Perhaps it is the negative possible self (feared self; Oyserman & Markus, 1990) that is central in avoidantly phrased student projects—"me, the out-of-shape, obnoxious procrastinator."

Continuative Action: Keep on Truckin' ...

Although potentially the same as "do more of," "keep doing X" or "continue to do X" may reflect the need to focus attention and effort on maintaining action that is not easily maintained, rather than a free choice to increase one's activity in a certain project. In other words, the inclusion of a lexical aspectual marker that implies continuity suggests effortful continuance: "Keep the house clean," "keep up on my reading," and so on. At the same time it also implies success to date (the house is clean and I am caught up on my reading), so we might expect such projects to show high efficacy, but lower enjoyment and higher stress, reflecting the effort required to maintain action.

Comparing the 94 continuative projects with a random sample of 150 (unmodified) projects along the key efficacy and affective dimensions in two discriminant function analyses, significant functions emerged in both cases: CANCORR = .46, $\chi^2(8)$ = 39.85, p < .001; and .45, $\chi^2(8)$ = 35.53, p < .001. "Keep on Xing" projects were characterized by lower stress and difficulty and increased control. Continuative projects were also seen as much further along (higher ratings on the stage dimension) than the comparison group.

Thus the greater efficacy we hypothesized to be associated with already doing something (and hence being able to continue it) was supported, but it seems that the valence, instead of being negative and reflecting effortful continuance, appears to reflect unstressful project pursuit. Such a view may be the result of the advanced stage associated with such projects, which does allow for judgments of goal proximity and adequate progress. Comparing the project dimension progress (success to date), which was not included in the discriminant function analysis as a result of too many missing ratings, we found "maintenance" projects are seen to have been much more successful to date (M = 7.13, SD = 2.42) than the comparison group (M = 5.16, SD = 3.12), $t(132.58)$ = –4.13, p < .001. In this single instance, then, it is not better to "just do it." If you have already done it, maintaining the action is, in fact, potentially less stressful and is associated with greater efficacy.

Limitations of Findings at the Project Level

This first exploration of action phrasing at the project level aimed at providing evidence that the language we use to express our actions reflects systematic nuanced differences in how we perceive that action, regardless of who we are and what other projects may make up our project system. If we take the generic project, "write a book chapter," we find that, on average, the explicitly conative variation "try to write a book chapter" reflects that the project is perceived as difficult, less likely to succeed, and that the actor is experiencing lower levels of control and competence. Such projects are clearly trying in their own right.

In contrast, projects of the sort "write more book chapters," which we call augmentative projects and which imply successful previous engagement, reflect the perception that the project is relatively unstressful and manageable, although it may not actually ever succeed. Our exam-

ple is somewhat misleading in that such projects are much more likely
to be leisure or health or body related and thus may reflect projects we
would like to do and that we associate with lower stress, but that we cannot seem to get around to doing (Hotson, 2001).

Evidence from this study supports previous findings in the literature
that avoidantly construed goals tend to be more negatively valenced. Indeed, projects of the sort "avoid putting off writing that book chapter"
tend to be viewed as less likely to succeed, less enjoyable, and more difficult than approach projects, and the actor perceives himself or herself
as being less competent. It does seem more pernicious to avoid doing X
than to just do Y. We have also seen that what I have termed reductively
phrased projects (do less of) function very much as avoidant projects, so
that the quantitative difference (less vs. not at all) does not mitigate perceptions of inefficacy and experiences of negative valence.

Finally we found that maintaining action (keep *on* writing book chapters) was associated primarily with increased efficacy and modestly with
lower stress. It would seem, then, that it may be better to be in a position
to "keep doing it" than to be "just doing it."

Taken together these results provide a baseline for understanding
how people appraise their ongoing or planned actions from the choice
of words they use to describe those actions. This is a first broad-brush
look at action phrasing within a relatively homogeneous population
(North American, English-speaking university students) and generalization outside of that population is not warranted. Further testing will be
required to ascertain how many of these phrasing–appraisal linkages
are universal in English (in other populations) or across various
languages (in other cultures).

These results also emerged from within heterogeneous archival data,
which did not allow for a test of a full range of the appraisals that can
possibly be reflected in nuanced project phrasing. The various
operationalizations of efficacy available (competence, control, likelihood of success, etc.) were expected and shown to differ in relation to
project phrasing, but this does not exclude the possibility that other factors in project pursuit (social meaning or support, for instance) may not
further distinguish these variations in phrasing.

We have been comparing projects without regard for domain or level
of action identification, each of which may increase or attenuate the
strength of the relations between certain appraisals and phrasing. For
instance, "try to be a better person" (high level of identification) may be
much more stressful and less likely to succeed than "try to be nice to Jim

the next time I see him" (lower level). Likewise "don't leave my socks on the floor" (maintenance avoidant) may be much more manageable and likely to succeed than "avoid failing first-year psychology" (academic avoidant). Such fine-grained comparisons are becoming possible as the volume of projects in SEAbank (Little, 1989) grows and will provide for the first time an empirical test of consistencies between how we as humans phrase our actions and how we think and feel about them.

INDIVIDUAL PHRASING TENDENCIES

We have shown that there do appear to be commonly shared links between how we talk about our actions and how we think and feel about those actions. The research outlined next explores whether certain individuals show a consistent tendency to phrase their projects using one or more of these variations in action phrasing and whether such tendencies, if they do exist, are associated with individual differences in well-being, project system appraisal, or personality traits. For instance, at the project level, we saw that explicitly conative phrasing ("try to …") was associated with lower efficacy and marginally lower project enjoyment. Does it follow that individuals who tend to phrase most or many of their projects as attempts will experience lower well-being and generally lower perceived efficacy? Perhaps they are less conscientious by nature?

In addition to the archival data described in the context of the preceding analyses of project-level phrasing, which were reanalyzed here at the level of the individual, 412 undergraduate university students enrolled in first-year psychology were given course credit to complete a package of questionnaires relating to a study on language and time perception (Chambers, 2001). In all, after excluding missing data and nonfluency in English, this provided a sample of 279 university students, of whom 28% were male and 72% were female, with a mean age of 21.

All projects listed in the individual's project elicitation module (i.e., where they are first asked to list as many projects as they can in 10–15 minutes) were coded. It was felt that the elicitation, which is not constrained in any way and is the first and most complete enumeration of projects in PPA, would serve as a much better representation of an individual's action phrasing tendencies than a nonrandom selection of 10 rated projects. Because the number of projects generated in the first module can vary from 7 to more than 50, the ratio of phrasing tendencies to the overall number of projects was calculated by dividing the frequency of each tendency by the total number of projects generated. These ratios were converted to z scores and any individual with a standardized ratio of greater than 1 was considered to have that particular phrasing tendency. Approximately 72% ($n = 159$) and 58% ($n = 161$) of respondents in both samples, respectively, did show at least one phrasing tendency, suggesting that these are common variations in how humans tend to express their actions.

Frequency and Stability

Table 5.2 provides the frequencies of phrasing tendencies for the two samples. With the possible exception of individuals who "do more of," who were noticeably more numerous in Sample 1, the frequency of individuals with a given phrasing tendency was relatively consistent across the two samples. Note that there were no gender differences in phrasing.

Are phrasing tendencies stable across time? An individual difference measure with no stability clearly cannot predict reliably; at the same time, personal action is dynamic and we would expect that the projects of individuals would vary as a function of the current concerns of the individual (Klinger, 1975) as well as time of year (McGregor, McAdams, & Little, 2004), health, and a host of variables from the social ecology that may impinge on personal action. Indeed the PPA perspective has largely arisen to better capture the dynamic nature of personality precisely because our behavior does change as a result of temporal and spatial contexts (Little, 1998, 1999a).

The personal projects listed in the elicitation of a second administration of PPA for 47 participants in Sample 1 were coded using the same parameters as the first administration. The same variables were calculated and the data compared between Time 1 (January) and Time 2 (March). Because there were a significantly lower number of projects per person in Time 2 than in Time 1, correlations between the two administrations are based on ratios. For example, the total number of try projects divided by the total number of projects was calculated for each time period and then compared (see Table 5.2).

It should be noted that this is a relatively conservative test of stability over time, given that the second administration of the package was done not long before exams at the "crunch" period of the term when the tendency of individuals was clearly to want to complete yet another required project. The lower overall number of projects suggests greater

TABLE 5.2
Frequency of Action Phrasing Use at the Individual Level and Test–Retest Reliability

Phrasing type	Sample 1[a] phrasing tendency (%)	Sample 2[b] phrasing tendency (%)	Time 1 M	Time 1 SD	Time 2 M	Time 2 SD	Pearson's r[c]
Total # of projects			30	12.2	25.2	12.1	0.71***
Explicitly conative (try)	9	8.2	0.8	1.41	0.51	0.97	0.45**
Augmentative (more/better)	33.3	15.8	5.7	4.71	3.08	3.37	0.63***
Avoidant (not)	14	11.8	1.5	1.78	0.89	1.43	0.28, ns
Reductive (less)	17.6	13.6	1.3	1.95	0.77	1.09	0.58***
Avoidant + reductive (not/less)	31.6	25.4	2.7	3.02	1.62	2.11	0.46***
Continuative (keep on)	13.1	11.5	1	1.44	0.87	1.32	0.34*

[a]$n = 222$; [b]$n = 279$; [c]calculated on the basis of ratio to total number of projects for both administrations.
*$p < .05$.
**$p < .01$.
***$p < .001$.

haste and this may translate into more telegraphic writing, in which not only are fewer projects generated but helping verbs and adverbs may be elided for speed. Nonetheless, there were significant correlations in language usage from Time 1 to Time 2, suggesting stable phrasing tendencies. Among these, the tendency to formulate "not" projects (i.e., in the purely avoidant category) was less stable, although this was offset in this investigation by combining not and less, based on the rationale outlined in the context of the project-level analyses outlined earlier.

The Trying Personality

At the individual level, we would expect the tendency to phrase projects as attempts will negatively impact the well-being of the individual by reflecting a sense of project system-wide impaired efficacy. Self-efficacy has been shown to be a strong predictor of well-being in social learning theory (Bandura, 1997) and in cybernetic models of action (Carver & Scheier, 1990; Hsee & Abelson, 1991), but also in the personal projects literature (Little et al., 2005; Wilson, 1990). In project analytic terms, a tendency to see several projects as attempts at action rather than action per se will likely reflect a lower sense of efficacy through impaired project outcome perceptions, and ultimately lower well-being. We also hypothesize that a tendency to phrase projects using "try to" as an out may also reflect a somewhat lower level of conscientiousness in the individual: "Oh well, I didn't finish the chapter, but at least I tried."

The 8% to 9% of both samples who showed a tendency to phrase projects as attempts also showed significantly lower SWB and higher depression than those with no phrasing tendency.[6] Thus the pernicious effects of trying too much do appear to emerge at the individual level, but are much more salient in terms of their association with SWB.

Examining the two samples as a whole in a discriminant function analysis ($n = 251$) to determine which among the key project appraisal dimensions best distinguish those who try too much from those who just do, the two groups were significantly distinguished, CANCORR = .33, $\chi^2(9) = 28.31, p < .001$, on a discriminant function that emphasized the general lower expectations of success and competence among those who try, as well as a perception that their projects were, on aver-

---

[6]We had also hypothesized that the trying individual would tend to show higher neuroticism and lower conscientiousness; however, neither of the Big Five traits differed significantly between groups.

age, more difficult and stressful. The "trying" personality does experience generalized lower efficacy in relation to his or her projects as a whole.[7] At the project system level, as measured by the PPSRS, this was supported in Sample 1 by the perception of lower global project efficacy ($M = 5.95, SD = 1.82$) than the comparison group ($M = 7.4, SD = 1.53$), $t(81) = 3.52, p < .001$.

The Morish Individual

At the project level we found, somewhat counterintuitively, that "doing more of" projects were less stressful than the norm, but were often seen as less likely to succeed. This disjuncture between efficacy and positive valence was explained as possibly the result of the projects themselves engendering positive affect (in thinking about them), whereas the attendant lack of efficacy is associated instead with environmental constraints on engaging in the project. We would expect that having many such projects in one's system may, in fact, imply that there are many projects that one would like to be doing but currently cannot. Thus both SWB and efficacy at the individual level may be lower for these individuals. We also hypothesize an association with lower openness to experience among the Big Five trait domains. Rather than doing something new, "morish" individuals would rather do more of what they have already done.

No significant differences emerged in either well-being or depression for these individuals, and project system level efficacy ratings were only marginally lower among those with a tendency to do more than those with no phrasing tendency.

Are individuals with a tendency "to do more of" distinguishable from those who have no clear action phrasing tendencies—who "just do it"? Examining the two samples as a whole in a discriminant function analysis ($n = 309$), the two groups were significantly distinguished, CANCORR = .27, $\chi^2(9, N = XXX) = 28.31, p < .01$, being with the dimensions of competence and likelihood of success were most salient. That is, people who do more tend to feel less competent overall in their projects and see their projects, on the whole, as less likely to succeed. At the individual level, it is thus the lack of efficacy associated with "doing more" that is most characteristic, despite the low stress associated with

---

[7]Again, statistics are available from the author, neilchambers@sympatico.ca.

such projects.[8] Perhaps at the individual level, the unstressful nature of "do more of" projects is offset by the lack of efficacy in actually being able to get around to engaging in them, resulting in a neutral effect on overall well-being, but a noticeably lower generalized efficacy. It seems that individuals who (want) to do more of it are not as well off as individuals who just do it.

The Avoidant Personality

We would expect the findings in the literature to hold at the individual level; that is, individuals with a tendency to phrase their goals as end states to be avoided will tend to have lower well-being (Elliot et al., 1997). We also expect higher neuroticism among these individuals, reflecting a general withdrawal orientation, moving away from what I do not like, rather than moving toward what I do. Perceived efficacy is also expected to be impaired given the findings at the project level that support the problematic nature of perpetually trying to avoid a state as opposed to reaching a single desired goal (Carver, 1996).

At the individual level, 52 (37%) respondents in Sample 1 and 64 (28%) in Sample 2 were found to have the tendency to phrase their projects either avoidantly or as "doing less of." Comparing these groups to those with no phrasing tendency, we found, somewhat surprisingly, that there was no significant difference in SWB or depression between the two groups in either sample. Given the demonstrated negative affect associated with both avoidant and "doing less of" phrasing found at the project level and noted in the literature, this result suggests that the avoidant phrasing tendencies must be particularly strong before the effects are evident at the level of overall well-being.

Recoding both groups so that only those with standardized ratio scores over 1.5 were classed as having the phrasing tendency, we found only modest evidence to support this view. Those in Sample 1, who had the tendency to phrase projects avoidantly or as "doing less of," showed marginally significant lower SWB, $t(103) = 2.12$, $p < .05$, than those with no phrasing tendency. No differences were evident in Sample 2.

It is noteworthy that the trying personality appears to be generally worse off affectively than the avoidant personality, in that it is individuals in the former group who show lower SWB and marginally higher rates of depression, whereas those in the latter group do not differ on

---

[8]No differences in openness to new experience were found in either sample.

these variables from the controls, or only marginally so. It certainly seems that it is not better to try and fail than never to try at all, at least not if one insists on phrasing one's doings as explicit tryings.

Examining the two samples of avoidant individuals as a whole in a discriminant function analysis ($n = 316$) to determine which among the key project appraisal dimensions best distinguish those who do so as to avoid, rather than those who just do, the two groups were significantly distinguished on a discriminant function, CANCORR = .27, $\chi^2(9)$ = 23.87, $p < .005$, which was most strongly characterized by low perceptions of competency and lower likelihood of success, as well as somewhat greater difficulty.[9] Thus, like the individual who tries and the one who tends to "do more of," the avoidant personality suffers from impaired efficacy, although in this case it is personal perceived competency that is most salient, rather than the more task-oriented likelihood of success.

Examining the dimension of self-identity of project pursuit (how much is this project "you") we find individuals with avoidant phrasing tendencies to identify significantly less with their actions ($M = 6.29$, SD = 1.38) than those with no phrasing tendency, mirroring the findings at the project level discussed earlier. This is consonant with Sheldon and Kasser's (1998) work, in which they found that if the project is not that meaningful (here, identified with self) then its successful completion is not that central to overall well-being.

The Maintainer

Having several projects that involve maintaining the same action would suggest a generally efficacious project system, because the actions are familiar and, as we saw at the project level, have been successful to date. Well-being will thus be higher and we might find such individuals rate themselves as more conscientious: "I want to make sure I keep up my end."

In Sample 1, 29 individuals (13%) and in Sample 2, 32 individuals (11.5%) were classed as having a tendency to keep on doing. Given the positive associations with this phrasing tendency at the project level, we expected generally higher SWB, lower depression, and higher efficacy in project pursuit. There was, however, no significant difference in either sample for the affective outcome measures, although personal pro-

---

[9]No trait-level differences were evident for the avoidant personality.

ject efficacy and structure were significantly higher for those who keep on doing than for those with no phrasing tendency (this was significant only in Sample 2).

Examining the two samples as a whole (n = 266) to determine which among the key project appraisal dimensions best distinguish those who prefer to keep on from those who just do, the two groups were significantly distinguished, CANCORR = .32, $\chi^2(9)$ = 28.51, p < .001, on a discriminant function that emphasized having projects that were seen as further along, $F_{(1, 264)}$ = 5.77, p < .05, as was the case at the project level, but also as more important, $F_{(1, 264)}$ = 5.75, p < .05. Strikingly different at the individual level, however, was the lower efficacy associated with keeping on, with lower perceived competence in project pursuit as a whole emerging as the best discriminating variable, $F_{(1, 264)}$ = 7.48, p < .01. Individuals who keep on also tended to see their project systems as somewhat less under control, $F_{(1, 264)}$ = 3.49, p = .06. This is striking because project-level perceptions of "keeping on with X" were associated with significantly greater control. Perhaps phrasing certain projects as "keep on doing X" functions as an attempt to provide a sense of control in individual projects that is missing in the project system as a whole.

We have seen across two distinct samples that the way in which an individual habitually phrases his or her projects can be a marker or an indication of project system-wide efficacy, affect, and even general well-being and depression. Phrasing tendencies were seen as relatively stable even when tested at two different times of the year when external impingements on students' project systems were significantly different from Time 1 to Time 2.

Interestingly, all four phrasing tendencies explored at the individual level appeared to reflect some problems with project pursuit in general. In all four discriminant function analyses, projects that were not simple statements of intended actions, but were couched in terms of "keeping on with," "doing more of," "trying to," or "avoiding so as to" reflected to greater or lesser degrees perceptions of impaired competence at the aggregate level. In three of the four tendencies (trying to, avoiding, and doing more of), individuals considered their projects as less likely to succeed on average, whereas individuals with both avoidant and explicitly conative phrasing tendencies found their projects to be more difficult than the comparison groups. The evidence to date would suggest, then, that it is indeed better to be "just doing it." A simple statement of volition carries with it, by comparison, a sense of efficacy, whether in relation to the actions undertaken in general (e.g., likelihood of success) or the self (e.g., competency).

The most pernicious propensity appears to be the tendency to describe one's actions as attempts. Individuals who "try to do" too often not only suffer from impaired efficacy, but are also likely to enjoy lower levels of overall well-being and be more prone to depression. Why this is so is clearly a question for further study. It cannot solely be the effect of lower perceived efficacy, as that was found in other turns of phrase. We might speculate that for these individuals action completion has been traditionally problematic, perhaps even from childhood (Kuhl, 1994), so that consistent use of the word *try* is a reflection of depressive realism (Alloy & Abramson, 1979) or, at least, the lack of positive illusion (Taylor & Brown, 1988). Alternatively it may reflect a defensive pessimism that has been shown to have costs in terms of well-being, although not in terms of actual achievement (Cantor, Norem, Niedenthal, Langston, & Brower, 1987). It is clear, though, that clinicians (and maybe even parents) are wise to exhort clients and offspring to phrase desired goals not as explicit attempts but as definitive actions to be undertaken.

The lack of any significant relation between the Big Five and the linguistic parameters studied here mirrors the weak relation found by Pennebaker and King (1999) in their study of language as an individual difference. They suggested, and we would like to reiterate, that language style may be "an independent and meaningful way of exploring personality" (p. 1296). In a study exploring the different relations between active and inactive projects and well-being, Hotson (2001) found that inactive projects, unlike active projects (Little, Lecci, & Watkinson, 1992), show no clear relation to the Big Five. We may find on further study that projects phrased more circumspectly such as those investigated here are more likely to be inactive.

CONCLUSION

These findings suggest it is important to attend not only to what individuals are saying about their planned and ongoing action, but how they say it (Allport, 1961). This is true whether the phrasing reflects individual differences, such as appears to be the case with the trying personality, or captures dynamic perceptions of variable environmental contingencies, reflecting the constantly changing social ecology of project pursuit (Little, 1999a) that emerged for most of the phrasing variables explored here. Although preliminary, the consistent associations between project phrasing and appraisal suggest that an empirically based understanding of common meanings assigned to the phrasing of our actions may provide useful insight into how individuals feel about what they are planning to do that goes beyond impressions or intuition. This may be of particular help to clinicians working with action constructs in a clinical setting (Little & Chambers, 2000, 2004) in initially recognizing linguistic markers of problematic project pursuit. Further research is required to shed light on whether modifying how we speak about what we are doing can change how we think and feel about our actions.

ACKNOWLEDGMENTS

Some of the research reported in this chapter was conducted for the author's doctoral dissertation and was supported by both a Doctoral Fellowship and Post Doctoral Fellowship from the Social Sciences and Humanities Research Council of Canada. Initial results were presented at the 62nd Annual Conference of the Canadian Psychological Association in Ottawa, Canada.

REFERENCES

Alloy, L. B., & Abramson, L. Y. (1979). Judgement of contingency in depressed and non-depressed students: Sadder but wiser? *Journal of Experimental Psychology: General, 108,* 441–485.

Allport, G. W. (1961). *Pattern and growth in personality.* New York: Holt, Rinehart & Winston.

Allport, G. W., & Odbert, H. S. (1936). Trait-names: A psycho-lexical study. *Psychological Monographs, 47*(211).

Bandura, A. (1997). *Self-efficacy: The exercise of control.* New York: Freeman.

Bernstein, B. (1971). *Class, codes and control* (Vol. 1). London: Routledge.

Buss, D. M. (1999). Human nature and individual differences: The evolution of human personality. In L. A. Pervin & O. P. John (Eds.), *Handbook of personality: Theory and research* (2nd ed., pp. 31–56). New York: Guilford.

Cantor, N., Norem, J. K., Niedenthal, P. M., Langton, C. A., & Brower, A. M. (1987). Lifetasks, self-concept ideals, and cognitive strategies in a life transition. *Journal of Personality and Social Psychology, 53,* 1178–1191.

Carver, C. S. (1996). Some ways in which goals differ and some implications of those differences. In P. Gollwitzer & J. Bargh (Eds.), *The psychology of action: Linking cognition and motivation to behavior* (pp. 645–672). New York: Guilford.

Carver, C. S., & Scheier, M. F. (1990). Origins and functions of positive and negative affect: A control-process view. *Psychological Review, 97,* 19–35.

Chambers, N. C. (1997). Personal projects analysis: The maturation of a multidimensional methodology. Retrieved May 1, 2005, from http://www.brianlittle.com/research/index.htm

Chambers, N. C., (2001). Time and personal action: Tenses and aspects of project pursuit (Doctoral dissertation, Carleton University, 2000). *Dissertation Abstracts International, 62*(2B), 1130.

Costa, P. T., & McCrae, R. R. (1992). *NEO PI–R professional manual.* Odessa, FL: Psychological Assessment Resources.

Diener, E., & Emmons, R. (1985). The independence of positive and negative affect. *Journal of Personality and Social Psychology, 47,* 1105–1117.

Diener, E., Suh, E. M., Lucas, R. E., & Smith, H. L. (1999). Subjective well-being: Three decades of progress. *Psychological Bulletin, 125,* 276–302.

Elliot, A. J., & Sheldon, K. M. (1997). Avoidance achievement motivation: A personal goals analysis. *Journal of Personality and Social Psychology, 73,* 171–185.

Elliot, A. J., Sheldon, K. M., & Church, M. A. (1997). Avoidance personal goals and subjective well-being. *Personality and Social Psychology Bulletin, 23,* 915–927.

Emmons, R. A. (1986). Personal strivings: An approach to personality and subjective well-being. *Journal of Personality and Social Psychology, 51,* 1058–1068.

Gee, T. L. (1999). Individual and joint-level properties of personal project matrices: An exploration of the nature of project spaces (Doctoral dissertation, Carleton University, 1998). *Dissertation Abstracts International, 59*(10B), 5609.

Goodine, L. A. (1986). *Anorexics, bulimics and highly weight preoccupied women: A comparison of personal project systems and personality factors.* Unpublished master's thesis, Carleton University, Ottawa, ON, Canada.

Hotson, H. (2001). *Lives interrupted: The impact of inactive personal projects on well-being.* Unpublished master's thesis, Carleton University, Ottawa, ON, Canada.

Hsee, C. K., & Abelson, R. P. (1991). Velocity relation: Satisfaction as a function of the first derivative of outcome over time. *Journal of Personality and Social Psychology, 60,* 341–347.

Kelly, G. A. (1955). *The psychology of personal constructs* (Vol. 1). New York: Norton.

Klinger, E. (1975). Consequences of commitment to and disengagement from incentives. *Psychological Review, 82,* 1–25.

Klinger, E., Barta, S. G., & Maxeiner, M. E. (1981). Current concerns: Assessing therapeutically relevant motivation. In P. C. Kendall & S. D. Hollon (Eds.), Assessment strategies for cognitive behavioral interventions (pp. 161–196). New York: Academic.

Kuhl, J. (1994). A theory of action and state orientations. In J. Kuhl & J. Beckman (Eds.), Personality and volition (pp. 9–46). Toronto: Hogrete & Huber.

Lakoff, G. (1987). *Women, fire and dangerous things: What categories reveal about the mind.* Chicago: University of Chicago Press.

Little, B. R. (1983). Personal projects: A rationale and method for investigation. *Environment and Behavior, 15,* 273–309.

Little, B. R. (1988). *Personal projects analysis: Theory, method and research.* Ottawa, ON: Social Sciences and Humanities Research Council of Canada.

Little, B. R. (1989). Personal projects analysis: Trivial pursuits, magnificent obsessions and the search for coherence. In D. M. Buss & N. Cantor (Eds.), *Personality psychology: Recent trends and emerging directions* (pp. 15–31). New York: Springer-Verlag.

Little, B. R. (1993). Personal projects and the distributed self: Aspects of a conative psychology. In J. M. Suls (Ed.), *The self in social perspective: Psychological per-*

spectives on the self (Vol. 4, pp. 157–185). Hillsdale, NJ: Lawrence Erlbaum Associates.

Little, B. R. (1996). Free traits, personal projects and idio-tapes: Three tiers for personality psychology. *Psychological Inquiry, 7,* 340–344.

Little, B. R. (1998). Personal project pursuit: Dimensions and dynamics of personal meaning. In P. T. P. Wong & P. S. Fry (Eds.), *The human quest for meaning: A handbook of psychological research and clinical applications* (pp. 193–212). Mahwah, NJ: Lawrence Erlbaum Associates.

Little, B. R. (1999a). Personal projects and social ecology: Themes and variation across the life span. In J. Brandtstädter & R. M. Lerner (Eds.), *Action and self-development: Theory and research through the life span* (pp. 197–221). Thousand Oaks, CA: Sage.

Little, B. R. (1999b). Personality and motivation: Personal action and the conative evolution. In L. A. Pervin & O. P. John (Eds.), *Handbook of personality: Theory and research* (2nd ed., pp. 501–524). New York: Guilford.

Little, B. R., & Chambers, N. C. (2000). Analyse des projets personnels: Un cadre intégratif pour la psychologie clinique et le counselling [Personal projects analysis: An integrative framework for clinical and counseling psychology]. *Revue Québécoise de Psychologie, 21,* 153–190.

Little, B. R., & Chambers, N. C. (2004). Personal project pursuit: On human doings and well-beings. In W. M. Cox & E. Klinger (Eds.), *Handbook of motivational counseling: Concepts, approaches and assessment* (pp. 65–82). Chichester, UK: Wiley.

Little, B. R., Dowden, C., Chambers, N. C., Hunt, J., Richardson, K., Hargrave, A., et al. (2005). *Personal projects and depressive affect: A meta-analysis.* Unpublished manuscript, Carleton University, Social Ecology Laboratory, Ottawa, ON, Canada

Little, B. R., Lecci, L., & Watkinson, B. (1992). Personality and personal projects: Linking Big Five and PAC units of analysis. *Journal of Personality, 60,* 501–525.

McAdams, D. P. (1996). Personality, modernity, and the storied self: A contemporary framework for studying persons. *Psychological Inquiry, 7,* 295–321.

McGregor, I., McAdams, D. P., & Little, B. R. (2004). *Personal projects, life-stories, and well-being: The benefits of acting and being true to one's traits.* Unpublished manuscript.

Melia-Gordon, M. (1992). *Lose ten pounds and decide what to do with the rest of my life: Health projects, intrapersonal projects and five-factor correlations.* Unpublished bachelor's thesis, Carleton University, Ottawa, ON, Canada.

Omodei, M. M., & Wearing, A. J. (1990). Need satisfaction and involvement in personal projects: Toward an integrative model of subjective well-being. *Journal of Personality and Social Psychology, 59,* 762–769.

Oyserman, D., & Markus, H. (1990). Possible selves in balance: Implications for delinquency. *Journal of Social Issues, 46,* 141–157.

Palys, T. S., & Little, B. R. (1983). Perceived life satisfaction and the organization of personal project systems. *Journal of Personality and Social Psychology, 44,* 1221–1230.

Pennebaker, J. (2001, February). *Emotional experiences and changes in natural language.* Presentation at the annual conference of the Society for Personality and Social Psychology, San Antonio, Texas.

Pennebaker, J., & King, L. (1999). Linguistic styles: Language use as an individual difference. *Journal of Personality and Social Psychology, 77,* 1296–1312.

Radloff, L. S. (1977). The CES–D Scale: A self-report depression scale for research in the general population. *Applied Psychological Measurement, 1,* 385–401.

Salmela-Aro, K. (1992). Struggling with self: The personal projects of students seeking psychological counselling. *Scandinavian Journal of Psychology, 33,* 330–338.

Sapir, E. (1921). *Language: An introduction to the study of speech.* New York: Harcourt.

Sarbin, T. R. (1994). The narrative as the root metaphor for contextualism. In T. R. Sarbin & J. I. Kitsuse (Eds.), *Constructing the social* (pp. 51–69). London: Sage.

Sheldon, K. M., & Kasser, T. (1998). Pursuing personal goals: Skills enable progress, but not all progress is beneficial. *Personality and Social Psychology Bulletin, 24,* 1319–1331.

Taylor, S. & Brown, J. (1988). Illusion and well-being: A social psychology perspective on mental health. *Psychological Bulletin, 103,* 193–210.

Wierzbicka, A. (1996). *Semantics, primes and universals.* Oxford, UK: Oxford University Press.

Wilson, D. A. (1990). *Personal project dimensions and perceived life satisfaction: A quantitative synthesis.* Unpublished master's thesis, Carleton University, Ottawa, ON, Canada.

Zomer, L. (2000). *Creativity, depression and intrapersonal projects: Resolving the paradox.* Unpublished bachelor's thesis, Carleton University, Ottawa, ON, Canada.

6

Personal Projects as Compensatory Convictions: Passionate Pursuit and the Fugitive Self

Ian McGregor

His unaffected piety and unremitting zeal in the discharge of sacred duties ... gained him the respect and esteem of all who knew him; ... the cathedral and orphanage are enduring monuments to his zeal and charity.
—Memorial plaque, St. John's Basilica, Newfoundland, Canada

B y the early 19th century a wind-battered rock in the icy Newfoundland Atlantic had evolved into an important first-stop port on the European-American trade route. Waves of wobbly legged sailors came and went from this easternmost crag of Canada after enduring weeks of exposure at sea. Local fishermen eked out a similarly precarious existence at the mercy of the implacable maritime elements. Against this backdrop of human uncertainty and vulnerability, in 1831, a remarkably passionate project arose. Inhabitants single-mindedly threw themselves into the project of building what was to be the largest basilica in North America. In a frenzy of conviction and generosity, locals donated their savings, stripped building materials from their own property, and helped en masse in any way they could, even if it meant transporting gravel in their aprons. The clergy found themselves in the strange position of having to remind the faithful helpers not to neglect their own families in their zeal to help.

This chapter presents theory and experimental research on causes of such passionate conviction, which throughout history has fueled some of the most inspiring but also some of the most horrible of human pursuits. Why do people adhere to their convictions so tenaciously? People's convictions (especially other peoples') can seem bizarre, whether they be about a sports team, personality research methods, national pride, or religious zeal. Most matters of opinion have extremists on both sides, avidly maintaining their positions even when confronted with diametrically opposing claims. What motivates black and white conviction in the face of usually gray social reality? This chapter proposes that conviction is appealing and prevalent because it alleviates distress about what to do, restores single-mindedness, and liberates action.

The chapter begins with a review of neuropsychological and cultural factors that incline Western individuals toward passionate conviction. After exploring the central role of conviction in Western philosophy and religion, it reviews research showing that some people react to experimentally induced uncertainties with compensatory conviction about unrelated concerns. Experimental results that illuminate the psychological appeal of conviction are then reviewed. Conviction confers a kind of cognitive myopia that helps distress-inducing uncertainties fade from awareness. The chapter concludes with two experiments showing that uncertainty also causes alcohol consumption. Conviction and alcohol are seen as alternative routes to cognitive myopia. Both invigorate passionate pursuit by dissolving uncertainty and restoring single-mindedness. It may not be purely coincidental that residents of St. John's, Newfoundland, were as famous for their love of Screech rum as for their religious conviction.

UNCERTAINTY, CULTURE, AND THE BRAIN

As long as I did not know why, I could do nothing and could not live ... I did not know what I wanted, I could give no reasonable meaning to any actions of my life.
(Tolstoy veering close to suicide, 1884/2005)

Lets go. OK lets go.
They remain motionless ...
(The culturally bereft characters in Waiting
for Godot, Beckett, 1948/2005)

Our human brains are jointly wired for uncertainty and for culture. Uncertainty was adaptive because it liberated us from our primate ancestors' fixed instincts. It gave us the capacity to consider multiple alternatives for accomplishing goals and enabled simulation and selection of optimal courses of action. Thus, the evolution of uncertainty allowed for a human explosion in creative possibilities for achieving goals. However the evolution of uncertainty also left meaning as an open question. In the face of awareness of our finite and apparently absurd existence, what is most worth doing? What are the meanings toward which we shrunken-snouted cortically impressive humans should direct our impressive means?

Necessarily, the capacity for culture symbiotically coevolved with our bulging frontal lobes to provide an authoritative guidance system to constrain human uncertainty. Together, the symbiotic coevolution of capacity for culture and personal uncertainty afforded an immense adaptive advantage. Culture could harness multiple creativities in service of consensual convictions. In addition to supporting communal efficiencies, culture also facilitated agency by saving individuals from the potential mire of personal ambivalence and interpersonal conflict about what to do. When culture breaks down, fertile imaginations can become malignant. Unconstrained individuals become tangled and paralyzed by uncertainty (Durkheim, 1897/1952).

Insight into why uncertainty about what to do should be so problematic comes from research on the behavioral inhibition system (BIS; Gray, 1982) in people and animals. Brain lesion and drug studies indicate that the BIS, centered in the septho-hippocampal circuits of all mammals, produces anxiety when a focal action is seriously impeded by failure, conflict, or uncertainty. For most animals, the typical kind of BIS activation scenario involves either a blocked or conflicted goal, or a novel and uncertain situation in which it is not clear what to do. The BIS responds to such action-impedance scenarios with anxiety to discourage persistence at the focal activity, direct motor suppression of the focal activity, and scan for alternative courses of action. The animal becomes anxious, immobilized, and vigilantly preoccupied until the problematic situation is either overcome or abandoned.

Like other animals, humans rely on the basic self-regulatory function of the BIS. It prevents overpersistence and facilitates disengagement from untenable focal goals. However, the human ability to promiscuously imagine alternative courses of action raises goal conflict and uncertainty as potentially chronic BIS activators. The human BIS has direct links to the prefrontal cortex, and so multiple imagined alternatives can activate approach–approach conflicts. As Lewin (1935) noted, approach– approach conflicts can become uncomfortable double approach–avoidance conflicts if approaching one alternative means losing out on others. Lewin's protégé, Festinger (1957), and other cognitive consistency theorists (Abelson et al., 1968) extended and popularized the view that conflicting or nonfitting thoughts can be as aversive as more concrete conflicting goals, especially if they are self-relevant. More recently, self-regulation theorists have similarly emphasized the importance of having clear, nonconflicting self-guides for organizing and directing action (Beckman & Irle, 1984; Carver & Scheier, 1990; Higgins, 1996). From this independent-self perspective, individuals need inner meaning to lend direction to the self and action (McGregor & Little, 1998). Without it, wandering uncertainties and approach–approach conflicts chronically activate BIS anxiety and motor inhibition, adding resistance to action as if the cognitive brake pedal were always depressed.

Imagine fictitious Lance, a proud young Newfoundland cod fisherman looking out at sea in the morning fog and contemplating the government's recently announced ban on cod fishing due to decimated stocks. As he ponders the question, "What will I do?" he is bewildered by the flurry of ideas that come to his mind. Start an internet business? Take his family's advice and become a priest? Follow his more bohemian bliss, and travel in Europe, trusting that something would come up? Refit his boat with lobster traps? Or get a simple job as a clerk and be poor but happy, as in his childhood? Or maybe get rich working at sea on an oil rig like his uncle Ishmael?

As Lance's confusion grows, he realizes that he is sitting motionless, staring at the gray horizon with a lump in his throat. He calls his brother Lorne, who earnestly reflects that Lance sounds bewildered. He probes Lance about what he really wanted to do and what kind of person he really wants to be. Lance snaps back that he has many ideas, but no way to decide. In frustration, he hangs up and heads to the local bookstore to peruse the self-help section (the whole second floor). Book after book chants the same theme: Follow your bliss, do your own thing, be yourself, to thine own self be true, look out for number one, love yourself, be real, find your authentic path, and so on.

To Western sensibilities, Lance's quest for true self is a familiar part of human development. Classic psychological theorists have advocated individuation, becoming, integration, self-acceptance, identity achievement, authenticity, and self-actualization as hallmarks of mental health. However, as desirable as such exhortations sound, self-discovery can be a bewildering task. It is not clear how to look for a true self, and some theorists have even concluded there is no true self to find (Cushman, 1990; Gergen, 1991). Indeed, the quest for a unique, self-fashioned identity is a relatively recent cultural phenomenon.

CULTURAL MEANINGS AND THE WESTERN MUTATION

Meanings were historically provided by consensual cultural worldviews. People turned to their cultures to help untangle uncertainties about what to think and do because self and social reality are ambiguous and often have no objective referents for truth. The validity of social and moral truth has traditionally depended on a kind of interrater reliability. Accordingly, humans have typically clung to consensually agreed on beacons to navigate the bewildering horizon. Shared meanings can guide us through the welter of possibilities, freeing us from debilitating ambivalence and conflict. As such, the capacity for culture and uncertainty symbiotically evolved. The capacity for culture supported the evolution of uncertainty's creative advantages, and the evolution of uncertainty promoted the evolution of culture and its collateral collective advantages.

Early human civilizations appear to have had a relatively easy time harnessing human imaginations with consensual cultural worldviews that were authoritatively legitimized by a local deity or leader. However, in what has been referred to as the Axial Age, between around 800 and 200 BCE, perhaps due to growing affluence and freedom from necessity, along with increased intercultural mobility and dissent, grand philosophical and religious systems emerged bearing authoritative codes of conduct. Hindu, Buddhist, Judaic, Zoroastrian, Taoist, Confucian, and Greek worldviews flowered with prescribed morals for how to live and what to do. The Greek response is particularly germane to this chapter, because it spawned our hyperindividualistic and zeal-prone Western worldview.

In contrast to the relatively stable economic, political, and geographical factors that enabled the development of consensual Confusian norms for guiding behavior in China, the social ecology of ancient Greece was less conducive to consensus. The rocky Greek terrain did not support stable agricultural communities that can foster shared norms, and cross-cultural exposure brought by trade and war highlighted competing perspectives (Diamond, 1997). As a result, a paradoxical quasi-culture of rugged individualism emerged, and the rational, internally consistent, bounded self replaced consensual norms as the appropriate guide for behavior. Accordingly, Greek thought came to emphasize separation of parts (i.e., self from others), national argument, personal agency, and introspective appreciation of essential truths (Nisbett, Peng, Choi, & Norenazayan, 2001).

In this individualistic ethos, Pythagoras (c. 580 BCE) devoted himself to knowledge, and the transcendent perfection of natural laws. He zealously practiced and taught an ascetic and introverted idealism that involved harmony of the soul through quiet understanding of underlying truths. This introspective theme of Greek philosophy (Tarnas, 1991) reverberates in phrases attributed to Socrates, such as know thyself, the unexamined life is not worth living, and the truth shall set you free. Plato similarly advocated that an individual should keep "his eye ever directed toward fixed and immutable principles ... all in order moving according to reason; these he imitates, and on these, so far as he can, he will mold his life" (Durant, 1939, p. 519). Even Aristotle's philosophy, although ostensibly less idealistic, is suffused with the same premium on personal integrity, claiming that the highest happiness comes from acting in accordance with one's essence, and because human essence is rationality, "the proper working of man is the working of the soul in accordance with reason" (Durant, 1939, p. 534).

It is important to emphasize, also, that integrity and the zealous quest for truth were not just grim moral directives. Greek philosophers were passionate lovers of truth. Plato's experience of philosophical unity and transcendent ideas was intensely emotional, even resembling mystical rapture (Tarnas, 1991). For the Greeks, rational, true essences, forms, or ideas that exist behind the jumble of phenomenal reality were not merely correct, they were experienced as delightfully beautiful and worthy of religious devotion. Divine truth in this perfect spiritual realm was brilliantly transcendent. Once one was oriented to it, the shadowy phenomenal world of change, conflict, and uncertainty felt banal and false by contrast.

Why did the Greeks love truth so zealously? Perhaps it was because their culture lacked consensual norms for guiding behavior. Perhaps they needed a surrogate guide for their actions that could keep them from being chronically mired in BIS-activating uncertainty about what to do, and personal conviction was that surrogate. As described later, the zealous legacies of all three monotheistic religions are supported by this highly individualistic Greek foundation.

RELIGIOUS PASSION IN THE WEST

The Greek premium on ideal truth was imported to feature prominently in Jewish and later Islamic thought via philosophers such as Philo, Plotinus, Avicenna, Averroes, and Maimonides. A prevalent neoplatonic theme was the identification of God with Logos—timeless, perfect, supreme intelligence. Saints Paul, John, Augustine, and Thomas Aquinas also gave this theme a central focus in the Greek version of Christian theology that undergirds evangelical Christianity to this day. Salvation from the chaos of the world comes from union with transcendent, divine truth.

James (1902/1958), in his survey of Christian mystical and religious experiences, concluded that "the absolute determinability of our mind by abstractions is one of the cardinal facts in our human constitution" (p. 65) and that "passionate enthusiasms make one feelingless to evil" (p. 92). Religious conviction can have a "polarizing and magnetizing" effect on one's experience (pp. 65–66). When in the grips of fervent zeal, true believers bubble over with descriptions of their experiences of joy, such as, "My soul was so captivated and delighted with the excellency of God that I was even swallowed up in him ... in the state of inward joy, peace, and astonishing" (p. 190).

The metaphors typically used to describe zealous religious experience are of illumination, unity, and clarity. Life is no longer murky, all is unified, and all paths clearly merge in the same direction. One convert, for example, recounted that on conversion there was "a strange seizure on my spirit ... brought light with it, and commanded a silence in my heart of all those tumultuous thoughts that before did use, like masterless hellhounds, to roar and bellow and make a hideous noise within me" (James, 1902/1958, p. 168). James's believers' accounts of fervor also often involved reports of increased energy, courage, and buoyancy for action. One convert reported, "I was amazed at my increased energy and vigor of mind" (p. 164); others likened the feeling to being "as light as if walking on air" and "soaring on the wings of faith" (p. 193).

James (1902/1958) presciently accounted for these testimonials of joy, clarity, and energy from a cognitive associationist perspective, noting that activated groups of ideas may have very little overlap with other groups of ideas, such that "when one group is present and engrosses the interest, all the ideas connected with other groups may be excluded from the mental field" (p. 174). He concluded that religious rapture and moral enthusiasm are "unifying states of mind, in which the sand and grit of the selfhood incline to disappear" (p. 240). They unify the "discordant self" (p. 399).

From a contemporary social cognitive perspective it makes sense that competing ideas would recede when one is gripped by passionate conviction. Highly important focal thoughts trivialize the importance of other thoughts by contrast (Simon, Greenberg, & Brehm, 1995), and reduced importance translates into reduced accessibility to awareness (Krosnick, 1989). Thus, with one dominant, internally consistent group of ideas salient to the individual, and other competing thoughts relegated to inaccessibility, the self feels unitary, clear, and poised for decisive action.

Further, convictions usually refer to highly desirable and familiar ideals that may placate the BIS. Even if goals in the external world are in a shambles, zealous devotion to favorite ideals in the privacy of one's mind may serve as a haven of coherence where soothingly untainted perfection can seize attention and down regulate BIS activation. Decreased BIS activation might further decrease ruminative self-focus (which may be the neo-cortical version of the BIS's vigilant scanning for alternative courses of action), and allow the individual to become all the more myopically focused on the zeal.

Another possibility is that idealistic zeal may be a way for people to distract attention from their anxiety-ridden, avoidance-motivated right hemisphere, and shift it to a more implemental approach-motivated left hemisphere. Focus on approaching incentives such as imagined certainty, worth, togetherness, symbolic immortality, or any variation of such potent approach motivations may accomplish a kind of "approach myopia." Left hemisphere activation is associated with approach-motivation, narrowed cognition to thoughts that support focal goals, and suppression of inconsistent cognitions (Drake, 1993; Harmon-Jones, 2004; Harmon-Jones & Allen, 1997; Sutton & Davidson, 1997; Tomarken & Davidson, 1994). Perhaps approach-mediated escape from the anxiety of conflicting thoughts partially accounts for the psychological and health benefits of approach-motivation (cf. Elliot & Friedman, chap. 3, this volume).

Passionate convictions may thereby allow individuals to become intoxicated by their zeal. The word *intoxication* comes from the root word meaning poison. The dictionary meanings refer jointly to blissful liberation and unrestrained action. Convictions may be intoxicating because they mask accessibility of BIS-activating goal disruptions that sap vital energy from action. Like weed-killer in a choked garden, conviction may allow the will to grow forth in a singular direction by quelling the tangle of conflicting alternatives that deplete and constrain the self. With the BIS deactivated, anxiety recedes, the cognitive brake pedal is released, and one is ready to roll with uninhibited vigor toward zealous goals. One feels holy.

Zealous single-mindedness is associated with spiritual enlightenment in all three Western monotheistic systems (Armstrong, 2000). Indeed, the first three of the Ten Commandments revered in Judaism, Christianity, and Islam refer to the importance of single-minded devotion to God. From the present perspective, this is because being captured by conviction liberates the individual from the torment and drag of uncertainty. When in the grips of zeal, no active self-regulation is required, no inhibition of thoughts and competing impulses necessary. One can find peace in a hermetically sealed conative universe of ideals, unsullied (and unchecked) by the grime of reality. Just as thought conflict produces the same kind of anxiety as action conflict (Festinger, 1957; Lewin, 1935), so should absorption in harmonious thoughts provide the same kind of bliss as flow in harmonious action (Csikszentmihalyi, 1999).

When under the spell of zeal, related personal projects are infused with buoyancy and vigor. Obstacles that would seem insurmountable to the nonzealous seem relatively trivial (Lydon & Zanna, 1990). James's accounts of religious converts caught up in the glow of conviction typically involve imagery of effortlessness—of floating, gliding, soaring, and bursting with vital energy. Zealots like John the Baptist indulge hardships like eating vermin and abject solitude willingly, and other famous saints have been known to engage in gratuitous acts of self-denial and hardship, such as joyfully kissing lepers and cleansing the suppurating boils of hospital patients with their tongues (James, 1902/1958). If passionate conviction can insulate one from worldly anxieties, then this helps to explain the naming of St. John's, Newfoundland, and why it was chosen as the site of what was to be the largest basilica in North America. Life was particularly uncertain and precarious for the fishermen and sailors of St. John's. Atop the gateway to St. John's basilica, a towering statue of St. John the Baptist overlooks the city and the ocean harbor, and calls the shaken to come for salvation. John the Baptist is referred to in the bible as "the voice of one crying in the wilderness." He lived semi-naked and alone on a diet of grasshoppers, and preached that worldly suffering could be transcended by zealous faith and devoted action. The naming of St. John's is a testimony to the power of conviction.

OTHER DOMAINS FOR PASSIONATE CONVICTION

Religious passion shaped the Western world and continues to fuel patriotic and passionate pursuit today. In 2004 the religious right in the United States carried to victory a president with an arguably disastrous record of domestic and foreign policy, because of his comforting claim to be a man of unwavering conviction—a born-again Christian who believes in moral absolutes (and is in love with his wife). However, this chapter is not just about religious conviction. It is about conviction and passionate pursuit, more generally. For Westerners who are not passionately religious, what other conviction opportunities are there?

Idealized love, another predominantly Western phenomenon (Dion & Dion, 1993), has been a perennial favorite. Even during the Middle Ages, when a dour version of zealous Christianity gripped vulnerable Europe, the people demanded a Mary. The Trinitarian God of omniscience and judgment was too remote and scary for simple souls who preferred to idealize Mary's warmth and safety. After a period of objection the obliging Catholic Church absorbed the popular longing for a mother goddess into its dogma, and by the time of the Gothic flowering in the 12th and 13th centuries, many of Europe's most impressive cathedrals were dedicated to Mary (Durant, 1950). At the same time, chivalry introduced a lay worship of feminine perfection. Troubadours and Minnesingers sang about the ideal of courtly and romantic love, putting it on a pedestal where its purity could be revered from a preserving distance. Accordingly, Dante saved a rosy place of honor in the highest sphere of heaven (on cloud nine with Christ and Mary) for his idealized lover, Beatrice. Even today, if one were to judge by representation in the popular Western media, one might conclude that romantic love is the primary domain of passionate conviction. Indeed, readers may recognize in James's accounts of religious ecstasy the soaring experience of falling in love.

For more sober individualists, however, personal pride and self-confident understanding continue as other favorite Western domains for conviction (Heine, Lehman, Markus, & Kitayama, 1999; McGregor, Nail, Marigold, & Kang, 2005). As Catholic ideals began to fade under the light of an increasingly skeptical and affluent Europe, heady free thinkers like Abelard, Erasmus, and Voltaire came full circle, reidentified themselves with the Greeks' proudly passionate pursuit of unfettered knowledge, and ushered in the Age of Reason. As described earlier, for Greek philosophers, the individualistic pursuit of truth was as intoxicating as religious or romantic passion. What serious scholar, aglow with a flash of insight or recognition, would not place Socrates or Aristotle next to Mary and Beatrice on cloud nine?

Conviction, whether it be about religion, romance, self-satisfied knowledge, or any other passionate pursuit, has a particular appeal for Westerners, whose individualistic Greek heritage has left them twisting slowly in a void (Bellah, Madsen, Sullivan, Swidler, & Tipton, 1985). Westerners are uniquely unable to rely on consensual culture to guide their uncertainties. This chapter proposes that passionate pursuit of grand ideals about God, love, work, knowledge, self, country, or personal opinions can dissolve uncertainty and liberate action. The following experiments have tested this proposition.

LABORATORY EXPERIMENTS ON COMPENSATORY CONVICTION

The historical and theoretical account generated thus far might seem to present a somewhat cynical perspective on human strivings. On the one hand, it shows Westerners heroically reaching for magnificent meanings despite the sometimes chaotic and bleak conditions they have faced. On the other hand, it may seem to desecrate meaningful quests by framing them as pathetic defense mechanisms. It is important to emphasize that I am not implying that passionate human strivings are just defense mechanisms. I do hope, however, that experimental research on conviction might contribute to understanding or even loosening some of the more curiously rigid forms of zeal that can have important personal, interpersonal, and societal implications.

Experimental research may strike some readers as a rather sterile approach to understanding passionate conviction. However, experiments may be particularly appropriate when studying such highly charged topics as conviction and uncertainty. There is considerable research evidence that when the stakes are high, many people tend toward motivated thinking and are adept at believing their desired conclusions (e.g., Kunda, 1990; Landau et al., 2004). For example, if you ask them, over 90% of U.S. professors will tell you that they are better than average (Gilovich, 1991) and undergraduates who are highly motivated to think well of themselves automatically fill their minds with thoughts about their strengths and virtues, precisely when confronted with threats (Dodgson & Wood, 1998).

Accordingly, consider once again our bewildered fisherman Lance. According to the ideas presented in this chapter, his uncertainty about his future might well contribute to compensatory religious conviction. However, he would not admit that his heightened conviction was related to, or some kind of escape from, feelings of impotent uncertainty. According to the theory presented here, the purpose of Lance's zeal would be to mask his despair in the first place. Thus, one might expect Lance to blithely report that being laid off was not so bad, and that he was giving more time to the church because he had been meaning to do that anyway. With this in mind, I hope the reader will forgive the abrupt shift from rich theory to sterile experimentation.

The studies reported here were inspired by an attempt to bottle the phenomenon of compensatory conviction in the experimental social psychology lab. The guiding assumptions are that if convictions are indeed used as a refuge from topically unrelated anxieties, then there should be evidence that (a) people turn to compensatory conviction when faced with uncertainty, (b) compensatory conviction effectively takes people's minds off of their uncertainties, (c) compensatory conviction is most evident among people who are most bothered by uncertainty and adept at motivated thinking, and (d) uncertainty causes other cognitive escapes as well. Several studies investigate causes, consequences, and personality moderators of compensatory conviction. The final two studies probe commonalities between conviction and alcohol intoxication as escapes from uncertainty.

Does Personal Uncertainty Cause Compensatory Conviction?

Results from several experiments indicate that people do indeed cling more zealously to various convictions when faced with uncertainty-related threats. In one compensatory conviction study Haji and I (Haji & McGregor, 2002) randomly assigned Canadian undergraduates to either ruminate about a personal dilemma that they were currently grappling with (personal uncertainty condition), or to complete parallel but relatively neutral materials about friends' dilemmas (control condition). We then assessed Canadian national pride and opinions about Islam. As expected, participants in the uncertainty condition praised Canada more extremely and with more conviction than did those in the control condition. A darker side of this compensatory conviction was revealed in the evaluations of Islam, however. Participants in the uncertainty condition also reacted with more zealous disdain for Islam. Importantly, these results were most pronounced among participants with high scores on the Preference for Consistency (PFC) scale, which assesses discomfort with self-inconsistency (Cialdini, Trost, & Newsom, 1995). Thus, it appears that compensatory conviction is particularly appealing for people most sensitive to cognitive conflict.

A related study found a similar result using a different measure of conviction (McGregor, Zanna, Holmes, & Spencer, 2001, Study 1). As in the previous study, participants were assigned to uncertainty or control conditions. The main dependent variable then assessed participants' conviction about unrelated social issues (capital punishment and abortion). For each issue, participants selected an opinion statement from a diverse list ranging politically from far left to far right, and then rated their conviction for that opinion. Again, uncertainty caused apparently compensatory conviction for opinions. Moreover, the exaggerated conviction served to quell the agitated feelings that had been aroused by the dilemma in the uncertainty condition. Finally, participants who had been randomly assigned to a third condition in which the personal uncertainty manipulation was followed by instruction to express a core value conviction showed no evidence of subsequent compensatory conviction or agitated feelings. Thus, expressions of conviction, whether spontaneous or mandated, provided insulation from uncertainty-related discomfort.

Three further studies showed that various other kinds of personal-uncertainty-related threats caused a heightened quest for meaning in life, exaggerated conviction for communal values and identifications, and the passionate pursuit of personal projects related to cherished meanings (McGregor et al., 2001, Studies 2–4). In the personal projects studies (2 and 4) in which personal projects (Little, 1983) were used as the dependent variables, uncertainty caused participants to lace their projects with conviction. Participants in the uncertainty condition planned on doing more important, value-congruent, identity-consistent, and meaningful projects than participants in the control condition. Together these three studies indicate that personal uncertainty causes exaggerated conviction at all levels of action control in the self-system, from the most abstract meanings, communal values, and identifications, down to specific personal projects.

Dozens of related experiments show that thinking about one's own death similarly causes people to more rigidly cleave to their values, identifications, and worldviews (for partial review, see Greenberg, Solomon, & Pyszczynski, 1997). Recent evidence suggests that personal uncertainty may be a particularly active ingredient in mortality salience. In one study, focusing people on their personal uncertainties caused even stronger worldview defense of consensual values than mortality salience, and mortality salience only caused defensiveness when it reminded people of existential uncertainties (van den Bos, Poortvliet, Maas, Miedema, & van den Ham, 2005). In another study mortality salience caused compensatory conviction about social issue opinions (McGregor & Thakurdeen, 2004). Together, these findings indicate that threats related to personal uncertainty cause exaggerated zeal about aspects of the self, and a tendency to cleave to communal norms and identifications. Uncertainty seems to make people in individualistic Western cultures yearn to scaffold themselves with a quasi-cultural architecture of personal conviction.

In contrast, people in more collectivist, Eastern cultures, who tend to rely more on authoritative social norms and situational cues to guide their behavior (Markus & Kitayama, 1991; Nisbett et al., 2001), can be less defensive when confronted with uncertainty-related threats (e.g., Heine & Lehman, 1997). To the extent that the independent, internally consistent self is not relied on to decide what to do, awareness of self-disintegrity should not be threatening. Where action is validated by social norms and contextual cues, the coherent, independent self can be relatively epiphenomenal. The key issue is that the individual must have some authoritative arbiter for deciding what to do. The authority can be personal or social, as long as it provides unequivocal guidance for action.

Differential cultural reliance on self-consistency may help to explain why the history of zeal is predominantly a Western phenomenon. The passionate conviction that fueled the triumphs of Islam in the 7th and 8th centuries and the motley Christian crusades in the 11th, 12th, and 13th has no equivalent in East Asian cultures (Nisbett et al., 2001). Eastern cultures, being more perfused with authoritative collective norms, place relatively more emphasis on paradox, dialectical thinking, situationally malleable truths, and the preferences of others for guiding behavior (Markus & Kitayama, 1991; Nisbett et al., 2001). No wonder faith-based monotheism never flourished in the East. Where consensual culture is strong, zealous personal conviction is less necessary.

Implicit Self-Esteem and Compensatory Conviction

If Westerners rely on the authoritative self to guide behavior, then those with implicit confidence in their self-value should be able to remain most calm when faced with uncertainty about what to do. They would have experiential assurance that they could prevail, and so uncertainty and conflict situations would not seem desperate. Conversely, Westerners with shakier implicit selves should be more easily overwhelmed by uncertainty and in need of escape from it. Accordingly, when faced with uncertainty, individuals with low implicit self-esteem (low ISE) should be most inclined to lunge toward passionate convictions as a way to make threatening thoughts fade from awareness.

ISE can be assessed with the Implicit Association Test (IAT) that assesses experiential associations that are not necessarily accessible to conscious awareness (Greenwald & Farnham, 2000). Reaction times on cognitive tasks that jointly involve self and positive categories are compared to those that jointly involve self and negative categories. According to a rationale similar to that underlying the Stroop measure of cognitive interference, participants who are relatively slow at self/positive and fast at self/negative categorization tasks are considered to have relatively negative implicit self-evaluations.

We felt this IAT measure would be a better marker of functional self-confidence than explicitly reported self-esteem (ESE) because there is evidence that some people with high ESE use their lofty explicit self-evaluations to mask feelings of inferiority and are particularly inclined to distort reality to make themselves feel good (e.g., Baumeister, Campbell, Krueger, & Vohs, 2003; Dodgson & Wood, 1998; Jordan, Spencer, & Zanna, 2003).

These motivational factors associated with high ESE may explain the absence of correlations between ESE and objective measures of esteem-worthiness (Baumeister et al., 2003) or ISE (McGregor & Marigold, 2003; McGregor et al., 2005). Indeed, they lead to the hypothesis that the combination of low ISE and high ESE should be associated with the greatest tendency to react to self-threats with exaggerated conviction in the face of uncertainty. Uncertainty should be particularly bewildering for low-ISE individuals, and high-ESE individuals should be particularly adept at using motivated thinking to escape from it.

In two studies, my colleagues and I assessed both ISE and ESE, and investigated whether people with low ISE but high ESE would be most inclined to react to uncertainty with compensatory conviction. In one study (McGregor & Marigold, 2003, Study 3), participants were randomly assigned to either write about an uncertain personal relationship (uncertainty condition) or a friend's uncertain relationship that did not invoke feelings of personal uncertainty (control condition). The main dependent variable assessed conviction for opinions about social issues. As predicted, only participants with the combination of low ISE and high ESE reacted to the uncertainty threat with compensatory conviction.

A related study (McGregor et al., 2005, Study 3) assessed whether low-ISE and high-ESE participants would similarly react to a confusion threat by exaggerating another aspect of conviction. Undergraduate psychology majors were randomly assigned to summarize either an extremely confusing statistical passage from a graduate psychology text (confusion condition) or an easy passage about the usefulness of statistics (control condition), and were told that the passages were examples of the kinds of tools that psychologists frequently used in their work (which we expected would make the psychology majors' confusion self-relevant). As in the previous study, results revealed that only participants with low ISE and high ESE reacted to the confusion threat with defensive conviction. This time the measure of conviction assessed participants' confidence that a high percentage of people in general would agree with their opinions. Low-ISE/high-ESE participants in the confusion condition suddenly became convinced that their convictions were very popular.

Together, these two studies indicate that individuals with shaky experiential selves but a penchant for motivated thinking react to uncertainty and confusion threats by exaggerating two aspects of conviction: certainty and consensus. Certainty and consensus are the very ingredients missing from Western culture. Thus, defensive conviction appears to be a spontaneous attempt to patch the culture-shaped hole in uncertain Western selves.

Zealous Intoxication

The main idea in this chapter is that vulnerable Westerners exaggerate their conviction as a means of escaping from uncertainty about what to do. I have proposed that focusing on convictions can crowd other troubling uncertainties out of awareness, either by direct BIS deactivation or by trivialization of the offending thoughts. Is there evidence that convictions can effectively mask uncertainties that are unrelated to the topic of conviction?

In five experiments, my colleagues and I assessed the effects of conviction manipulations on the subjective salience of participants' topically unrelated personal uncertainties (reviewed in McGregor, 2004). The subjective salience scale assesses items such as the extent to which personal uncertainties feel important, big, hard to ignore, urgent, and pressing at the moment. In all studies, participants were first instructed to write about their personal uncertainties (i.e., about personal dilemmas, which, as the reader will recall, caused defensive reactions in the experiments reviewed earlier). Then participants were randomly assigned to write essays related to aspects of personal conviction, or in the control conditions, about related topics for which they did not hold particularly zealous thoughts. In the five experiments, writing about conviction related to opinions, values, successes, loves, or group identifications significantly decreased subjective salience of unrelated personal uncertainties. Importantly, in four of these five experiments, this effect was strongest among individuals with high ESE; that is, among participants who are most motivated to mask unpleasant topics with pleasant ones (Dodgson & Wood, 1998; Smith & Petty, 1995).

These findings provide some evidence for a kind of zealous intoxication, and may help explain why people exaggerate their conviction when troubled, and why mystical experiences with transcendent truths can feel so wonderful. As illustrated in Figure 6.1, when intoxicated with important and consensual convictions, the fluxing jumble of conflicting thoughts fades into an unimportant background. The individual becomes myopically fixed on a focal ideal that shines as essential reality.

Alcohol Intoxication

> *The sway of alcohol over mankind is unquestionably due to its*
> *power to stimulate the mystical faculties of human nature.*
> (James, 1902/1958, p. 324)

> *One can live only so long as one is intoxicated, drunk with life.*
> (Tolstoy, 1884/2005, p. 142)

The preceding defensive conviction studies demonstrate that Westerners with low ISE and high ESE use a kind of zeal intoxication to escape from uncertainty. Low ISE gives them the need to escape, and the high ESE can be used as a marker of ability to cognitively twist reality to support desired

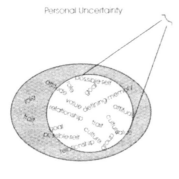

Personal Uncertainty

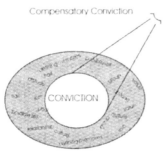

Compensatory Conviction

CONVICTION

Figure 6.1. Compensatory conviction decreases subjective salience of uncertainties.

conclusions. What strategies are available, however, for individuals whose low ISE inclines them to escape, but who do not have high ESE?

Alcohol may be a more democratic solution, available to individuals with low and high ESE alike. As cited earlier, James noted the similarities between zealous and alcoholic intoxication. His observation is corroborated by the recent research finding that meaningful personal projects and alcohol use are inversely related, which suggests the possibility that conviction and alcohol may serve a common function (Lecci, MacLean, & Croteau, 2002). I propose that cognitive myopia is the common function.

Steele and colleagues introduced the term *alcohol myopia* to refer to a kind of short-sighted information processing caused by alcohol intoxication, wherein only the most salient cues are accessible to awareness. Alcohol myopia effects relieve uncomfortable cognitive dissonance (Steele, Southwick, & Critchlow, 1981) by preventing individuals from noticing both sides of a cognitive conflict. This cognitive simplification associated with alcohol myopia can liberate vigorous and uninhibited action much in the same way that zeal myopia can (e.g., MacDonald, Zanna, & Fong, 1996). All but focal thoughts are relegated to the periphery of awareness. Importantly, in contrast to exaggerated conviction, motivated drinking does not require capacity for motivated thinking, and so should be available to low- and high-ESE individuals alike.

My lab has conducted two experiments to investigate alcohol intoxication as a defensive reaction to personal uncertainty. In the first study, Mills and I ran 199 undergraduates through a marketing study on personality and beer preferences. They began by describing their weekly alcohol consumption and completing personality scales including ESE and the PFC (which, recall, assesses preference for self-inconsistency). They were then randomly assigned to the dilemma-based uncertainty or control conditions described earlier. Finally, they were invited to sample two kinds of beer and a sports drink from chilled jugs. They were told to sample as often as necessary to form an opinion about how much they liked each. The main dependent variable was the amount of beer drunk (residualized on sports drink to ensure that it was beer drinking and not just drinking in general that was being assessed). The beer was actually nonalcoholic beer, but we sprayed the rim of the jug with pure alcohol, which convinced participants that it was alcoholic beer. Results revealed a significant three-way interaction among PFC, weekly consumption, and uncertainty condition. High-PFC participants who were relatively heavy habitual drinkers responded to the personal uncertainty manipulation with the highest beer consumption of all. These results indicate that people who are averse to cognitive conflict, and who have had experience with the myopia-inducing effects of alcohol (experienced drinkers), turn to alcohol when faced with cognitive conflict. Importantly, ESE did not moderate the results. Thus, alcohol appears to be an available way for the humble and the proud alike to flee from personal uncertainty.

This is the first laboratory experiment to causally demonstrate increased alcohol consumption as a means of coping with a prior psychological stressor. Past attempts may have failed because alcohol myopia is a particularly good solution to uncertainty and conflict, but also an aggravator of more singular threats and stressors. When singular threats, such as failure, humiliation, and separation loom, alcohol myopia could magnify the discomfort by highlighting the threat as the only thought on one's mind. Uncertainty threats, however, require the ability to think of multiple perspectives at the same time, and so should be uniquely soluble in alcohol.

Encouraged by this initial finding, Leon and I (Leon & McGregor, 2004) conducted a second study to explicitly link the self to use of alcohol as an escape from personal uncertainty. Recall that only individuals with shaky ISE (but high ESE) reacted to personal uncertainty with defensive conviction. We wondered whether all individuals with shaky ISE, regardless of ESE, would be drawn to alcohol when faced with personal uncertainty. Lack of implicit self-confidence would make the myopic escape particularly appealing.

The experimental setup in this second study was similar to that of the previous study, with the following changes. First, we recruited only female participants (N = 100) to evade male "drink to party" motives that additional analyses identified in the previous study (cf. Cooper, Frone, Russell, & Mudar, 1995). Second, we included a measure of ISE as well as ESE. Third, all participants began the study by writing a paragraph about relationship uncertainties that made uncertainty salient for them all. Fourth, we manipulated self-focused attention by randomly assigning participants to either complete the study in front of a large mirror or no mirror (e.g., Silvia, 2002). We expected that the primed uncertainty would be particularly aversive for low-ISE participants whose shaky self-concepts were highlighted by self-focus. Results indicate that this was the case. Beer consumption (again controlling for amount of sports drink consumed) was significantly highest among participants with low ISE in the self-focus condition. Importantly, as in the previous study, there were no effects of ESE.

SUMMARY AND CONCLUSION

This chapter began with the claim that humans are jointly wired for uncertainty and for culture. The symbiotic dialectic between individual uncertainty and consensual cultural norms allows for creative choices in the service of communal ends. Western "culture" paradoxically promotes individualism, however. It advises that actions should be based on personal convictions, and independent assessments of the true and good. This individualistic norm is potentially problematic because people are capable of imagining alternative ways of being good and true, and without consensual norms as arbiters of truth, people are at risk of being mired in uncertainty, conflict, and action paralysis. The Western solution to this predicament, promoted by the likes of Pythagoras, Plato, St. Paul, and St. Augustine, is passionate conviction. Conviction allows one to transcend the chaos of nonconsensual temporal life. It absorbs attention, masks conflicting thoughts, and invigorates singular action.

Several experiments showed participants exaggerating their conviction about religions, meanings, values, and personal projects in response to personal uncertainty. Moreover, other experiments found that this defensive zeal was most pronounced among individuals with low ISE. Western individuals lack consensual norms for behavior and those with low ISE also lack experiential confidence in the goodness of the self. Low-ISE Westerners are thus particularly vulnerable when faced with uncertainty. They have no arbiter, cultural or personal, for navigating it. As a means of escape, these individuals engage in defensive compensatory conviction, which achieves a kind of zeal myopia. As conviction and imagined agreement of others are exaggerated, uncertainties fade into relative unimportance. Several studies indicated that defensive conviction is a viable defense only for individuals with high ESE, however. Low-ESE individuals appear unable or unwilling to mount the cognitive distortion required to exaggerate personal certainty and imagined agreement of others. Accordingly, several studies demonstrated that conviction only reduced subjective salience of personal uncertainties among individuals with high ESE claims.

Two final studies showed that alcohol intoxication is another way that Westerners cope with personal uncertainty. Alcohol intoxication may be a popular antidote because, like zeal intoxication, it dulls awareness of the conflicting cognitions associated with the uncertainty. Both studies showed that people specifically increased their alcohol consumption when faced with uncertainty. Those particularly averse to uncertainty, or with low ISE highlighted by a self-focus manipulation were especially likely to react to uncertainty by drinking more alcohol. Thus, across the conviction and alcohol studies, individuals with shaky implicit selves were particularly defensive, perhaps because they have no confident resources, collectivistic or individualistic, for guiding action in the face of uncertainty. To escape from the cognitive conflict, they turn to exaggerated zeal or alcohol for intoxicated single-mindedness.

This chapter began with the suggestion that St. John's Newfoundlanders may have become famous for their passionate conviction because of the extraordinary amount of vulnerability and uncertainty there. Interestingly, St. John's is also famous for its love of bad tasting Screech—rum dregs with redeeming alcohol content. Today, Newfoundlanders are faced with considerable vulnerability and uncertainty from the elements, but also from the unemployment caused by the collapse of the cod fisheries. Consider once again, proud Christian Lance and his humbler brother Lorne, two unemployed cod fishermen huddled in a cabin waiting out the frigid St. John's winter. The research presented in this chapter suggests that since their layoffs, Lance and Lorne might find themselves drinking more hot toddies than usual, but Lance might be more likely than Lorne to get up in the morning for Mass.

More broadly, this chapter implies that the compensatory convictions of a lot of Lances have contributed to the uniquely passionate projects of the Western world. Admittedly, it is a far distance to travel in one's imagination, from random assignment and manipulation of independent variables, to Europe's cathedrals and the Crusades. However, group projects are often sustained by, and reflective of, the passionate pursuits of individual Lances. If it seems cynical to taint sublime human passions with the attribution of compensatory conviction, it may be easier to depict some of the West's more shocking and awful passionate projects as such.

When Pope Urban II went on a 9-month speaking tour in 1095 to rally support for the first Crusade, France had shrunk to a fraction of its former size and was in one of its darkest periods. The glory of Charlemagne had been immediately followed by wars of succession, wave after wave of Norse attacks in the 9th and 10th centuries, and a perceived threat from advancing Islam. By the end of the 11th century France was a fragmented tangle of mutually hostile principalities, independently ruled by despotic dukes. From a compensatory conviction perspective, it is not surprising that the bewildered and vulnerable French were the most numerous and zealous of the Crusaders. On his speaking tour, Urban proclaimed (with eerie familiarity):

> Oh race of Franks! race beloved and chosen by God! ... an accursed race, wholly alienated from God, has violently invaded the lands of these Christians, and has depopulated them by pillage and fire ... [be encouraged by] the glory and grandeur of Charlemagne ... wrest that land from a wicked race ... Undertake this journey eagerly ... and be assured of the reward of imperishable glory in the Kingdom of Heaven. (Durant, 1950, p. 587)

With a battle cry of "God wills it!" a first wave of 12,000 ill-prepared Crusaders independently broke from France without waiting for the decided date. In an orgy of zeal they attacked and pillaged Jews and Greek Christians on their way to the Holy Land. The first armed resistance they faced annihilated them.

REFERENCES

Abelson, R. P., Aronson, E., McGuire, W. J., Newcomb, T. M., Rosenberg, M. J., & Tannenbaum, P. H. (1968). *Theories of cognitive consistency: A sourcebook.* Chicago: Rand McNally.

Armstrong, K. (2000). *The battle for God: A history of fundamentalism.* New York: Ballantine.

Baumeister, R. F., Campbell, J. D., Krueger, J. I., & Vohs, K. D. (2003). Does high self-esteem cause better performance, interpersonal success, happiness, or healthier lifestyles? *Psychological Science in the Public Interest, 4,* 1–44.

Beckett, S. (2005). *Waiting for Godot.* Retrieved May 1, 2005, from http://samuel-beckett.net/Waiting_for_Godot_Part1.html. (Original work published 1948)

Beckmann, J. & Irle, M. (1984). Dissonance and action control. In J. Kuhl & J. Beckmann (eds.), Action control: From cognition to behavior (pp. 129–146). Berlin: Springer–Verlag.

Bellah, R. A., Madsen, R., Sullivan, W. M., Swidler, A., & Tipton, S. M. (1985). *Habits of the heart: Individualism and commitment in American life.* Berkeley: University of California Press.

Carver, C. S., & Scheier, M. F. (1990). Principles of self-regulation: Action and emotion. In E. T. Higgins & R. M. Sorrentino (Eds.), *Handbook of motivation and cognition* (pp. 3–52). New York: Guilford.

Cialdini, R. B., Trost, M. R., & Newsom, J. T. (1995). Preference for consistency: The development of a valid measure and the discovery of surprising behavioral implications. *Journal of Personality and Social Psychology, 69,* 318–328.

Cooper, M. L., Frone, M. R., Russell, M., & Mudar, P. (1995). Drinking to regulate positive and negative emotions: A motivational model of alcohol use. *Journal of Personality and Social Psychology, 69,* 990–1005.

Csikszentmihalyi, M. (1999). If we are so rich, why aren't we happy? *American Psychologist, 54,* 821–827.

Cushman, P. (1990). Why the self is empty. *American Psychologist, 45,* 599–611.

Diamond, J. (1997). *Guns, germs, and steel: The fates of human societies.* New York: Norton.

Dion, K. K., & Dion, K. L. (1993). Individualistic and collectivistic perspectives on gender and the cultural context of love and intimacy. *Journal of Social Issues, 49,* 53–69.

Dodgson, P. G., & Wood, J. V. (1998). Self-esteem and the cognitive accessibility of strengths and weaknesses after failure. *Journal of Personality and Social Psychology, 75,* 178–197.

Drake, R. A. (1993). Processing persuasive arguments: 2. Discounting of truth and relevance as a function of agreement and manipulated activation asymmetry. *Journal of Research in Personality, 27,* 184–196.

Durant, W. (1939). *The life of Greece.* New York: Simon & Schuster.

Durant, W. (1950). *The age of faith.* New York: Simon & Schuster.

Durkheim, E. (1952). Suicide: A study in sociology (J. A. Spaulding & G. Simpson, Trans.). London: Routledge & Kegan Paul. (Original work published 1897)

Festinger, L. (1957). *A theory of cognitive dissonance.* Evanston, IL: Row, Peterson.

Gergen, K. J. (1991). *The saturated self.* New York: Basic Books.

Gilovich, T. (1991). *How we know what isn't so: The fallibility of human reason in everyday life.* New York: The Free Press.

Gray, J. A. (1982). *The neuropsychology of anxiety: An enquiry into the functions of the septo-hippocampal system.* New York: Oxford University Press.

Greenberg, J., Solomon, S., & Pyszczynski, T. (1997). Terror management theory of self-esteem and cultural worldviews: Empirical assessments and conceptual refinements. In M. P. Zanna (Ed.), *Advances in experimental social psychology* (Vol. 29, pp. 61–139). Orlando, FL: Academic.

Greenwald, A. G., & Farnham, S. D. (2000). Using the implicit association test to measure self-esteem and self-concept. *Journal of Personality and Social Psychology, 79,* 1022–1038.

Haji, R., & McGregor, I. (2002, June). *Compensatory zeal and extremism about Canada and Islam: Responses to uncertainty and self-worth threats.* Poster presented at the annual meeting of the Society for the Psychological Study of Social Issues, Toronto.

Harmon-Jones, E. (2004, October). *The action-based model of cognitive dissonance and its links to self-regulation and affective and cognitive neuroscience.* Paper presented at the meeting of the Society for Experimental Social Psychology, Fort Worth, TX.

Harmon-Jones, E., & Allen, J. J. B. (1997). Behavioral activation sensitivity and resting frontal EEG asymmetry: Covariation of putative indicators related to risk for mood disorders. *Journal of Abnormal Psychology, 106,* 159–163.

Heine, S. J., & Lehman, D. R. (1997). Culture, dissonance, and self-affirmation. *Personality and Social Psychology Bulletin, 23,* 389–400.

Heine, S. J., Lehman, D. R., Markus, H. R., & Kitayama, S. (1999). Is there a universal need for positive self-regard? *Psychological Review, 106,* 766–794.

Higgins, E. T. (1996). The "Self Digest": Self-knowledge serving self-regulatory functions. *Journal of Personality and Social Psychology, 71,* 1062–1083.

James, W. (1958). *The varieties of religious experience.* New York: Penguin. (Original work published 1902)

Jordan, C. H., Spencer, S. J., & Zanna, M. P. (2003). I love me ... I love me not: Implicit self-esteem, explicit self-esteem, and defensiveness. In S. J. Spencer, S. Fein, & M. P. Zanna (Eds.), *Motivated social perception: The Ontario symposium* (Vol. 9, pp. 117–146). Mahwah, NJ: Lawrence Erlbaum Associates.

Krosnick, J. A. (1989). Attitude importance and attitude accessibility. *Personality and Social Psychology Bulletin, 15,* 297–308.

Kunda, Z. (1990). The case for motivated reasoning. *Psychological Bulletin, 108,* 480–498.

Landau, M. J., Solomon, S., Greenberg, J., Cohen, F., Pyszczynski, T., Arndt, J., et al. (2004). Deliver us from evil: The effects of mortality salience and reminders of 9/11 on support for president George W. Bush. *Personality and Social Psychology Bulletin, 30,* 1136–1150.

Lecci, L., MacLean, M. G., & Croteau, N. (2002). Personal goals as predictors of college student drinking motives, alcohol use and related problems. *Journal of Studies on Alcohol, 63,* 620-630.

Leon, C., & McGregor, I. (2004). Unpublished data. York University, Toronto, ON, Canada.

Lewin, K. (1935). *A dynamic theory of personality* (D. K. Adams & K. E. Zaner, Trans.). New York: McGraw-Hill.

Little, B. R. (1983). Personal projects: A rationale and method for investigation. *Environment and Behavior, 15,* 273–309.

Lydon, J. E., & Zanna, M. P. (1990). Commitment in the face of adversity: A value-affirmation approach. *Journal of Personality and Social Psychology, 58,* 1040–1047.

MacDonald, T. K., Zanna, M. P., & Fong, G. T. (1996). Why common sense goes out the window: Effects of alcohol on intentions to use condoms. *Personality and Social Psychology Bulletin, 22,* 763–775.

Markus, H. R., & Kitayama, S. (1991). Culture and the self: Implications for cognition, emotion, and motivation. *Journal of Personality and Social Psychology, 98,* 224–253.

McGregor, I. (2004). Zeal, identity, and meaning: Going to extremes to be one self. In J. Greenberg, S. Koole, & T. Pyszczynski (Eds.), *Handbook of experimental existential psychology* (pp. 182–189). New York: Guilford.

McGregor, I., & Little, B. R. (1998). Personal projects, happiness, and meaning: On doing well and being yourself. *Journal of Personality and Social Psychology, 74*, 494–512.

McGregor, I., & Marigold, D. C. (2003). Defensive zeal and the uncertain self: What makes you so sure? *Journal of Personality and Social Psychology, 85*, 838–852.

McGregor, I., Nail, P., Marigold, D. C., & Kang, S. J. (2005). Defensive pride and consensus: Strength in imaginary numbers. *Journal of Personality and Social Psychology, 89*, 978–996.

McGregor, I., & Thakurdeen, M. (2004, January). *Dissonant death and defensive zeal: The effect of mortality salience on compensatory conviction is moderated by preference for consistency.* Poster session presented at the annual meeting of the Society for Personality and Social Psychology, Austin, TX.

McGregor, I., Zanna, M. P., Holmes, J. G., & Spencer, S. J. (2001). Compensatory conviction in the face of personal uncertainty: Going to extremes and being oneself. *Journal of Personality and Social Psychology, 80*, 472–488.

Nisbett, R. E., Peng, K., Choi, I., & Norenzayan, A. (2001). Culture and systems of thought: Holistic versus analytic cognition. *Psychological Review, 108*, 291–310.

Silvia, P. J. (2002). Self awareness and the regulation of emotional intensity. *Self and Identity, 1*, 3–10.

Simon, L., Greenberg, J., & Brehm, J. (1995). Trivialization: The forgotten mode of dissonance reduction. *Journal of Personality and Social Psychology, 68*, 247–260.

Smith, S. M., & Petty, R. E. (1995). Personality moderators of mood congruency effects on cognition: The role of self-esteem and negative mood regulation. *Journal of Personality and Social Psychology, 68*, 1092–1107.

Steele, C. M., Southwick, L. L., & Critchlow, B. (1981). Dissonance and alcohol: Drinking your troubles away. *Journal of Personality and Social Psychology, 41*, 831–846.

Sutton, S. K., & Davidson, R. J. (1997). Prefrontal brain asymmetry: A biological substrate of the behavioral approach and inhibition systems. *Psychological Science, 8*, 204–210.

Tarnas, R. (1991). *The passion of the Western mind: Understanding the ideas that have shaped our world view.* New York: Ballantine.

Tolstoy, L. N. (2005). A confession. Retrieved May 1, 2005, from http://www.underthesun.cc/Classics/Tolstoy/confession/. (Original work published 1884)

Tomarken, A. J., & Davidson, R. J. (1994). Frontal brain activity in repressors and nonrepressors. *Journal of Abnormal Psychology, 103*, 339–349.

van den Bos, K., Poortvliet, P. M., Maas, M., Miedema, J., & van den Ham, E. J. (2005). An enquiry concerning the principles of cultural norms and values: The impact of uncertainty and mortality salience on reactions to violations and bolstering of cultural worldviews. *Journal of Experimental Social Psychology, 41*, 91–113.

III

Basic Processes of Project Pursuit: External-Contextual Functions

7

Relational Aspects of Project Pursuit

Katariina Salmela-Aro and Brian R. Little

From cradle to grave our lives are embedded in the activities of others. Indeed, even before birth and after death our presence or absence can have a profound effect on the passions and pursuits of other beings. Our births may be anticipated with joy or with dread. News of our death may elicit tears of grief or relief. Not infrequently, these positive and negative emotions may commingle, so that relational features of our comings and goings are both affectively charged and complex. In between our entries and exits, our lives are interwoven with others in ways that can range from ecstatic union to bland indifference to protracted enmity.

The study of personal and social relationships is focally concerned with exploring these relational aspects of human lives, and within this field increasing attention is being given to the motivational aspects of intimate and vital relationships. Similarly, research on motivation, although traditionally focused on individual project creation and appraisals, has recently witnessed increased interest in the interpersonal aspects of people's motivation. Consequently, there is a lively nexus of research where personality, motivational, and social psychologists explore goals and projects in their relational contexts (e.g., Berg, Meegan, & Deviney, 1998; Brunstein, Dangelmayer, & Schultheiss,

1996; Diener & Fujita, 1995; Harlow & Cantor, 1994; Little, 1987; Little & Ryan, 1979; Meegan & Berg, 1998).

At the most synoptic level, relational science (Reis, 2006), much like personality science (Little, 2005), embraces an extraordinary range of academic disciplines drawing from genetics, neuroscience, and evolutionary biology, but also from the rich traditions of the humanities. It is particularly important, then, that we develop conceptual bridges that help traverse these disparate domains (Little, 2005). Our purpose in this chapter is to illustrate how the personal projects perspective provides one such a bridge and offers a new vantage point for studying goals and actions in their relational context.

PERSONAL PROJECTS ARE NOT (MERELY) INDIVIDUALISTIC

At the outset, however, we need to clarify a definitional issue with respect to the term *personal projects.* As detailed in chapter 1, the term evolved from Kelly's (1955) personal constructs as a reflexive unit of analysis providing metaphorical parallels between the pursuits of scientists and those they study (Little, 1972). Whereas Kelly's constructs were focused on cognitive aspects of living, projects were more concerned with action in context (Little, 1972). Even though personal construct theory has a rich interpersonal component, its "focus of convenience," to use a Kellian term, was more on the construings than on the doings of daily life.

It may be tempting, nonetheless, for those concerned primarily with interpersonal and relational issues to think that personal projects implies primarily individualistic goals, actions, and pursuits. This would be a mistake.

It is true that personal projects are imbued by the motives, aspirations, and construals of individuals (indeed, Part II of this volume is largely devoted to these internal and self-regulatory processes). It is also true that some individuals may be primarily committed to the pursuit of self-focused goals and individualistic projects. Perhaps those individuals described as having the Dark Triad of personality—narcissism, psychopathy, and Macchiavellianism (Paulhus & Williams, 2002)—would be most likely to pursue projects that are individualistic, selfish, or designed to undermine the projects of others. However, it is important to emphasize that personal projects are not restricted to individualistic pursuits. Some people's lives are devoted to projects that are overwhelmingly focused on others and, as we demonstrate, interpersonal projects are among the most frequently evoked categories of projects that emerge when individuals list their current and future pursuits. Moreover, the role of the "other" in the evocation, shaping, affirmation, management, and termination of personal projects is a central component of our research perspective, and projects both draw from and contribute to the social ecological contexts within which they are embedded. Personal projects, in short, are inherently, deeply, and pervasively interpersonal.

THEORETICAL ROOTS OF A RELATIONAL PERSPECTIVE ON PERSONAL PROJECTS

Two related conceptual frameworks have stimulated our study of relational issues in the pursuits of daily life: the personal project framework (Little, 1983) and a more comprehensive social ecological framework in which personal projects are central analytic units (Little, 1980; Little & Ryan, 1979). Although other perspectives have augmented these frameworks over the years, they framed the initial explorations of personal projects as transactional endeavors. It will be helpful, therefore, to summarize briefly those aspects of the frameworks most relevant to interpersonal and relational issues.

Project Sequencing Model

In Little (1983) a sequential model was proposed in which the transition from an intimation of a possible pursuit to a completed project was postulated as passing through four major phases: inception, planning, action, and termination.

At the inception stage of projects, other individuals play a critical role. Cultural and role prescriptions may make awareness of a personal project vivid or may proscribe a whole domain of projects as something one literally should not even think about. Other people may help us identify precisely what a given project might be, subtly changing its nature even as we are formulating it. As part of the preevaluation process, we may find that we reject pursuing a project because it will have a negative impact on others, or we may shape the project to minimize conflict. When we finally resolve to ourselves that a project will commence, audiences—real or imagined—are often there to influence the subsequent path. We may decide and communicate to ourselves, for example, that we will go for a walk with the dog. The simple locution, "Do you want to go for a walk?" might lead to licks and leaps of affirmation and six legs will trot out into the cold. The same request of a thermally sensitive spouse may be met with a raised eyebrow and at best rather restrained licking. A potential joint project will be put on hold for a warmer day.

The pragmatics of planning some projects (e.g., obtaining material, space, and other resources) is almost invariably interlinked with others. Indeed, one of the reasons we can get projects launched is that others have provided the space (both in a political and practical sense) for us to proceed with impunity. Or they may be full-fledged partners in our projects. Of course, if we shift the positions of the actors in our examples, our personal projects may be primarily the pursuits envisaged and cherished by other people. In short my projects may be mine alone but they may be subtly or explicitly ours or yours. They may also be shaped by the projects of others in ways that may redound to our mutual benefit or stop us dead in our tracks.

During the action phase of projects, other people may serve to facilitate or frustrate our pursuit. As we report elsewhere in this volume (Grant, Little, & Phillips, chap. 8), there appear to be gender differences in the relative weight these interpersonal influences play in influencing well-being. Well-being is particularly compromised for men when others impede project progress; for women, well-being is enhanced if there is a facilitative and supportive network of others.

In the termination phase of a project, the role of other people may play an especially subtle role. Indeed, some projects may be interminable precisely because the price they may extract in a relationship seems too high. The inability to shut down a project that has lost personal meaning but is sustained because of an inability to disengage from it, often through its implications for others, can play a major role in depression (cf. Klinger, 1975, 1977).

Social Ecological Model

The social ecological model (Little, 2000, chap. 1, this volume; Little & Ryan, 1979) was a formal model of human development and human well-being based on the assumption that successful adaptation requires individuals to assume increasing control over balancing the claims of stable and dynamic personal features and stable and dynamic contextual features. Thus, relatively fixed traits, as well as the free traits (see Little & Joseph, chap. 14, this volume) that we enact, often in the interest of interpersonal goals, direct action, both helping a person to achieve goals and to contend with the costs incurred that might compromise physical and emotional well-being. Similarly, relatively fixed features of the environmental context, including the cultural and social climates within which a person lives need to be balanced against the personal propensities and aspirations of the individual. As we demonstrate in this chapter, personal contexts—the idiosyncratically constructed foci of our everyday contexts—are also important for adaptation and well-being, with research indicating that these personal contexts are particularly dominated by relational issues.

The central proposition of the social ecological perspective is that it is through personal projects that individuals gain coherence in their lives through the balancing and juggling of internal and external influences that impinge on them. These influences will change in nature and impact as the person ages, so the social ecological model is in essence a model for life-span developmental analysis. We describe several such adaptive influences in the research reviewed here.

PPA METHODOLOGICAL ROUTES FOR ASSESSING RELATIONAL ISSUES

Just as relational themes were rooted in the theoretical framework of personal projects analysis (PPA), the methodological components of PPA were designed, from the outset, to illuminate aspects of the interpersonal ecology in the individual's daily transactions. Because the PPA components were explained in chapter 2, we simply list here how each module has been used to examine interpersonal and relational issues in project pursuit.

PPA Modules

1. *Project elicitation.* After individuals generate their list of personal projects, content analyses can be done by judges or by the respondents themselves, and one of the most frequently mentioned and important content domains is that of interpersonal projects. Depending on the kind of respondents being studied, this category can be further subdivided into projects relating to friends, peers, family, parents, intimate others, children, relatives, or workmates (see, e.g., Cantor, Acker, & Cook-Flannagan, 1992; Langston & Cantor, 1989; Little, Lecci, & Watkinson, 1992; Salmela-Aro & Nurmi, 1996, 2004).

The number (or proportion) of interpersonal projects listed has been a major focus of research (see particularly Salmela-Aro & Nurmi, 1996, 2004).

2. *Priming for interpersonal projects.* Either before or after the free listing of personal projects, it is possible to ask participants to list interpersonal projects or personal projects related to specific social contexts, such as those concerned with family, partnerships, or friends (Nurmi, Salmela-Aro, & Koivisto, 2002; Salmela-Aro, Nurmi, & Näätänen, 2004).

3. *Appraisal dimensions.* Standard PPA dimensions and particularly the ad hoc dimensions have been deeply concerned with relational issues. In the original version of PPA (Little, 1983), two dimensions were directly related to interpersonal aspects of project management: how visible one felt one's projects were and how much importance other people accorded the projects. The assumption underlying the creation of these dimensions was that successful pursuit of some projects would need the active support of others and that, in contrast, projects that were kept to oneself or that were deemed to be of no value from the perspective of other people might be difficult to bring to fruition.

More recently, dimensions relating directly to project support have been explored as well as the project support or hindrance provided by others. Each of these dimensions can be phrased so as to elicit information related to specific categories of people such as spouses, parents, or managers. A compendium and thorough discussion of all ad hoc dimensions is available (Chambers, 1997).

4. *"Open column" data.* The original PPA matrix contained two columns in which individuals could provide information on "With Whom" and "Where" each project was undertaken (Little, 1983). These questions facilitated exploration of the project-related social network and spatial ecology.

5. *Joint cross-impact matrices.* This form of cross-impact matrix has individuals rate the extent to which each of their projects is impacted by another person's projects (particularly in intimate relationships). Measures of mutual support or conflict can be assessed through this technique. Variations on this method include the examination of projects that are regarded by two individuals as being joint projects and having each person appraise such projects independently (Hwang, 2004).

Each of these modular components of PPA is drawn on as we discuss the nature of interpersonal projects and their impact on human flourishing.

The Nature and Number of Interpersonal Projects

Interpersonal projects are those involving others on a personal level and include family, friends, and intimate others. Typical examples are "spend more time with my family," "hang out with Ellen," and "visit my uncle." When we simply examine the number of such projects generated during the elicitation phase of PPA, there is clear evidence that they are a ubiquitous form of project pursuit. Indeed, consistently and in the results of research groups using quite different forms of project elicitation, interpersonal projects are among the most frequent categories of projects reported, although as we shall see, there is research evidence suggesting both gender differences and subtle shifts in the kind of interpersonal projects that are engaged in at different points in the life cycle.

Among adolescents, friend-related personal projects are mentioned most often, after school and future education projects (Salmela-Aro, 2001; Salmela-Aro, Vuori, & Koivisto, 2003). During the transition from school to work life, family-related personal projects are the third most often mentioned after education and work-related projects (Nurmi & Salmela-Aro, 2002). During young adulthood, in college student populations, the two highest frequency categories of personal projects are interpersonal and academic (Little & Chambers, 2004; Salmela-Aro, 1992), whereas among adults the projects related to occupational and interpersonal projects are predominant (Little & Chambers, 2004; Salmela-Aro & Nurmi, 2004).

When university students were asked to produce three personal projects, 14% of the participants mentioned a project related to family, 21% mentioned a project related to the opposite sex, and 20% mentioned a project related to friends (Salmela-Aro & Nurmi, 1996). In an adult sample, projects related to the occupation were the largest group, and family-related projects were the second largest (Salmela-Aro & Nurmi, 2004). Similarly, among an adult sample 34.6% mentioned a project related to family (Nurmi, Pulliainen, & Salmela-Aro, 1992). In a recent study, Salmela-Aro and Nurmi (2004) found four clusters based on adults' personal projects: work, leisure, self, and family clusters. In this study, the family cluster included 29% of the adults. Moreover, it seems that interpersonal projects are particularly prevalent before middle

adulthood: 25- to 34-year-olds (30%) were more interested in family-related projects than were older participants (16% for 35–44, 9% for
45–54, 4% for 55–64-year-olds; Salmela-Aro, Nurmi, Aro, Poppius, &
Riste, 1992). In short, although the types of interpersonal projects differ
by age, the prevalence of interpersonal projects is notably high across
the life span.

Personal Project Appraisal Dimensions: The Development of Relational Themes

Again, from the outset, relational aspects of project pursuit were featured in the appraisal matrix used to examine how individuals think and
feel about their projects. In our early work we posited five general
themes that underlie project appraisals: meaning, structure, community, efficacy, and stress (see Little, chap. 1, this volume). The community theme was intended to tap into the relational aspects of project
pursuit.

Originally two dimensions tapped this: how visible and how valued
by others were one's projects. These dimensions consistently emerged
as highly correlated, in part because of the necessary dependency of
others knowing about one's projects to accord them value. However,
over the years, a diversity of ad hoc dimensions was used to explore additional relational aspects of projects. One clearly important dimension, and one now used in our standard PPA procedure, is project
support, which researchers have partitioned further to include dimensions relating to different kinds of support such as material or
emotional support for one's endeavors.

Other ad hoc dimensions provide a more subtle view of the relational
aspects of project pursuit. For example, guilt experienced when engaged in a project and the extent to which a project was consistent with
one's important roles in life (Burgess, 1982; MacDiarmid, 1990) are
among literally dozens of dimensions that have been used to tap into
the ways in which other people frame and shape, explicitly or implicitly,
the projects we perform in our daily lives (Chambers, 1997; Little,
1999).

Early research on project community placed a heavy emphasis on
what other people were doing in and with a person's own projects. We
needed to counterbalance this with dimensions tapping into the extent
to which projects were explicitly mounted to support others. For example, in studying senior executives in public and private management po-

sitions we asked two independent questions: To what extent was the project done for others and to what extent was it done for oneself? Interestingly, in several different groups these dimensions were orthogonal, suggesting that counterpoising self and others as contrasting foci for projects may be misleading (see Riediger, chap. 4, this volume, who makes a similar point about the positive and negative impact of projects). Supporting this is the finding that for adolescents, projects that involved relations with others (e.g., volunteering in the community, sports, boyfriend or girlfriend activities) were found to have the highest ratings on self-identity (Little, 1987), suggesting that finding "oneself" may be in concert with, not in opposition to, relating to others and being needed.

Examining Interpersonal Projects on Standard Dimensions

When we examine the standard project dimensions for different categories of projects, it is clear that for most people interpersonal projects are positive experiences (highly enjoyable, concordant with self, low in stress). For example, when we draw a random sample of 3,600 projects from SEAbank, which contains tens of thousands of personal projects and their appraisals gathered over a quarter-century, an interesting and theoretically compelling picture emerges of interpersonal projects, particularly when compared with other high-frequency categories. In terms of the original five themes underlying project appraisals, interpersonal projects are clearly high in meaning (e.g., high in enjoyment and importance) and high in community (both visible and valued by others). Interpersonal projects are also relatively low on stress and difficulty. Interestingly, they are not rated high on dimensions tapping into structure or manageability. The reason is clear. Among the key dimensions underlying structure or manageability are whether one initiated a project and how much control one has over it. Of all the major project categories, interpersonal projects are most likely to have been initiated by others and they are also comparatively low in perceived control. That said, the overall mean score for the manageability dimensions is still close to 7 on a 10-point scale.

As we shall see, when we start to look at specific categories of interpersonal projects, there are some differences in their appraisals. However, the most important conclusion that we can draw about interpersonal projects in general is that they are among the most valued and enjoyable pursuits in which people are engaged, despite the fact that many of these projects are the pursuits of others into whose swirl we find ourselves formally invited or excitedly swept.

It is precisely such projects—those that we share with others—that we turn to now as they cast light on some of the most central questions of a relational science.

THE VICISSITUDES OF INTERDEPENDENCE

From Mine to Our in Project Pursuit

As individuals, our personal projects may proceed unimpeded by and without impact on the projects of others, although short of being a hermit or recluse, it is difficult to imagine this as anything other than an exceptional state of affairs. As we have stressed in this chapter, personal projects are embedded in an interpersonal ecology that involves trade-offs and conflicts but also facilitation and support. This has been a subject of empirical research in personal projects analysis virtually since its inception (e.g., Brandtstädter, 1998; Palys & Little, 1983; Ruehlman & Wolchik, 1988; Salmela-Aro, Aunola, & Nurmi, 2005) and has revealed some subtleties in the ways in which personal projects are interdependent with those of others.

One early example is the study by Yard (1980) of the personal projects of members of the Royal Canadian Mounted Police (RCMP) and their spouses. He used an early version of the joint cross-impact matrix (see Little & Gee, chap. 2, this volume), in which individuals estimated the extent to which their spouses' projects had a positive, neutral, ambivalent, or negative impact on their own. Both the officers and their spouses completed the matrices independently of each other. Yard discovered a very high degree of congruency or reciprocity between spouses in their cross-impact scores. This was an exploratory study and it was not anticipated that such a high degree of reciprocity would be apparent. It would have been theoretically plausible, for example, for one spouse to have a strong impact (positive or negative) on a more passive spouse. However, for both positive and negative impact and a combined measure of overall positive impact, the couples showed strikingly high correlations: If one spouse had little impact on the other, this was reciprocated; if one had projects that kept knocking on the door of his spouse, she would be knocking right back with her own. One of several possibilities discussed in Yard's thesis was that this might represent the presence of shared or joint projects although this seemed to explain the correlation between positive mutual impact better than it did negative impact.

Almost a quarter-century later, two studies explored the nature of such shared or joint projects. Hebert (2003) adapted PPA to study university students who were involved in an intimate relationship and obtained ratings from both members of the couple on their own projects and those that both regarded as joint projects. One of the most interesting findings in Hebert's study was that for men, life satisfaction scores were very significantly related to their personal and joint project appraisals; for women, life satisfaction was not strongly related to their own personal project appraisals but was related to their romantic partner's personal project appraisals. In this sense "your" projects mattered more than "mine" for these women in determining life satisfaction.

Hwang (2004) explicitly examined such joint projects and their relation to the quality of romantic relationships. Using a Web-based version of PPA, specially designed to elicit projects shared by a diverse group of people who were involved in intimate relationships, Hwang showed that the sheer number of joint projects shared by a couple was, in itself, a strong predictor of the quality of the spousal relationship, after controlling for the influence of other relevant variables.

Interpersonal Projects and Life-Span Development

The interpersonal ecology of project pursuit is likely to vary across different stages of the life span and depend on the nature of transitional periods as individuals move through the different behavior settings that dominate phases of life. Two different transitional stages of life can be used to illustrate how a personal projects perspective casts light on relational aspects of development: entry into the world and entry into adulthood.

As intimated at the beginning of this chapter, birth itself is a project that involves, typically, although not always, a triadic relationship: the unborn child and each parent. It is the first transition in life, from intrauterine life to life in which parents greet the new child with delight or, sadly, with dread.

Again, one of the early studies with personal projects (McKeen, 1984) examined the relational factors that contributed to successful birth. Examining pregnancy from the expectant mother's perspective, McKeen (1984) found that the single best predictor of successful birth, using both soft and hard indicators of success (e.g., the mother's subjective experience and Apgar scores), was the extent to which the mother regarded her partner as supportive of her projects, particularly those related to the pregnancy. Interpersonal projects also bridge the transition from birth to the postdelivery home environment and here there are subtle differences between mothers and fathers and between families with different numbers of children in the family. For example, Salmela-Aro, Nurmi, Saisto, and Halmesmäki (2000, 2001) found that during the transition to parenthood, women become more interested in projects related to family life after the birth of a child. This change was more substantial among the primiparous than among the multiparous mothers. However, among men there were no changes in family-related projects during the transition to parenthood.

Considerable attention has also been given to the transitional period known as emerging adulthood (Arnett, 2000) and important aspects of this transition are changes in the nature of interpersonal projects (Salmela-Aro et al., 2005). Using latent growth curve analysis (Muthén & Muthén, 1998–2004), it was shown that the frequency of friend-related projects decreased across the time of emerging adulthood. Second, the number of family-related projects indicated an accelerating increase across emerging adulthood. The results showed further that there was both individual variation in the level of family-related projects and accelerating increase in them across this transitional period. These changes in interpersonal projects are important for effective adaptation. Cantor, Norem, Niedenthal, Langston, and Brower (1987) demonstrated that the sequencing and timing of interpersonal goals affects adaptation. Those university students who, over a course of a term, first give priority to interpersonal tasks and later to academic tasks are most likely to flourish.

INTERPERSONAL PROJECTS AND HUMAN FLOURISHING

We conceive of human flourishing as comprising three important functions: a sense of personal well-being, successful achievement of valued projects or tasks, and having impacts that enhance the well-being not only of intimate others but of the larger community. There is now an extensive research literature examining how interpersonal projects influence both personal well-being and effective performance and a growing awareness that personal projects can have an impact on the surrounding community so that personal investments in action may generate social capital. We consider each aspect of flourishing in turn.

Interpersonal Projects and Subjective Well-Being

In an early meta-analysis of the relations between personal projects dimensions and well-being (Wilson, 1990), interpersonal dimensions had only moderately strong relations with measures of subjective well-being; efficacy and stress were consistently stronger and less variable predictors of well-being. Indeed, project efficacy (positively) and stress (negatively) reliably account for 25% of the variance in subjective well-being (Little, 1989). There may have been several reasons for these results. First, most of the samples were university students who may have been primarily concerned about academic achievement, with efficacy and stress representing, respectively, success and failure in progressing in this domain. Second, there may have been insufficient sampling of dimensions relating to interpersonal themes in the early studies. However, even when attempts were made to increase the prediction of well-being by the addition of more sophisticated and detailed measures of relational support or communal themes, the incremental validity provided by these measures was not substantial (see James, 2000; Ruehlman & Wolchik, 1988). A third possible explanation for these findings is that the positive effects of project visibility, support, and value by others is indirect only and is primarily mediated by their impact on efficacy and stress.

When we turn again to the sheer frequency of interpersonal projects in the daily pursuits of individuals, however, a different picture emerges. There is a rapidly growing literature concerning how social and interpersonal projects are related to well-being. In a longitudinal study of university students, Salmela-Aro and Nurmi (1997) found that family-related projects predicted high self-esteem and low psychological distress in terms of subsequent depressive symptoms. In turn, self-esteem predicted having interpersonal projects later on (Salmela-Aro & Nurmi, 1997). Salmela-Aro (2001) showed that, during their transition from vocational school to work life, those young adults who had many social, interpersonal projects reported more positive mood states (using the PANAS scales) than those who had relatively few interpersonal projects. Emmons (1991) also reported that those young adults who sought to establish intimate relationships were more likely to experience positive well-being. Among adults in a recent study, Salmela-Aro and Nurmi (2004) found that those employees having a family orientation in terms of a high number of family-related projects reported high life satisfaction, high satisfaction with work life, and a low level of burnout. Finally, Salmela-Aro et al. (2001) found in a cross-lagged longitudinal study during transition to parenthood that an increase in family-related personal projects during pregnancy and after the birth of a child predicted a decline in women's depressive symptoms. Moreover, the results show that interpersonal projects are related to high subjective well-being, whereas intrapersonal or more self-oriented projects are related to low subjective well-being (Little, 1993; Salmela-Aro, 1992).

In summary, the mere presence of interpersonal projects in the lives of individuals at different stages of life seems to be predictive of subjective well-being, but their effect may be through their indirect role in mitigating stress and promoting a sense of efficacy in daily life.

Interpersonal Projects and Performance

Interpersonal projects not only lead to an increase in well-being but also better performance, in terms of both academic and social performance. Salmela-Aro (2001) found that those young adults who had many social, interpersonal projects had higher grades in high school. Reinforcing the link with performance, Nurmi and Salmela-Aro (2002) found that during the transition from vocational school to work, family-related projects predicted being in a professional work status rather than being unemployed later on in life.

Social projects also seem to be related to having important social contacts. The results showed, for example, that those young adults who were married, living in a cohabitation relationship, or had children reported more family-related projects than others (Nurmi & Salmela-Aro, 2002). Having children during young adulthood predicted reporting family projects later in life (Salmela-Aro & Nurmi, 1997). Moreover, family-related projects as a young adult predicted being married later on. Finally, among young adults, negative life events predicted having fewer family-related projects later in life (Salmela-Aro & Nurmi, 1997).

Examining the confidence that one has in interpersonal projects also reveals consequences for social relationships and well-being. Salmela-Aro and Nurmi (1996) identified two groups of female young adults: the socially confident group (75%), with positive and confident appraisals (high on outcome and low on negative affect) of their interpersonal projects, and the socially uncertain group (35%), with negative and uncertain appraisals (low on outcome and high on negative affect). The results showed that the young women in the socially uncertain group reported more negative interactions with their parents and with their intimate relationships, and also fewer new acquaintances than the socially confident young women. Moreover, those women who appraised their interpersonal projects in negative and uncertain ways showed higher levels of depressive symptoms, stress, and loneliness, and lower levels of self-esteem. In addition, their results revealed that young females with uncertain interpersonal projects become more depressed during the transitional period of starting university studies.

Taken together, the research evidence suggests that being engaged and confident in interpersonal projects has a salutary effect on individuals. Both in terms of achievement and affiliative outcomes, they contribute to human flourishing.

Personal Investment and Social Capital: Having Impact on Others in Project Pursuit

As we noted in the introductory caveat, not all personal projects are individualistic pursuits focused on the goals of the person initiating the project. We have also reviewed the subtleties of research on the nature of projects undertaken jointly with intimate others. However, there is another aspect of human flourishing that has to do with projects that impact others who are not part of our immediate family or network of friends. Some individuals have considerable personal investment in projects that generate social capital (Phillips, Little, & Goodine, 1997; Putnam, 2000). Conversely, individuals can be the recipients of social capital that is generated by others. Recent research has examined these aspects of interpersonal projects and their impact (see also Grant et al., chap. 8, this volume).

Phillips et al. (1997) conducted an extensive study of volunteering projects—personal investments in activities of direct benefit to others not necessarily known personally to them. In extensive interviews, we explored the nature of their projects, the reasons for undertaking them, and their intention to continue in volunteer activities. Two groups of participants showed an intriguing difference in the relation between motives and intentions to continue volunteering: students and young retirees. There were individuals in both groups whose primary motivations for volunteering were self-oriented or for the benefit of others. It was expected that the intention to continue volunteering, and hence increase social capital, would be linked with having more altruistic motives. This was indeed the case with the young retirees. However, with students, the reverse was found. It was those students who were engaged in voluntary projects primarily to enhance their own skills and satisfy their needs and interests who were more likely to indicate a willingness to continue with such activities.

Finally, the relation between social networks and social capital was explored recently by Jokisaari and Nurmi (2005). After eliciting personal goals relating to work with a group of Finnish students in the school-to-work transition period, the respondents completed a module that asked them to list people associated with the most important work goal, including an assessment of the strength of relationship to them, their occupation, and whether they helped or hindered acquisition of the work goals. The results indicated that students who had networks containing people of higher socioeconomic status and weaker ties with them were more successful than others in this transition. In a similar study with slightly younger adolescents, Salmela-Aro (2004) found somewhat different results, however, regarding educational projects. In this case, the evidence was that close ties, rather than weak ties, were of greater benefit, and this was particularly so for girls relative to boys.

Clearly the research agenda on personal projects, networks, and social capital is both rich and complex. It underscores the fact that personal projects are not just private pursuits nor intimate undertakings, but also actions with impact, enabling both individuals and communities to flourish.

CONCLUSION

We have shown that personal projects, far from being individualistic private pursuits are pervasively relational in nature. The inception and planning stages of project pursuit are deeply influenced by the expectation and mere presence of other people also pursuing projects. Apart from hermits, project pursuit is almost always played out in a world where negotiation of project space (sometimes quite literally) is constantly negotiated, sometimes for better, sometimes for worse. The termination of projects may be prevented because one realizes that, at the root, the project is really motivated by the concerns and needs of other people. So one perseveres.

Personal projects methodology has been shown to be able to access a number of aspects of relational concerns by flexible adaptation of several of its core modules. In the project elicitation module, interpersonal projects have consistently been found to be among the most frequently elicited projects; only academic projects for students and work projects for those in the labor force rival them as pervasive features of everyday project pursuit. They are also consistently found to be rated among the most rewarding of projects. Indeed, when they are not rewarding they serve as a red flag that something may be awry in a person's life. The use of the joint cross-impact matrices has highlighted the importance of shared projects on relational well-being. Finally, personal projects can serve as sources of social capital. Volunteering projects have been shown to redound to the benefit of the project pursuer and the recipients, although, particularly with young people, we have seen that such projects may well have motivational force that includes personal growth and challenge, not merely altruistic concerns for others.

In short, from birth to death, my projects are pervasively influenced by the real or imagined presence of other project pursuers. The mere presence of others in our projects appears salutary: Interpersonal projects are among the most joyous of our pursuits. On the other hand, when our interpersonal projects are fractious or when our shared projects are actually coercive, human flourishing is diminished. When we conceive projects not as mine but as ours, we move into the domain of relational intimacy. Once again, harmonious shared projects have been found to enhance well-being, although there may be some asymmetries between men and women in terms of who is the greater beneficiary. Finally, reaching out into the larger community, projects done for others—not necessarily intimate others—creates the kind of social capital that we now know helps enhance the sustainability of the larger societies within which we pursue our own concerns.

Personal projects, be they mine, ours, yours, or theirs, can only fully be understood by taking others into account. Personal projects, therefore, we conclude are profoundly and pervasively interpersonal phenomena.

REFERENCES

Arnett, J. (2000). Emerging adulthood: A theory of development from the late teens through the twenties. *American Psychologist, 55,* 469–480.

Berg, C., Meegan, S., & Deviney, F. (1998). A social-contextual model of coping with everyday problems across the life-span. *International Journal of Behavioral Development, 22,* 239–261.

SALMELA-ARO AND LITTLE

Brandtstädter, J. (1998). Action perspective on human development. In W. Damon (Series Ed.) & R. Lerner (Vol. Ed.), *Handbook of child psychology: Vol. 1. Theoretical models of human development* (5th ed., pp. 807–863). New York: Wiley.

Brunstein, J., Dangelmayer, G., & Schultheiss, O. (1996). Personal goals and social support in close relationships: Effects on relationship mood and marital satisfaction. *Journal of Personality and Social Psychology, 71,* 1006–1019.

Burgess, P. D. (1982). *The wife/mother/student: Impact of the student role on personal project systems.* Unpublished master's thesis, Carleton University, Ottawa, ON, Canada.

Cantor, N., Acker, M., & Cook-Flannagan, C. (1992). Conflict and preoccupation in the intimacy life task. *Journal of Personality and Social Psychology, 63,* 644–655.

Cantor, N., Norem, J. K., Niedenthal, P. M., Langston, C. A., & Brower, A. M. (1987). Life tasks, self-concept ideals, and cognitive strategies in a life transition. *Journal of Personality and Social Psychology, 53,* 1178–1191.

Chambers, N. C. (1997). *Personal projects analysis: The maturation of a multidimensional methodology.* Retrieved May 1, 2005, from http:// www.brianrlittle.com/ research/index.htm

Diener, E., & Fujita, F. (1995). Resources, personal strivings, and subjective well-being: A nomothetic and idiographic approach. *Journal of Personality and Social Psychology, 68,* 926–935.

Emmons, R. A. (1991). Personal strivings, daily life events, and psychological and physical well-being. *Journal of Personality, 59,* 453–472.

Harlow, R., & Cantor, N. (1994). Social pursuits of academics: Side effects and spillover of strategic reassurance seeking. *Journal of Personality and Social Psychology, 66,* 386–397.

Hebert, S. (2003). *Personal and joint system appraisal as correlates of relationship and life satisfaction in romantic relationships: An exploratory study.* Unpublished bachelor's thesis, Carleton University, Ottawa, ON, Canada.

Hwang, A. A. (2004). *Yours, mine, ours: The role of joint personal projects in close relationships.* Unpublished doctoral dissertation, Harvard University, Cambridge, MA.

James, D. S. (2000). *The nature of the self and well-being: A relational analysis using personal projects.* Unpublished doctoral dissertation, Carleton University, Ottawa, ON, Canada.

Jokisaari, M., & Nurmi, J.-E. (2005). Company matters: Goal-related social capital in the transition to working life. *Journal of Vocational Behavior, 67,* 413–428.

Kelly, G. A. (1955). *The psychology of personal constructs* (Vol. 1). New York: Norton.

Klinger, E. (1975). Consequences of commitment to and disengagement from incentives. *Psychological Review, 82,* 1–25.

Klinger, E. (1977). *Meaning and void: Inner experience and the incentives in people's lives.* Minneapolis: University of Minnesota Press.

Langston, C. A., & Cantor, N. (1989). Ups and downs of life tasks in a life transition. In L. A. Pervin (Ed.), *Goal concepts in personality and social psychology* (pp. 127–167). Hillsdale, NJ: Lawrence Erlbaum Associates.

Little, B. R. (1972). Psychological man as scientist, humanist and specialist. *Journal of Experimental Research in Personality, 6,* 95–118.

Little, B. R. (1983). Personal projects: A rationale and method for investigation. *Environment and Behavior, 15,* 273–309.

Little, B. R. (1980). The social ecology of children's nothings. *Ekistics, 47,* 93–95.

Little, B. R. (1987). Personality and the environment. In D. Stokols & I. Altman (Eds.), *Handbook of environmental psychology* (pp. 206–244). New York: Wiley.

Little, B. R. (1989). Personal projects analysis: Trivial pursuits, magnificent obsessions, and the search for coherence. In D. M. Buss & N. Cantor (Eds.), *Personality psychology: Recent trends and emerging directions* (pp. 15–31). New York: Springer.

Little, B. R. (1993). Personal projects and the distributed self: Aspects of a conative psychology. In J. M. Suls (Ed.), *The self in social perspective: Psychological perspectives on the self* (Vol. 4, pp. 157–185). Hillsdale, NJ: Lawrence Erlbaum Associates.

Little, B. R. (1999). Personality and motivation: Personal action and the conative evolution. In L. A. Pervin & O. P. John (Eds.), *Handbook of personality: Theory and research* (2nd ed., pp. 501–524). New York: Guilford.

Little, B. R. (2000). Free traits and personal contexts: Expanding a social ecological model of well-being. In W. B. Walsh, K. H. Craik, & R. H. Price (Eds.), *Person–environment psychology: New directions and perspectives* (2nd ed., pp. 87–116). Mahwah, NJ: Lawrence Erlbaum Associates.

Little, B. R. (2005). Personality science and personal projects: Six impossible things before breakfast. *Journal of Research in Personality, 39,* 4–21.

Little, B. R., & Chambers, N. C. (2004). Personal project pursuit: On human doings and well-beings. In W. M. Cox & E. Klinger (Eds.), *Handbook of motivational counseling: Concepts, approaches and assessment* (pp. 65–82). Chichester, UK: Wiley.

Little, B. R., Lecci, L., & Watkinson, B. (1992). Personality and personal projects: Linking big five and PAC units of analysis. *Journal of Personality, 60,* 501–525.

Little, B. R., & Ryan, T. J. (1979). A social ecological model of development. In K. Ishwaren (Ed.), *Childhood and adolescence in Canada* (pp. 273–301). Toronto: McGraw-Hill Ryerson.

MacDiarmid, E. W. (1990). *Level of molarity, project cross impact and resistance to change in personal project systems.* Unpublished master's thesis, Carleton University, Ottawa, ON, Canada.

McKeen, N. A. (1984). *The personal projects of pregnant women.* Unpublished bachelor's thesis, Carleton University, Ottawa, ON, Canada.

Meegan, S., & Berg, C. (1998). *The interpersonal context of appraisal and coping with developmental life tasks.* Unpublished manuscript, University of Utah, Salt Lake City.

Muthén, L. K., & Muthén, B. O. (1998–2004). *Mplus user's guide.* Los Angeles: Muthén & Muthén.

Nurmi, J.-E., Pulliainen, H., & Salmela-Aro, K. (1992). Age differences in adults' control beliefs related to life goals and concerns. *Psychology and Aging, 7,* 194–196.

Nurmi, J.-E., & Salmela-Aro, K. (2002). Goal construction, reconstruction and depressive symptoms in a life-span context: The transition from school to work. *Journal of Personality, 70,* 385–420.

Nurmi, J.-E., Salmela-Aro, K., & Koivisto, P. (2002). Goal importance, and related agency-beliefs and emotions during the transition from vocational school to work: Antecedents and consequences. *Journal of Vocational Behavior, 60,* 241–261.

Palys, T. S., & Little, B. R. (1983). Perceived life satisfaction and the organization of personal project systems. *Journal of Personality and Social Psychology, 44,* 1221–1230.

Paulhus, D. L., & Williams, K. M. (2002). The dark triad of personality: Narcissism, Machiavellianism and psychopathy. *Journal of Research in Personality, 36,* 556–563.

Phillips, S. D., Little, B. R., & Goodine, L. A. (1997). Reconsidering gender and public administration: Five steps beyond conventional research. *Canadian Journal of Public Administration, 40,* 563–581.

Putnam, R. D. (2000). *Bowling alone: The collapse and revival of American community.* New York: Touchstone Books/Simon & Schuster.

Reis, H. (2006). The relationship context of social psychology. In P. Van Lange (Ed.), *Bridging social psychology: Benefits of transdisciplinary approaches.* Mahwah, NJ: Lawrence Erlbaum Associates.

Ruehlman, L. S., & Wolchik, S. (1988). Personal goals and interpersonal support and hindrance as factors in psychological distress and well-being. *Journal of Personality and Social Psychology, 55,* 293–301.

Salmela-Aro, K. (1992). Struggling with self: The personal projects of students seeking psychological counselling. *Scandinavian Journal of Psychology, 33,* 330–338.

Salmela-Aro, K. (2001). Personal goals during a transition to adulthood. In J.-E. Nurmi (Ed.), *Navigation through adolescence* (pp. 59–84). New York: Routledge Falmer.

Salmela-Aro, K. (2003). *Personal goals during emerging adulthood.* Poster session presented at the First Emerging Adulthood congress, Society for Adolescent Research, Cambridge, MA.

Salmela-Aro, K. (2004, September). *Motivational orientation among adolescents.* Presentation at the 9th International Conference on Motivation, Lisbon, Portugal.

Salmela-Aro, K., Aunola, K., & Nurmi, J.-E. (2005). *Personal goals, role transitions, and depressive symptoms during university studies: A 10-year follow-up.* Manuscript submitted for publication.

Salmela-Aro, K., & Nurmi, J.-E. (1996). Uncertainty and confidence in interpersonal projects—Consequences for social life and well-being. *Journal of Social and Personal Relationships, 13,* 109–122.

Salmela-Aro, K., & Nurmi, J.-E. (1997). Goal contents, well-being, and life context during transition to university: A longitudinal study. *International Journal of Behavioral Development, 20,* 471–491.

Salmela-Aro, K., & Nurmi, J.-E. (2004). Motivational orientation and well-being at work: A person-oriented approach. *Journal of Change Management, 17,* 471–489.

Salmela-Aro, K., Nurmi, J.-E., Aro, A., Poppius, E., & Riste, J. (1992). Age differences in adults' personal projects. *Journal of Social Psychology, 133,* 415–417.

Salmela-Aro, K., Nurmi, J.-E., & Näätänen, P. (2004). The role of work-related personal projects during two burnout interventions: A longitudinal study. *Work & Stress, 18,* 208–230.

Salmela-Aro, K., Nurmi, J.-E., Saisto, T., & Halmesmäki, E. (2000). Women's and men's personal goals during the transition to parenthood. *Journal of Family Psychology, 14,* 171–186.

Salmela-Aro, K., Nurmi, J.-E., Saisto, T., & Halmesmäki, E. (2001). Goal construction and depressive symptoms during transition to motherhood: Evidence from two longitudinal studies. *Journal of Personality and Social Psychology, 81,* 1144–1159.

Salmela-Aro, K., Vuori, J., & Koivisto, P. (2003). Adolescent's socialization and self-direction towards the work life. In *People and work* (Research Rep. No. 58, pp. 71–76). Helsinki: Finnish Institute of Occupational Health.

Wilson, D. A. (1990). *Personal project dimensions and perceived life satisfaction: A quantitative synthesis.* Unpublished master's thesis, Carleton University, Ottawa, ON, Canada.

Yard, G. F. (1980). *Personal project system variables as predictors of job satisfaction and performance effectiveness in members of the Royal Canadian Mounted Police.* Unpublished master's thesis, Carleton University, Ottawa, ON, Canada.

8

Personal Projects
and Organizational Lives

Adam M. Grant, Brian R. Little, and Susan D. Phillips

Emily loves her job as a software developer. She looks forward to work each morning, excels in her endeavors, enjoys and admires her supportive team members, and is delighted with her working life. In contrast, Robert, a manager in a large accounting firm, despises his job. He trudges reluctantly to the office day after day, works halfheartedly, feels isolated from his colleagues, and knows deeply and with some desperation that his work life is devoid of meaning. Why is one employee so satisfied and performing well, and the other neither content nor productive? Why are some Emilies and Roberts of organizations flourishing and some floundering?

The field of organizational behavior provides four alternative perspectives that help explain such differences. One focuses on personal features, a second on environmental or contextual features, and a third on the interaction of persons and their contexts. A fourth perspective, also interactional, provides a distinctive vantage point that will be the central concern of this chapter (compare with the social ecological model in Little, chap. 1, this volume).

The study of personal features as the source of delight and discontent in organizations has had a strong tradition in both personality and organizational psychology. Perhaps Emily possesses more "positive" personality traits (Judge, Heller, & Mount, 2002) and more positive beliefs about and orientations toward work (Wrzesniewski, McCauley, Rozin, & Schwartz, 1997) so that she is bound to be happy in most tasks and surroundings. Robert, on the other hand, may be just plain miserable, no matter where he trudges.

The environmental or contextual perspective detects the sources of differential flourishing at work as being due to forces ranging from the overall macrolevel features of organizations to the microlevel aspects of work design. At the macro level, the culture and climate of Emily's smaller, more decentralized organization may be more favorable than Robert's (Ashkanasy, Wilderom, & Peterson, 2000; Rousseau, 1978). At a middle or *meso* level of analysis, we might find that the social context provides Emily with more constructive relationships with supervisors and coworkers (Gerstner & Day, 1997; Karasek & Theorell, 1990) and more appealing information (Salancik & Pfeffer, 1978). Alternatively, the reward system might play a major role: Emily may receive more favorable incentives, such as compensation, benefits, promotions, and job security, than does Robert (Gerhart & Rynes, 2003). At the micro level, Emily's job may provide more autonomy, feedback, skill variety, and significance (Hackman & Oldham, 1980), and Robert's role may be ambiguous, conflicted, and straining (Katz & Kahn, 1978). In short, Emily is flourishing because her work context is maximally supportive; Robert is floundering because his environment is toxic (Danna & Griffin, 1999; Frost, 2003).

Each of these explanations can only take us so far. Taken collectively, they serve to illustrate that influences on psychological experiences and behaviors in organizations are often overdetermined and change in response to multiple simultaneous causes (Hackman, 1985; Weick, 1974). However, each focuses exclusively on either attributes of the person (P) or the environment (E). A third perspective examines the interaction of persons and environments, comprising a P × E lens on people in organizations. The rise of an interactional or person–environment perspective in personality, environmental, community, and organizational psychology (e.g., Argyle & Little, 1972; Little, 1987; Mischel, 2004; Ostroff, 1993; Walsh, Craik, & Price, 2000) emphasized that as well as the "main effects" of P and E in influencing everyday behavior, the interaction (P × E) was critical. Emily may thrive at work primarily because there is a fine fit between her sociable, excitement-seeking personality and the rather open and tolerant policies at her boutique software firm. Robert might, in fact, be even more miserable in such an environment because at least he can get lost where he currently works. Having to appear sociable on top of suffering the indignities of being underpaid and unappreciated would be a sure prescription for exhaustion. Under this view of interactionism, a good P × E fit is central to understanding the qualities of organizational life (Caplan, 1987; Pervin, 1989).

In this chapter, we apply a fourth perspective to organizational lives. It, too, is an interactional approach, but is distinctive in that it comprises a dynamic interactionist rather than mechanical interactionist perspective (Little, 1987; see Magnusson, 1999). The latter essentially adopts an analysis of variance approach to looking at person–environment interaction, whereas the former attempts to locate the interaction within a dynamic unit of analysis that carries the features of both persons and their contexts. That unit is the personal project.

The personal project (Little, 1983, chap. 1, this volume) serves as a conceptual carrier unit and as a measurement unit that inherently links persons and contexts. At work, the personal project connects individuals to their groups and organizations by examining individual pursuits that occur in conjunction with, are directed toward, and are enacted on behalf of other individuals, groups, and the organization as a whole. That is, the personal project captures cognitions, affect, and behaviors that influence and are influenced by the contexts in which they take place (Little, 2000). The personal project allows us to see Emily engaged in goal-oriented action that both expresses her characteristics and impacts her context. It affords us glimpses of Robert in action or inaction, cunningly avoiding engagement in a context he sees as demeaning.

Our goal, then, is to explore the relevance of personal projects to organizational lives. First, we define personal projects at work and explore their potential advantages over the more traditional units of tasks and jobs. Second, we draw on extant research on personal projects and related units to illustrate how projects address some of the central themes in organizational life. We show how projects enrich our understanding of work processes, contexts, and outcomes, and how projects can be both predictors of job satisfaction and performance and outcome measures in their own right. Finally, we discuss future directions for organizational research on personal projects and the applied implications of personal projects for redesigning work to enhance satisfaction and performance. Are projects replacing jobs? If so, does the quest for increased satisfaction and improved performance entail redesigning projects rather than jobs?

DEFINING AND DISTINGUISHING THE PERSONAL PROJECT AT WORK

Defined as an "extended set of personally relevant action" (Little, Lecci, & Watkinson, 1992, p. 502; see also Little, 1989, chap. 1, this volume), the personal project encompasses both goals—cognitive representations of desired outcomes (Austin & Vancouver, 1996)—and behaviors undertaken in pursuit of goals. In the organizational context, it is important to distinguish the personal project from that described in the project management literature (e.g., Thompson, 1967). In the project management literature, a project is a formal endeavor undertaken by members of the organization, whereas a personal project is an individual's subjective construal of his or her pursuit or activity. For example, Emily's formal project, one that could be found in her job description, might be to "provide liaison with the business development team," whereas her personal project might be to "get the BD Team off our case, once and for all."

In organizational settings, we propose that the personal project offers advantages over traditional units of measurement of work processes and actions, notably tasks and jobs. A *task*, the most basic building block of work, is an assigned piece of work that an employee carries out (Griffin, 1987). A *job* is an aggregation of assigned tasks designed to be performed by one employee (Ilgen & Hollenbeck, 1992; Wong & Campion, 1991). We believe that personal projects, which derive from and are embedded in a social ecological model of human behavior (Little, 2000, chap. 1, this volume), have the advantage of being both personally salient and pitched at a middle scale of action that situates them somewhere between tasks and jobs, as outlined in Table 8.1.

Personal Saliency

The first advantage of the personal project is its personal saliency. Because tasks and jobs are defined externally from a manager's perspective or by an organization's requirements, they may not encapsulate the actions that are personally salient and important to the employee (Taber & Alliger, 1995). In contrast, the personal project represents the actions that are most significant and relevant in the employee's experience.

TABLE 8.1
The Personal Project as a Unit of Work

Construct	Definition	Personal Saliency	Scale of Action
Personal Project	Extended set of personally relevant action.	Personally defined. Encompasses personally relevant actions, both assigned and voluntary.	Middle-range unit; encompasses processes and outcomes of behavior, and multiple acts and goals.
Task	Assigned piece of work that an employee carries out.	Externally defined. Encompasses only assigned actions.	Microscopic unit; focuses on the basic building blocks of work that employees carry out.
Job	Aggregation of assigned tasks designed to be performed by one employee.	Externally defined. Encompasses only assigned actions.	Macroscopic unit; focuses on the collection of activities that employees carry out.

This is important for two reasons. First, people can identify the same actions at many different levels of analysis (Vallacher & Wegner, 1987). At a low level of analysis, people identify their actions in terms of how they are performed, and at a high level, they identify their actions in terms of why they are performed. For instance, some marketers describe their actions at work in terms of selling products, whereas others describe them in terms of making the world a better place (Pratt, 2000).

Second, employees in identical jobs assigned to carry out the same tasks differ substantially in their definitions of what activities are part of their jobs (Morrison, 1994; see also Parker, Wall, & Jackson, 1997). It appears that these differences arise when employees cognitively redefine and behaviorally reshape the boundaries of their tasks and jobs. Wrzesniewski and Dutton (2001) described several studies that illustrate how employees carry out these "job crafting" activities. For example, hospital janitors assigned identical tasks and jobs often differ markedly in the activities that they actually carry out at work: Some janitors incorporate voluntary actions into their daily activities at work, offering help to patients and timing their work to increase efficiency for nurses, whereas others stick to narrowly defined and prescribed responsibilities.

Accordingly, an examination of employees' assigned tasks and jobs may overlook the activities that occupy the majority of their time, energy, and attention. Because employees can identify the same actions at different levels, and reshape their tasks and jobs, assessing an employee's experience on the basis of an external definition of a task or a job may not accurately capture the employee's activities, pursuits, and experiences. Conversely, a focus on the personal projects of employees highlights the activities and pursuits that are most salient in their work experiences. Whereas tasks and jobs only capture activities assigned to an employee, personal projects can include any activity in which an employee is engaged at work. Projects thus allow researchers to understand discretionary, extrarole activities as well as the assigned activities that tasks and jobs involve (Roberson, Houston, & Diddams, 1989). Indeed, Pomaki, Maes, and ter Doest (2004) found that studies based on personally salient open elicitation formats (see Little & Gee, chap. 2, this volume) have additional power to detect moderators of the relations between work variables and outcomes. Therefore, personal projects may enable researchers to understand a broader range of actions than tasks and jobs permit, and to understand the actions that are most significant in the employee's life.

Scale of Action

A second advantage of the personal project is its scale of action. Tasks are typically microscopic units of work, whereas jobs are global, macroscopic units. The macroscopic nature of jobs can pose conceptual, methodological, and practical challenges. In particular, the job unit of measurement can obscure important variations in work experiences (Mintzberg, 1973). If we merely measured job attitudes and perceptions, we might fail to notice that Emily may have a project or two that she finds discouraging, and we would fail to learn why this is the case. We might also overlook the fact that Robert, although generally miserable, seems to love one aspect of his work, which serves as his primary source of motivation. Moreover, jobs are a sufficiently global unit that employees' evaluations of them can fluctuate substantially depending on which aspects of the job are in focus at the moment of evaluation (see Schwarz, 1999). Conceptually, these findings make it difficult for researchers to discern employees' feelings from their ratings of jobs (Taber & Alliger, 1995). Methodologically, these findings leave ambiguous how job evaluations should be measured with precision. Practically, it remains uncertain whether employees' ratings of their jobs are accurate representations of their work experiences.

More molecular units of work may therefore be advantageous. Indeed, measuring employees' ratings of tasks can predict outcomes over and above their ratings of jobs (Taber & Alliger, 1995). However, the microscopic nature of tasks poses a different set of challenges. At a conceptual level, employees carry out many tasks, and it is not clear which tasks are relevant to understanding their behaviors and experiences. At a methodological level, it is not evident how employees' ratings of tasks should be aggregated. At a practical level, it can take several hours for employees to provide ratings of their tasks (Taber & Alliger, 1995).

What organizational science may find of value are units of measurement that are more global than tasks, yet not so global that they prevent researchers from capturing important variations in cognition, affect, and behavior. We believe personal projects meet these criteria. Personal projects are middle-range units (Little, 1983, 1989) that are generally more molecular than jobs and more molar than tasks.[1] Personal projects aggregate employees' experiences into personally salient chunks and allow a large proportion of their work experiences to be encapsulated by examining the systems of activities in which they are engaged. Thorngate (1976) argued that no explanation of social behavior can be concurrently simple, general, and accurate. We believe the same is true for units of measurement of social behavior. Assessments of jobs are simple and general, but potentially inaccurate. Assessments of tasks may be simple and accurate, but tedious to elicit and not sufficiently general. These trade-offs between simplicity and accuracy involved in measuring jobs and tasks may be partially mitigated in assessments of personal projects, which enables researchers to study action at a level less global—and therefore more accurate—than jobs, but at a level more global—and therefore more generalizable and representative—than tasks.

RESEARCH ON PERSONAL PROJECTS AT WORK

We have proposed that personal projects can capture a broader range of action that is more personally salient to employees and is more amenable to accurate measurement than jobs and tasks. In line with this no-

---

[1]Although the personal project's home is as a middle-level unit between a task and a job, the personal project unit can be used to move up and down levels, from trivial pursuits to magnificent obsessions (Little, 1989).

tion, Cropanzano, James, and Citera (1993) argued that examining an employee's personal projects provides a wealth of information about the employe's cognition, affect, and behaviors. To explore some of this information, we turn to recent research on personal projects at work and illustrate the ways in which personal projects inform our understanding of four key issues in organizational behavior.[2] The first is how work is described and appraised: How do people identify what they are really doing? What do they find meaningful, stressful, or value congruent? Second, personal projects enable us to examine the relationships between action and context: For instance, what influence does organizational climate have on employees' goals and projects? Third, personal projects can inform an understanding of work outcomes relevant to employees: to what extent do our appraisals of work influence job satisfaction and performance? Fourth, we consider the notion that the personal projects methodology can be scaled up to explore organizational projects, not merely personal ones.

The Nature of Work: "What's Up? How's It Going?"

In this section, we describe research suggesting that the personal project unit allows us to assess the content of work, its identity and meaning, and the reciprocal impact of work on the self and the social and organizational environment.

Project Content. What people think they are doing and how they describe what they are doing are the starting points for personal projects analysis (PPA). As described in chapter 2, the first step in PPA is to elicit the projects in which people say they are engaged. Projects can then be classified in a variety of ways, enabling assessment of different aspects of work. One type of classification involves different phrasings of projects. For example, describing projects in terms of avoidance rather than approach (Elliot, Sheldon, & Church, 1997) or in terms of trying rather than doing (Chambers, chap. 5, this volume; Little & Chambers, 2004) has been found to be associated with lower levels of well-being. A second approach to describing and classifying projects is

---

[2]Our review addresses research on personal projects at work and personal goals at work. Although the goal-setting research in organizational behavior has focused primarily on externally assigned goals (Locke & Latham, 1990, 2002), a series of important and relevant studies have been conducted on personal goals (see also Pomaki & Maes, 2002).

according to the domain or type of activity (Little et al., 1992).[3] For example, Phillips, Little, and Goodine (1996, 1997) studied the impact of reform in the Canadian government during the early 1990s that was intended to evoke a culture change to encourage greater attention to the management of human resources. They used PPA to explore assessments of the work projects of 120 managers, classifying these projects into nine activity domains.[4] If the attempts at reengineering the organizational culture were taking hold, it would be expected that projects related to managing people would be considered not only important but also personally meaningful, efficacious, and supported by colleagues and the culture generally. The analysis reflected poorly on the reform attempts and revealed some significant gender differences. Although women managers rated managing people projects higher in personal meaning, they also perceived that they had much less support for them from coworkers, superiors, or the organizational climate than did their male counterparts. Ironically, and in contrast to male managers, they felt that there was less support for managing people projects than almost any other type of project. This suggests that any culture change that was taking place was far from having the desired effects, and was likely to lead to disillusionment on the part of women managers before affecting their male colleagues (Phillips et al., 1996).

Project Identity and Meaning. Weick (1999, 2004) argued that how projects are formulated has important implications for an employee's identity and experience of meaning (see also Morrison, 1994; Roberson, 1990; Taber & Alliger, 1995; Vallacher & Wegner, 1987; Wrzesniewski & Dutton, 2001). Weick described how firefighters in the

---

[3]The actions that compose tasks can also be physical, psychological, and social (Wong & Campion, 1991). In studying personal projects, we can examine the physical, psychological, and social activities that are salient to the employee. For example, Taber and Alliger (1995) provided an informative demonstration of this idea by asking employees to describe what they are doing in different tasks. This suggests that employees may sometimes devote the majority of their time and attention to particular types of projects and expend little energy and effort on others.

[4]Respondents were asked in the project dump to list both work and nonwork projects. In the PPA matrix, they were asked to select five work and five nonwork projects for closer consideration. The work projects were then classified into nine domains: self-development, managing people, administration, dealing with superiors and colleagues, political and public liaison, financial management, policy or program development, policy or program implementation, and strategic planning. The PPA was also modified to include several dimensions that related directly to the supportiveness, on the one hand, and the hindrance of the organization climate, on the other hand.

Mann Gulch disaster perished because they refused to drop their tools as they attempted to escape from an unmanageable fire:

> Thus, when I ask why firefighters keep their tools and lose their lives, I may be posing the issue in a way that precludes a meaningful answer. My question fails to address their ready-to-hand mode in which tools disappear into equipment defined by its use and availableness … . If I want them to drop their tools, then I need to understand what *their* project is and then intervene in a manner that changes that project convincingly. If they are unable to see beyond their project of fire suppression, then perhaps the leader has to stop that project cold, create a defining moment, confirm that they face an exploding fire, and reset the project clearly and firmly as a race. And if the project of a race replaces the project of suppression, then speed and lightness and rapid movement toward a safe zone become the new relevancies, and anything that interferes with the project of a race now becomes visible and is discarded … . Some holdover from their prior project of suppression, or some inability or unwillingness to shift projects under pressure, may constitute absorbed coping in the world of a wall of fire. (Weick, 1999, p. 137)

This example illustrates that personal projects, not merely formal organizational projects, play an important role in shaping the meaning of an employee's actions. Firefighters clung to their role identities and defined their projects in terms of suppressing the fire. Alternatively, changing the project to escaping the fire may have transformed the meaning of their actions and saved their lives. Even for those who are not literally putting out fires, the capacity to shift perspectives on one's project in the heat of the moment may well be salutary. A key aspect of this capacity is the extent to which one has committed to a particular course of action (Staw, 1997). Indeed, the subtleties of how people commit to projects in the first place, what keeps them motivated to carry out their projects, and how they divest themselves of ones that are not going well are central topics in contemporary research on projects in organizational life (Goodine, 2000).

Further, just as Hackman and Oldham (1980) conducted job design research to ascertain the characteristics of meaningful work by analyzing data at the job level, analysis at the project level can be used to consider the characteristics of meaningful projects. Hackman and Oldham (1980) found that three core job characteristics influenced employees' experiences of meaning. One of these is task identity, the extent to which individuals were working on a whole and identifiable piece of work from start to finish. Are the same characteristics important at the project level, or do other factors emerge as crucial? Does Emily need to feel that each of her projects is a whole, identifiable piece of work that she works on from beginning to end? Does she only need a project or two to meet this standard? Or does she need to feel that her projects combine to provide her work with a clear identity? The project level of analysis lends itself to these types of questions that—although important—have been largely neglected in organizational research.

Project Cross-Impact.   In an age of multitasking, organizational researchers have devoted surprisingly little attention to understanding how individuals manage multiple activities and competing demands (Ashford & Northcraft, 2003; Locke & Latham, 1990; see also Riediger, chap. 4, this volume; Shah, Friedman, & Kruglanski, 2002). The personal project offers one potential remedy to this conundrum. The cross-impact matrix in PPA asks individuals to evaluate the impact that their projects have on each other. In an examination of an employee's project system, this technique can be used to investigate the ways in which one project hinders another, a second project advances another, and so forth. For instance, Robert's project of "keeping his boss at bay" has a strong negative impact on the rest of his projects; he is so frequently attending to his corrosive relationship with his boss that he cannot effectively manage the rest of his work.

The main cross-impact challenges may not lie within work projects, but rather as spillover effects from work to the rest of one's life, or vice versa (see Rothbard, 2001). For instance, does Emily's stress in helping her mother get adjusted to a nursing home affect how she goes about her projects at work, or her desire to become more involved in her community? For Robert, who is hoping to retire soon, is the finding that his work projects have a strong negative impact on his other projects an encouraging sign that he will make a successful transition to retirement? Research applying the cross-impact matrix to investigate the interactions of project pursuit in individuals' work, home, and community lives has gone beyond time management implications to health and other effects. For instance, Karoly and Ruehlman (1996) found that conflict between personal work goals and other personal goals predicted the amount of pain that managers experienced. In a variety of ways then, personal projects can be used to understand the interrelations between different domains of work and life and to inform policy discussions around work–life balance.

Projects in Context: "How Are Things Going Around Here?"

One explanation for Emily's ability to get on with and actually enjoy her projects at work may be that she has the benefit of a supportive organizational climate. Organizations are certainly "strong" situations that have a considerable effect on employees' behaviors and perceptions of their contexts (Davis-Blake & Pfeffer, 1989; cf. House, Shane, & Herold, 1996; Staw & Cohen-Charash, 2005). As units of analysis, personal projects capture what individuals think they are doing in the context of their social ecology and thus inherently integrate persons and situations into measurement. Accordingly, personal projects have been used to understand the effects of organizational climate on employees.

In the 1990s, much of the work on gender differences in the organizational science literature focused on glass ceilings and chilly climates—in particular, the notion that climates in many large organizations were less welcoming for women than men. It was in this context that Phillips et al. (1996, 1997) examined the relations between organizational climate and 112 managers' perceptions of their projects in the Canadian government, anticipating that there would be significant gender differences in how the climate was described and experienced.

Gender differences were indeed found, but not as expected. Although the climate was not described in significantly different ways by male and female managers (controlling for level in the organization), the relation between women's perceptions of the climate and perceptions of their personal projects was more than three times stronger than the relation for men. That is, women managers' feelings about their projects at work were far more sensitive to the organizational climate than men's. This could be seen as a gender effect—that women are more attuned to their environments—or as a gendered acculturation or newcomer effect (Stewart, 1982). As minorities in the senior ranks of the organization who were both younger and newer to their positions than their male colleagues, it was probably advantageous for women to be highly attentive to the norms of conduct in the organization. As Maier and Brunstein (2001) argued, "a mismatch between personal goals and behavioral opportunities at the workplace may impair newcomers' satisfaction and organizational commitment" (p. 1039; see also Rollag, 2004).[5]

---

[5]Further support for this acculturation effect was provided by examining the linkage effect in two municipal governments and a high-tech firm. In the two municipal governments, where women were not numerical minorities, the project–climate linkage effect decreased considerably. In the high-tech firm, where the proportion of women was even lower than in the original federal government study, the linkage effect increased (Phillips et al., 1997).

Projects and Outcomes: "How Did You Do?"

Satisfaction and performance are perhaps the two most widely studied dependent variables in organizational behavior research. Particular attention has been devoted to the nature, causes, and boundary conditions of the relation between satisfaction and performance, sometimes described as the Holy Grail of industrial-organizational psychology (Landy, 1989). Evidence on the relation between satisfaction and performance is mixed, however, indicating that this relation is sometimes positive, sometimes negative, and sometimes nonexistent (for reviews, see Cropanzano & Wright, 2001; Fisher, 2003; Judge, Thoresen, Bono, & Patton, 2001). In organizational research, the personal project unit opens several new doors for understanding important questions about the determinants of satisfaction and performance as outcome variables. Further, personal projects can be used as more than predictors of other outcome measures; rather, they can be treated as outcome measures themselves.

Projects Predicting Job Satisfaction.   The central tenet of the social ecological model is that well-being depends on the sustainable pursuit of core personal projects (Little, 2000). Job satisfaction is perhaps the most common measure of well-being at work (Weiss, 2002), and both well-being and job satisfaction were among the earliest foci of research adopting personal projects methods (Slack-Appotive, 1982; Yard, 1980). These studies clearly indicated that project control, efficacy, and absence of stress were key correlates of well-being and satisfaction at work.

     More recent research has examined the effect of goal or project achievement on job satisfaction.[6] For example, Harris, Daniels, and Briner (2003) conducted a daily diary study and found that successful attainment of personal goals at work was associated with higher positive

---

[6]Job satisfaction is, of course, not the only relevant measure of subjective well-being in the organizational context. Salmela-Aro and Nurmi (2004) found that burnout increased with excessively high levels of work commitment, measured in terms of the number of personal work goals. Karoly and Ruehlman (1996) found that emotional arousal, self-criticism, and goal conflict in personal goals was a significant predictor of managers' anxiety levels. Christiansen, Backman, Little, and Nguyen (1999) found that employees who perceived their projects as low in stress, high in positive cross-impact, congruent with their identities, and likely to progress successfully reported higher levels of subjective well-being. Finally, Pichanick (2003) provided a clear example of how the construal of personal projects at work may impact aspects of human flourishing. She showed that well-being was higher among hospital workers who saw their projects as providing personal growth, rather than familiar routine, and who actively pursued projects rather than passively waiting for assignments.

affect activation at the end of the day. The relation between goal achievement and positive affect was moderated by goal importance, however,
such that the relation was most robust when the individuals found the
goals personally important. As Pomaki and Maes (in press) also demonstrate, the relation between goal achievement and work-related well-being is not a simple one. In a longitudinal study of nurses, they reveal an
adaptive self-regulatory process at play in which perceived controllability over and efficacy in personal goals moderated the effect of goal attainment on job satisfaction, emotional exhaustion, and work stress.
When employees perceived their goals as controllable and likely to succeed, goal attainment increased satisfaction and decreased exhaustion
and stress. When employees perceived their goals as uncontrollable and
unlikely to succeed, goal attainment decreased satisfaction and
increased exhaustion and stress.

Another important theme in recent research has been the importance
of commitment in project pursuit. Roberson (1989, 1990) found that
goal commitment was related to frequency of goal-directed behaviors
and to job satisfaction. Similarly, Goodine (2000) found that project commitment mediated the positive relation between competence and work
satisfaction; executives in her study who felt competent in and committed to their projects tended to be highly satisfied with their work. Finally,
as Phillips et al. (1996, 1997) showed, the routes to job satisfaction
through project pursuit may differ somewhat by gender. In their study of
managers in the public sector, they found that for women, the most important factors promoting job satisfaction were the support of coworkers, supervisors, and the organizational climate (producing a sense that
"we're in this together"). Although support was not unimportant for male
managers, a substantially more important factor was the perceived absence of impedance ("just get out of my way").

The differential role of support can be further understood in relation
to perceptions of project control (see also Bell & Staw, 1989). Although
for both men and women managers a sense of control over work projects was positively correlated with work satisfaction, for men, control
was highly correlated with support, whereas for women, control and
support were not closely related (Phillips et al., 1996, 1997). This may
mean that "the strategy for men is first to achieve control over their projects and then to build or bring along support of others in the organization. Women, in contrast, tend to seek out and value organizational
support even if they do not control a project" (Phillips et al., 1996, p.
33). The implication is that a work environment in which there is an ab-

sence of collegial and cultural support may have a more deleterious effect on women's work-related well-being than on that of men. The fact that Emily may work in a supportive team may be of considerable consequence then. The fact that Robert is blocked at every turn, similarly, may be a key factor in understanding his bitterness.

Projects Predicting Performance.   Whereas job satisfaction research focuses on subjective experience, performance is concerned with behavior and its value to the organization. Georgopoulos, Mahoney, and Jones (1957) conducted what appears to be the earliest study of employees' personal work goals and performance. They found that employees were more productive when they saw productivity as a path toward achieving their personal goals, there were few barriers to following this path, and their personal goals were salient and important to them. Thus, it seems to be not only the saliency of personal projects or goals, but also how they are construed, that matters. More recently, Audia, Kristof-Brown, Brown, and Locke (1996) conducted an ambitious laboratory experiment observing work processes and outcomes and assessing the personal goals of individuals performing a multistage assembly task. They found that when individuals set quantity goals, they were more likely to utilize work processes that allowed them to increase their production output during the work stages. Further, setting process goals predicted a higher number of process changes but lower levels of performance than setting outcome goals.

Here, too, organizational contexts have an effect. Probst, Baxley, Schell, Cleghorn, and Bogdewic (1998) found that residents and staff members in a family medicine program who perceived that their organizations supported autonomy and progress toward personal goals were rated as more effective in their teaching.[7] Their findings indicate that the organizational contexts in which personal projects and goals are carried out can play an important role in influencing employee performance.

As research indicates, there is also a temporal dimension to the relation of projects and goals to performance outcomes. Focusing on academic research projects, Daft, Griffin, and Yates (1987) interviewed researchers about their significant (those that received awards; high ci-

---

[7]See also Barrick, Mount, and Strauss (1993), who found that the effect of conscientiousness on job performance was mediated by autonomous goal setting and goal commitment. VandeWalle, Brown, Cron, and Slocum (1999) conducted a study of the personal goals and performance of salespeople. They found that goal intentions (level, planning, and effort) predicted sales performance, and that personal goals mediated the effect of goal orientation on performance.

tation counts; and favorable responses from colleagues, reviewers, and readers) and insignificant research projects. They found considerable variation by project stage. Significant projects were characterized by low levels of clarity and certainty in beginning stages, high excitement and commitment throughout, and the reduction of equivocality or uncertainty during the process.[8]

Finally, personal projects have been used to predict team performance as well as individual performance. Grant (2003) conducted a longitudinal study of 22 publishing teams. The teams ranged in size from two to seven members, and each team was charged with revamping, rewriting, and reorganizing a book in the span of 3 months. Grant asked the editors and associate editors who comprised these teams to generate and rate their work projects on a series of dimensions, and also asked these employees to treat their work overall as a superordinate project and rate it on the same dimensions. Because one objective of this research was to predict each team's performance in the superordinate project of creating a book, supervisors evaluated the performance of each team in this project.[9] The commitment of team leaders to this superordinate project early in the work process was a strong positive predictor of the final overall effectiveness of the entire team. Thus, Grant (2003) found that individuals' project perceptions can be predictive of the performance of teams.[10]

Projects as Outcomes.   In some cases, the assessment of project pursuit is more than a predictor of performance, satisfaction, or other indicators of well-being; it is itself an outcome measure. Such measurement, as we illustrate, has been undertaken at the system, the domain, and the dimensions levels. At the system level, we might ask what effects

---

[8]Another outcome variable studied in relation to personal projects and work is success in finding jobs. Nurmi, Salmela-Aro, and Koivisto (2002) studied individuals in the transition to jobs from vocational school. They found that the greater their emphases on personal work goals, and the greater their perceptions of progress toward achieving personal work goals, the more likely the students were to find a job that matched their education and the less likely they were to be unemployed. Individuals who found a job that matched their education later rated their work goals as highly achievable and as stimulating positive emotions; individuals who were unemployed saw their work goals as less achievable and less related to positive emotions.

[9]Along these lines, Kristof-Brown and Stevens (2001) conducted a study to demonstrate the utility of examining the personal goals of individuals in project teams. They found that congruence in members' perceptions of performance goals was associated with higher satisfaction and contributions, and the strength of mastery or learning goals was an even stronger predictor of individual satisfaction.

[10]Future research should take into account the hierarchical structure of projects. Analytical methods such as hierarchical linear modeling make it possible to understand projects at different levels, from the microlevel of personal projects, to the mesolevel of dyadic, team, and group projects, to the macrolevel of departmental, organizational, and industry projects.

certain kinds of interventions, such as attempts at burnout prevention or the redesign of work, have on project pursuit. Salmela-Aro, Näätänen, and Nurmi (2004), for example, conducted a longitudinal study on the effects of two psychotherapy interventions on burnout and work personal projects. Measures of burnout were one obvious outcome measure, and the interventions did decrease burnout. However, the interventions also had interesting effects on personal projects. Compared to participants in a control group, participants in the intervention group showed an increase in perceived progress on personal projects, social support for personal projects, and effectiveness in managing emotions related to personal projects. The decrease in burnout was particularly significant for the participants who experienced a reduction in negative emotions in projects.

An alternative approach is to consider whether certain factors or interventions affect project pursuit in a particular domain. For example, in assessing the performance of a work team, a key measure undoubtedly relates to the quality of its output, but how well individuals work together as a team is also an important measure (Hackman, 1987). What enables employees to be effective in the interpersonal projects involved in teamwork? In addressing this question in his study of publishing teams, Grant (2003) used supervisor ratings of employee effectiveness in a specific project domain (interpersonal projects) as measures of performance. Although commitment of the team leader was predictive of team performance in the collective, superordinate project, Grant found that commitment was not related to performance in interpersonal projects at the individual level of analysis. Rather, a different set of factors predicted effectiveness for interpersonal projects. Team members who rated their interpersonal projects as beneficial to themselves and to others were seen by their supervisors as being effective in interpersonal projects. Notably, these factors did not turn out to be significant predictors of overall individual performance; they were only predictive of individual performance in interpersonal projects. This finding suggests that different factors may enable effective performance at different levels and in different domains of analysis.

Scaling Up: From Personal to Organizational Projects

As organizational science naturally reminds us, projects are not merely personal. We have made a careful and important distinction between personal and formal, organizational projects. Nevertheless, the projects methodology can be used to study the latter, thereby crossing, levels of analysis, as Hackman (2003) urged us to do. An illustration of the use of PPA to scale up to organizational projects is a study of 33 women's social movement organizations (Phillips, 1992). A key issue at this level of analysis is whose projects we are measuring. When different respondents rate their organization's projects, they might have quite disparate understandings of what these projects are in the first place, making any further analysis difficult. However, Phillips (1992) found quite remarkable independent consensus between the senior staff and elected board members of these women's groups regarding what constituted the project systems of their organizations. As with personal projects, organizational projects were classified by domains appropriate to this type of organization (e.g., lobbying and advocacy, image building, membership service, fund raising, etc.) and were compared on project factors similar to those derived for the analysis of personal projects. What stood out for these types of organizations were enormous difficulties experienced in one particular domain—fund raising—that was low in efficacy, support, and visibility, and particularly high in stress.

In organizational science, there is obviously considerable opportunity for taking such an approach much further. For instance, the projects methodology could be used to compare members' or employees' ideal or "ought" projects—what they think their collective's or their organization's projects could or should be—with their perceptions of what its core projects actually are. This may reveal important information about the sources of the organization's progress, satisfaction, and discontent. In addition, this approach could be adapted to study the interdependencies of group members' pursuits by applying the cross-impact matrix to understand how employees support and undermine each other's projects.

WHEN ORGANIZATIONS BECOME PROJECTS: NEW DIRECTIONS AND APPLIED RESEARCH

We have explored the implications of the project unit of measurement for understanding organizational behavior. The illustrations provided in this chapter suggest that personal projects offer several advantages in organizational research. First, projects can be fruitful in predicting outcomes of relevance to individuals and organizations. Second, they can be measured as outcomes of relevance to individuals and organizations. Third, in line with Hackman's (2003) recommendations, projects allow researchers to cross, span, link, and integrate multiple levels of analysis.

We now turn in a more speculative manner to the applied implications of the project for changing, as well as understanding, organizational behavior. We believe that the distinctions among projects, jobs, groups, and organizations are becoming increasingly blurred. For example, much work is now organized around projects, rather than jobs. An employee's "job" may often be a collection of disparate or sequential projects that are performed under the auspices of an organizational context. In addition, intraorganizational and interorganizational networks and advances in communication allow for project groups to be formed beyond the boundaries of departments and organizations.

Our own work in academia is an instructive example of this phenomenon. Each of our organizational lives is comprised of a collection of research, teaching, writing, advising, consulting, and administrative projects. We collaborate with scholars at universities across the country and the globe, and we form project groups on an ad hoc basis at conferences. This very volume, a work project about projects, fits this description. It was formed across the boundaries of universities, nations, and oceans. Although the book began as a set of individual personal projects, it grew beyond the personal into a dyadic, group, and organizational project.

Our observations about the ways in which projects have affected jobs, groups, and organizations give rise to ideas for redesigning work that venture beyond understanding, predicting, and explaining organizational phenomena into the territory of change. Rather than merely explaining such change, how can project redesign help individuals, groups, and organizations accommodate to the newly project-oriented world of work?

From Job Redesign to Project Redesign

According to Hackman and Oldham (1980), due to the challenges of changing the person and the context, redesigning the job is more feasible. However, researchers have found that restructuring an entire job is also challenging, and it often entails trade-offs between individual and organizational objectives, particularly in terms of satisfaction and performance (Morgeson & Campion, 2002).

Imagine that we were to promise to the CEO of an automotive company that we could enhance car quality and employee satisfaction by redesigning jobs to provide employees with task identity. Each employee will work on a whole car, rather than merely a small component. That CEO has no doubt that the employees will be more motivated, satisfied, and careful, as various experiments in such forms of production have shown (Maccoby, 1997), but would probably reject our proposal. Even if the quality of the company's products increased, the concern would be that decreased productivity might cause the quantity to suffer drastically. Relinquishing the efficiency of specialization and division of labor would entail considerable organizational sacrifices in terms of profitability. The redesign of work thus poses a conundrum, particularly once we move from standardized production lines to more complex work environments. How is it possible for an organization to improve employees' work experiences without sacrificing its performance objectives?[11]

We propose project redesign interventions as a potential solution to this dilemma. The project is a tractable construct (Little, 2000); people regularly change, complete, and discard existing projects, and adopt new ones. Project redesign may involve the adoption of new projects or the tweaking of some aspects of existing ones. As such, it may be more feasible to redesign individuals' projects than their entire jobs, which are considerably less malleable. Instead of redesigning Robert's entire job, we can examine his system of projects to determine which projects are most flexible. We might begin by determining whether we can eliminate any of his most stressful or frustrating projects without undermining his performance. We could also encourage him to proactively take on extrarole projects that benefit others and the organization (see Grant, in press) without detracting from assigned responsibilities. Project redesign is a practical alternative to job redesign that may facilitate the improvement of individuals' work experiences without detracting from their performance.

CONCLUSION

We have pursued several projects in this chapter. First, we described potential advantages of personal projects over the traditional units of tasks

---

[11] Task redesign may be a viable alternative to job redesign. However, we see two problems with this idea. First, like jobs, tasks are often designed toward optimal efficiency. The redesign of tasks thus faces constraints similar to the aforementioned limitations of job redesign. Second, because an individual's work often subsumes a large number of tasks, the practical challenges of redesigning a large enough proportion of tasks to make a difference would likely be overwhelming.

and jobs. Second, we reviewed existing research relevant to personal projects at work. These studies illustrate the relevance of personal projects to understanding the nature, the contexts, and the outcomes of work. Third, we discussed new directions for the project in a changing world of work.

By applying the project unit of measurement to organizational research, we begin to understand the complexities, intricacies, and nuances of Emily's and Robert's thoughts, moods, preferences, and behaviors at work. The social ecological framework within which projects have a central role accords a place for stable trait influences and stable contextual elements (Little, 2000). More important, it calls attention to the way in which projects are in dynamic interaction with both of these sources of influence and offers a way in which some traction might be gained in trying to enhance the quality of lives in organizations.

The framework also calls attention to the small, but potentially vital exceptions to the general trend of an individual's stance toward work. Emily may be a delightfully engaged and productive employee, but we should be alert to any project that might serve as a tipping point for overall system change. For example, buoyant as she may be, to really understand Emily, we need to be aware of the continuing importance of her "take care of Mom" project or the newfound saliency of her "take care of my health" project. Like many core interpersonal projects, they may pulse into significance at unpredictable times, putting both Emily and her work team at risk.

What about Bob? Although Robert might be known throughout his organization as a miserable, bitter old man, a close friend may see a side of him that only emerges when he is engaged in certain projects; these pursuits, despite his overall misery at work, help him to muddle through. These projects may be furtive or far out, but they may also form the foundation for his retirement years. Were Robert to let his guard down and let Bob emerge occasionally, or were the climate of his firm to engender greater openness, his core projects might have a chance to be enacted before the day his coworkers toast his departure with raised glasses and strained smiles.

In the final analysis, personal projects provide meaning, structure, and community in the lives of people in organizations, and they also have impacts on those organizations. Personal projects, in short, are acts that have impacts and leave imprints. Personal projects, in this sense, are not merely personal. They are the connective tissue that keeps organizations functioning, for better or for worse.

REFERENCES

Argyle, M., & Little, B. R. (1972). Do personality traits apply to social behaviour? *Journal for the Theory of Social Behaviour, 2,* 1–35.

Ashford, S. J., & Northcraft, G. (2003). Robbing Peter to pay Paul: Feedback environments and enacted priorities in response to competing task demands. *Human Resource Management Review, 13,* 537–559.

Ashkanasy, N., Wilderom, C., & Peterson, M. F. (Eds.). (2000). *Handbook of organizational culture and climate.* Thousand Oaks, CA: Sage.

Audia, G., Kristof-Brown, A., Brown, K. G., & Locke, E. A. (1996). Relationship of goals and micro level work processes to performance on a multi-path manual task. *Journal of Applied Psychology, 81,* 483–497.

Austin, J. T., & Vancouver, J. B. (1996). Goal constructs in psychology: Structure, process, and content. *Psychological Bulletin, 120,* 338–375.

Barrick, M. R., Mount, M. K., & Strauss, J. P. (1993). Conscientiousness and performance of sales representatives: Test of the mediating effects of goal setting. *Journal of Applied Psychology, 78,* 715–722.

Bell, N. E., & Staw, B. M. (1989). People as sculptors versus sculpture: The roles of personality and personal control in organizations. In M. B. Arthur, D. T. Hall, & B. S. Lawrence (Eds.), *Handbook of career theory* (pp. 634–643). New York: Cambridge University Press.

Caplan, R. D. (1987). Person–environment fit theory and organizations: Commensurate dimensions, time perspectives, and mechanisms. *Journal of Vocational Behavior, 31,* 248–267.

Christiansen, C. H., Backman, C., Little, B. R., & Nguyen, A. (1999). Occupations and well-being: A study of personal projects. *American Journal of Occupational Therapy, 53,* 91–100.

Cropanzano, R., James, K., & Citera, M. (1993). A goal-hierarchy model of personality, motivation, and leadership. *Research in Organizational Behavior, 15,* 267–322.

Cropanzano, R., & Wright, T. A. (2001). When a "happy" worker is really a "productive" worker: A review and further refinement of the happy-productive worker thesis. *Consulting Psychology Journal: Practice & Research, 53,* 182–199.

Daft, R. V., Griffin, R. W., & Yates, V. (1987). Retrospective accounts of research factors associated with significant and not-so-significant research outcomes. *Academy of Management Journal, 30,* 763–785.

Danna, K., & Griffin, R. W. (1999). Health and well-being in the workplace: A review and synthesis of the literature. *Journal of Management, 25,* 357–384.

Davis-Blake, A., & Pfeffer, J. (1989). Just a mirage: The search for dispositional effects in organizational research. *Academy of Management Review, 14,* 385–400.

Elliot, A. J., Sheldon, K. M., & Church, M. A. (1997). Avoidance personal goals and subjective well-being. *Personality and Social Psychology Bulletin, 23,* 915–927.

Fisher, C. D. (2003). Why do lay people believe that satisfaction and performance are correlated? Possible sources of a commonsense theory. *Journal of Organizational Behavior, 24,* 753–777.

Frost, P. J. (2003). *Toxic emotions at work: How compassionate managers handle pain and conflict.* Boston: Harvard Business School Press.

Georgopoulos, B. S., Mahoney, G. M., & Jones, N. W., Jr. (1957). A path-goal approach to productivity. *Journal of Applied Psychology, 41,* 345–353.

Gerhart, B., & Rynes, S. L. (2003). *Compensation: Theory, evidence and strategic implications.* Thousand Oaks, CA: Sage.

Gerstner, C. R., & Day, D. V. (1997). Meta-analytic review of leader–member exchange theory: Correlates and consequences. *Journal of Applied Psychology, 82*, 827–844.

Goodine, L. A. (2000). An analysis of personal project commitment (Doctoral dissertation, Carleton University, 2000). *Dissertation Abstracts International, 61*(4-B), 2260.

Grant, A. M. (2003). *Working hard, or hardly working? Predicting group, individual, and project effectiveness at work.* Unpublished bachelor's thesis, Harvard University, Cambridge, MA.

Grant, A. M. (in press). Relational job design and the motivation to make a prosocial difference. *Academy of Management Review.*

Griffin, R. W. (1987). Toward an integrated theory of task design. *Research in Organizational Behavior, 9*, 79–120.

Hackman, J. R. (1985). Doing research that makes a difference. In E. E. Lawler, A. M. Mohrman, S. A. Mohrman, G. E. Ledford, & T. G. Cummings (Eds.), *Doing research that is useful for theory and practice* (pp. 126–175). San Francisco: Jossey-Bass.

Hackman, J. R. (1987). The design of work teams. In J. Lorsch (Ed.), *Handbook of organizational behavior* (pp. 315–342). Englewood Cliffs, NJ: Prentice-Hall.

Hackman, J. R. (2003). Learning more by crossing levels: Evidence from airplanes, orchestras, and hospitals. *Journal of Organizational Behavior, 24*, 1–18.

Hackman, J. R., & Oldham, G. (1980). *Work redesign.* Reading, MA: Addison-Wesley.

Harris, C., Daniels, K., & Briner, R. (2003). A daily diary study of goals and affective well-being at work. *Journal of Occupational and Organizational Psychology, 76*, 401–410.

House, R. J., Shane, S. A., & Herold, D. M. (1996). Rumors of the death of dispositional research are vastly exaggerated. *Academy of Management Review, 21*, 203–224.

Ilgen, D. R., & Hollenbeck, J. R. (1992). The structure of work: Job design and roles. In M. Dunnette & L. Hough (Eds.), *Handbook of industrial and organizational psychology* (pp. 165–207). Palo Alto, CA: Consulting Psychologists Press.

Judge, T. A., Heller, D., & Mount, M. K. (2002). Five-factor model of personality and job satisfaction. *Journal of Applied Psychology, 87*, 530–541.

Judge, T. A., Thoresen, C. J., Bono, J. E., & Patton, G. K. (2001). The job satisfaction–job performance relationship: A qualitative and quantitative review. *Psychological Bulletin, 127*, 376–407.

Karasek, R., & Theorell, T. (1990). *Healthy work: Stress, productivity and the reconstruction of working life.* New York: Basic Books.

Karoly, P., & Ruehlman, L. S. (1996). Motivational implications of pain: Chronicity, psychological distress, and work goal construal in a national sample of adults. *Health Psychology, 15*, 383–390.

Katz, D., & Kahn, R. L. (1978). *The social psychology of organizations* (2nd ed.). New York: Wiley.

Kristof-Brown, A. L., & Stevens, C. K. (2001). Goal congruence in project teams: Does the fit between members' personal mastery and performance goals matter? *Journal of Applied Psychology, 86*, 1083–1095.

Landy, F. J. (1989). *Psychology of work behavior.* Pacific Grove, CA: Brooks/Cole.

Little, B. R. (1983). Personal projects: A rationale and method for investigation. *Environment and Behavior, 15*, 273–309.

Little, B. R. (1987). Personality and the environment. In D. Stokols & I. Altman (Eds.), *Handbook of environmental psychology* (Vol. 1, pp. 206–244). New York: Wiley.

Little, B. R. (1989). Personal projects analysis: Trivial pursuits, magnificent obsessions, and the search for coherence. In D. M. Buss & N. Cantor (Eds.), *Personality psychology: Recent trends and emerging directions* (pp. 15–31). New York: Springer-Verlag.

Little, B. R. (2000). Free traits and personal contexts: Expanding a social ecological model of well-being. In W. B. Walsh, K. H. Craik, & R. H. Price (Eds.), *Person–environment psychology: New directions and perspectives* (2nd ed., pp. 87–116). Mahwah, NJ: Lawrence Erlbaum Associates.

Little, B. R., & Chambers, N. C. (2004). Personal project pursuit: On human doings and well beings. In W. M. Cox & E. Klinger (Eds.), *Handbook of motivational counseling: Concepts, approaches, and assessment* (pp. 65–82). London: Wiley.

Little, B. R., Lecci, L., & Watkinson, B. (1992). Personality and personal projects: Linking big five and PAC units of analysis. *Journal of Personality, 60,* 501–525.

Locke, E. A., & Latham, G. P. (1990). *A theory of goal setting and task performance.* Englewood Cliffs, NJ: Prentice-Hall.

Locke, E. A., & Latham, G. P. (2002). Building a practically useful theory of goal setting and task motivation: A 35-year odyssey. *American Psychologist, 57,* 705–717.

Maccoby, M. (1997, November–December). Is there a better way to build a car? *Harvard Business Review, 161–170.*

Magnusson, D. (1999). Holistic interactionism: A perspective for research on personality development. In L. A. Pervin & O. P. John (Eds.), *Handbook of personality: Theory and research* (2nd ed., pp. 219–247). New York: Guilford.

Maier, G. W., & Brunstein, J. C. (2001). The role of personal work goals in newcomers' job satisfaction and organizational commitment: A longitudinal analysis. *Journal of Applied Psychology, 86,* 1034–1042.

Mintzberg, H. (1973). *The nature of managerial work.* New York: Harper & Row.

Mischel, W. (2004). Toward an integrative science of the person. *Annual Review of Psychology, 55,* 1–22.

Morgeson, F. P., & Campion, M. A. (2002). Avoiding tradeoffs when redesigning work: Evidence from a longitudinal quasi-experiment. *Personnel Psychology, 55,* 589–612.

Morrison, E. W. (1994). Role definitions and organizational citizenship behavior: The importance of employee's perspective. *Academy of Management Journal, 37,* 1543–1567.

Nurmi, J.-E., Salmela-Aro, K., & Koivisto, P. (2002). Goal importance, and related agency-beliefs and emotions during the transition from vocational school to work: Antecedents and consequences. *Journal of Vocational Behavior, 60,* 241–261.

Ostroff, C. (1993). The effects of climate and personal influences on individual behavior and attitudes in organizations. *Organizational Behavior and Human Decision Processes, 56,* 56–60.

Parker, S. K., Wall, T. D., & Jackson, P. R. (1997). "That's not my job": Developing flexible employee work orientations. *Academy of Management Journal, 40,* 899–929.

Pervin, L. A. (1989). Persons, situations, interactions: The history of a controversy and a discussion of theoretical models. *Academy of Management Review, 14,* 350–360.

Phillips, S. D. (1992). Projects, pressure and perceptions of effectiveness: An organizational analysis of national Canadian women's groups (Doctoral dissertation, Carleton University, 1990). *Dissertation Abstracts International, 52*(11-A), 4075.

Phillips, S. D., Little, B. R., & Goodine, L. A. (1996). Organizational climate and personal projects: Gender differences in the public service (Research Paper No. 20, Canadian Centre for Management Development). Ottawa, ON, Canada: Minister of Supply and Services.

Phillips, S. D., Little, B. R., & Goodine, L. A. (1997). Reconsidering gender and public administration: Five steps beyond conventional research. *Canadian Journal of Public Administration, 40,* 563–581.

Pichanick, J. S. (2003). The regulation of well-being: Growth and action orientations (Doctoral dissertation, Harvard University, 2003). *Dissertation Abstracts International, 64*(5-A), 1739.

Pomaki, G., & Maes, S. (2002). Predicting quality of work life: From work conditions to self-regulation. In E. Gullone & R. A. Cummins (Eds.), *The universality of subjective wellbeing indicators* (pp. 151–173). Dordrecht, Netherlands: Kluwer.

Pomaki, G., & Maes, S. (in press). Beneficial and detrimental effects of goal attainment and goal disengagement on nurses' well-being. *Applied Psychology: An International Review.*

Pomaki, G., Maes, S., & ter Doest, L. (2004). Work conditions and employees' self-set goals: Goal processes enhance prediction of psychological distress and well-being. *Personality and Social Psychology Bulletin, 30,* 685–694.

Pratt, M. G. (2000). The good, the bad, and the ambivalent: Managing identification among Amway distributors. *Administrative Science Quarterly, 45,* 456–493.

Probst, J. C., Baxley, E. G., Schell, B. J., Cleghorn, G. D., & Bogdewic, S. P. (1998). Organizational environment and perceptions of teaching quality in seven South Carolina family medicine residency programs. *Academic Medicine, 73,* 887–893.

Roberson, L. (1989). Assessing personal work goals in the organizational setting: Development and evaluation of the Work Concerns Inventory. *Organizational Behavior and Human Decision Processes, 44,* 345–367.

Roberson, L. (1990). Prediction of job satisfaction from characteristics of personal work goals. *Journal of Organizational Behavior, 11,* 29–41.

Roberson, L., Houston, J. M., & Diddams, M. D. (1989). Identifying valued work outcomes through a content analysis of personal goals. *Journal of Vocational Behavior, 35,* 30–45.

Rollag, K. (2004). The impact of relative tenure on newcomer socialization dynamics. *Journal of Organizational Behavior, 25,* 283–872.

Rothbard, N. P. (2001). Enriching or depleting? The dynamics of engagement in work and family roles. *Administrative Science Quarterly, 46,* 655–684.

Rousseau, D. M. (1978). Characteristics of departments, positions, and individuals: Contexts for attitudes and behavior. *Administrative Science Quarterly, 23,* 521–540.

Salancik, G. R., & Pfeffer, J. (1978). A social information processing approach to job attitudes and task design. *Administrative Science Quarterly, 23,* 224–253.

Salmela-Aro, K., Näätänen, P., & Nurmi, J.-E. (2004). The role of work-related personal projects during two burnout interventions: A longitudinal study. *Work & Stress, 18,* 208–230.

Salmela-Aro, K., & Nurmi, J.-E. (2004). Employees' motivational orientations and well-being at work. *Journal of Change Management, 17,* 471–489.

Schwarz, N. (1999). Self-reports: How the questions shape the answers. *American Psychologist, 54,* 93–105.

Shah, J. Y., Friedman, R., & Kruglanski, A. W. (2002). Forgetting all else: On the antecedents and consequents of goal shielding. *Journal of Personality and Social Psychology, 83,* 1261–1280.

Slack-Appotive, S. (1982). *Sex differences in the relationship between personal projects and job satisfaction.* Unpublished master's thesis, Carleton University, Ottawa, ON, Canada.

Staw, B. M. (1997). The escalation of commitment: An update and appraisal. In Z. Shapira (Ed.), *Organizational decision making* (pp. 191–215). New York: Cambridge University Press.

Staw, B. M., & Cohen-Charash, Y. (2005). The dispositional approach to job satisfaction: More than a mirage, but not yet an oasis. *Journal of Organizational Behavior, 26,* 59–78.

Stewart, A. J. (1982). The course of individual adaptation to life change. *Journal of Personality and Social Psychology, 42,* 1100–1113.

Taber, T. D., & Alliger, G. M. (1995). A task-level assessment of job satisfaction. *Journal of Organizational Behavior, 16,* 101–121.

Thompson, J. (1967). *Organizations in action.* New York: McGraw-Hill.

Thorngate, W. (1976). Possible limits on a science of social behavior. In J. H. Strickland, F. E. Aboud, & K. J. Gergen (Eds.), *Social psychology in transition* (pp. 121–139). New York: Plenum.

Vallacher, R. R., & Wegner, D. M. (1987). What do people think they're doing? Action identification and human behavior. *Psychological Review, 94,* 3–15.

VandeWalle, D., Brown, S. P., Cron, W. L., & Slocum, J. W. (1999). The influence of goal orientation and self-regulation tactics on sales performance: A longitudinal field test. *Journal of Applied Psychology, 84,* 249–259.

Walsh, W. B., Craik, K. H., & Price, R. H. (Eds.). (2000). *Person–environment psychology: New directions and perspectives.* Mahwah, NJ: Lawrence Erlbaum Associates.

Weick, K. E. (1974). Middle range theories of social systems. *Behavioral Science, 19,* 357–367.

Weick, K. E. (1999). That's moving: Theories that matter. *Journal of Management Inquiry, 8,* 134–142.

Weick, K. E. (2004). How projects lose meaning: The dynamics of renewal. In R. Stablein & P. Frost (Eds.), *Renewing research practice* (pp. 183–204). Stanford, CA: Stanford Business Books.

Weiss, H. M. (2002). Deconstructing job satisfaction: Separating evaluations, beliefs and affective experiences. *Human Resource Management Review, 12,* 173–194.

Wong, C. S., & Campion, M. A. (1991). Development and test of a task level model of motivational job design. *Journal of Applied Psychology, 76,* 825–837.

Wrzesniewski, A., & Dutton, J. E. (2001). Crafting a job: Revisioning employees as active crafters of their work. *Academy of Management Review, 26,* 179–201.

Wrzesniewski, A., McCauley, C. R., Rozin, P., & Schwartz, B. (1997). Jobs, careers, and callings: People's relations to their work. *Journal of Research in Personality, 31,* 21–33.

Yard, G. F. (1980). *Personal project system variables as predictors of job satisfaction and performance effectiveness in members of the Royal Canadian Mounted Police.* Unpublished master's thesis, Carleton University, Ottawa, ON, Canada.

9

Differentiating and Integrating Levels of Goal Representation: A Life-Span Perspective

Alexandra M. Freund

When interviewing for a position some years ago, I was asked what my goals were: Where would I want to be in 10 years from now? What kind of research would I want to pursue in the future? What did I want to contribute to the discipline? I had just finished trying to provide answers to these questions on my future goals, when the interviewer asked me something along the following lines: "So, in your research, you focus on goals. I am wondering how much of our lives has anything to do with goals. Most people do not have goals. And even if they do, goals do not predict behavior very well." I was somewhat puzzled by the apparent contradiction—hadn't I just been asked about my goals? Was this just chit-chat or was there something diagnostic about my goals for how well I was suited for the job? Maybe because I was not offered the job or perhaps due to my bewilderment in the situation, the question has become a sort of theme for me since this interview. How much of our lives has anything to do with goals? Are goals constructions that participants in our studies have to build on the spot because we ask them to? Are goals an epiphenomenon, protecting the belief of free will or choice where, in actuality, cognition, behavior, emotions, and motivation are under the control of the environment (e.g., Bargh & Ferguson, 2000; Wegner, 2002)? How do goals develop and how are they embedded into the social context? Finally, do goals predict anything?

LEVELS OF GOALS

In attempting to address some of these questions, I propose a heuristic model of different levels of goals. This model assumes that goals—that is, anticipated states a person, group, or society values as either desirable (approach goals) or undesirable (avoidance goals)—play an important role in individual development. To address the question of how goals influence development, two broad levels of goal representations are distinguished: (a) age-related expectations, and (b) personal goals. Goals are seen as being represented on different levels, only one of which is the person, and not all aspects of goals are consciously represented all of the time.

In this context, the term *level* refers to neither the concreteness of personal goals (e.g., Carver & Scheier, 1999) or personal projects (e.g., Little, 1989), nor to McAdams's (1995) model of three levels of personality (moving from basic personality traits to narrative identities; see Sheldon, chap. 13, this volume, for expanding this framework to include an organismic foundation of personality), nor to Little's (1996) three tiers of personality, which distinguishes havings, doings, and beings (see also Chambers, chap. 5, this volume, for a linguistic approach to Little's conceptualization of tiers of personality in terms of personal projects analysis). Instead, in the model used here, the term *level* denotes (a) the level of representation of goals in society as norms and expectations and as personal age-related beliefs, (b) personal projects or goals, and (c) nonconscious goals and motives.

On a societal level, goals are represented in the form of *social norms* (Level 1-1) that reflect age-related expectations (e.g., age for starting school) and that inform age-related opportunity structures and goal-relevant resources. *Personal beliefs* (Level 1-2) about the appropriate timing and sequencing of goals are informed but not determined by social norms and expectations. They also reflect individual values and experiences (e.g., appropriate age to start dating). On Level 1, then, goals are represented as social and as personal age-related expectations. The second level denotes the *personal projects* or *goals* (Level 2-1) an individual selects or pursues (e.g., being successful in one's profession). What does a person want to achieve, maintain, or avoid? In addition to consciously represented personal projects or goals, *nonconscious goals* and *motives* (Level 2-2; e.g., achievement motivation) influence behavior and development by organizing behavior over time and situations into meaningful action units.

On each of these levels, goals can be represented as more or less concrete (e.g., the personal goal of being a good person vs. helping the homeless in the soup kitchen every Thursday), and as referring to actions (e.g., social norms about completing high school around the age of 18 years), more general traits (e.g., personal age-related expectations that older people should be generative), or identity (e.g., personal project or goal to feel good about myself). These levels of goals also interact in complex ways. For instance, age-related social expectations might directly influence behavior, which, via self-observational processes, might contribute to conscious personal projects or goals that direct future behavior. The different levels of goals codetermine the direction of development and individual level of functioning. In this chapter, I elaborate on this heuristic model of levels of goals.

Levels of Goals and Their Importance for Development

One of the central assumptions of life-span developmental psychology is that development is a dynamic process involving the interplay of proactively creating and reacting to one's environment (Baltes, 1987; Baltes, Lindenberger, & Staudinger, 2006; Brandtstädter, 1998). The role of a person in his or her development is seen not only in reacting to a changing environment and opportunity structures. Instead, a person also proactively shapes and selects his or her environment. From this perspective, a person is neither seen as only reacting to external stimuli, nor as a closed, self-sufficient system. A person creates an environment as a function of the given social, cultural, and biological constraints in a way that it best fits with his or her personal goals (Lerner & Busch-Rossnagel, 1981). An adequate description of development thus needs to take the social (and physical) environment as well as the active role of the person into account. Figure 9.1 presents how these different levels of analysis are reflected in a model of goals.

In the following sections, each level of goal representation is elaborated in more detail. Note that the levels are not conceptualized as clear-cut categories that show no overlap. Their boundaries are fuzzy

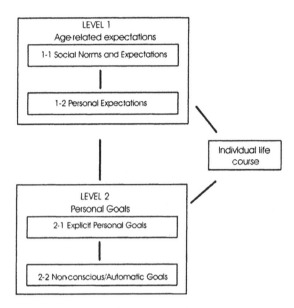

Figure 9.1. Heuristic model of two levels of goal representation influencing the individual life course.

and, moreover, they interact with each other. Together, these levels of goal representation are proposed to guide individual behavior over time and situations.

Age-Related Expectations: Social Norms and Expectations (Level 1)

Age-related expectations are represented on two distinct but interrelated levels, namely on the societal and on the personal level. Both influence individual development.

Social Norms and Expectations as Indicators of Age-Related Resources.   According to Mayer (1986), modern societies are characterized by an institutionalization of the life course. Age-related institutional structures of a society are reflected in social norms and expectations about developmental transitions (e.g., age of starting school). Moreover, social norms and expectations express societal values (e.g., positive evaluation of education) as well as biological conditions such as physical maturation for starting school (Hagestad &

Neugarten, 1985). Age-related norms define on the one hand age limitations for developmental trajectories in the individual life course. On the other hand, they indicate institutional or social opportunity structures such as the age-dependent availability of resources. An example of age-related institutional opportunity structures is the modern school system that typically offers children and adolescents free access to education, whereas this is not true for middle-aged or older adults. In this sense, then, age-related social expectations or norms such as getting a basic education during childhood and adolescence are indicators of the availability of resources in certain life domains for a specific age group (Freund, 2003; Heckhausen, 1999).

Another way in which social norms and expectations influence individual development are social sanctions (e.g., social approval or disapproval) for the appropriate timing of developmental transitions. Social expectations about the age(s) at which a person should or should not do something serve as an orientation for the development, selection, pursuit, and maintenance of personal projects or goals (Cantor, 1994; Freund, 1997; Nurmi, 1992).

Age-Related Social Expectations and Individual Development. Age-related social expectations provide a comparison standard for judging if a person is on time or off time (Neugarten, 1968). Being off time is not necessarily negatively valued. For instance, if the discrepancy from the socially expected timing is advanced, it is often evaluated as positive (e.g., graduating from high school at the age of 16). If a person is delayed in his or her development, the likelihood of negative evaluation is much higher. The result of comparisons with age-related norms or expectations depends on the life domain under consideration and whether the discrepancy implies a gain or a loss (Heckhausen, 1999; Wrosch & Heckhausen, 1999). As a large body of research suggests that people generally avoid negative outcomes of social comparisons (e.g., Wood & Taylor, 1991), it is likely that people strive to set and pursue age-appropriate personal projects or goals that prevent unfavorable social comparisons.

Personal beliefs or expectations about the life course are not independent of generally shared, social expectations. One of the questions that has not yet been studied is the consequence of sharing as compared to opposing social expectations on development. There is, however, some empirical support for the hypothesis that social norms and expectations influence the setting of personal projects or goals (Freund &

Smith, 1999; Staudinger, Freund, Linden, & Maas, 1996). For young adulthood, two central developmental tasks have been identified: work and family. In accordance with these developmental tasks, Settersten and Hagestad (1996a, 1996b) found high social consensus for the expectations of founding a family and starting a career in young adulthood. These social expectations are, in turn, also reflected in personal projects or goals. In a study by Wiese and Freund (2001), most young adults (more than 85%) reported personal projects or goals in the family and work domain. Such high social consensus about the importance of family and work in young adulthood is probably related to the fact that young adults have clear developmental deadlines (Heckhausen, 1999). For instance, in Germany there are official or unofficial institutional regulations about the maximum age for entering certain professional positions. Biological constraints—more clearly on the part of women—pose clear developmental deadlines for fertility. Setting personal projects or goals in accordance with social norms and expectations may in these instances help to take advantage of available resources and also to ensure later access to resources (e.g., to certain jobs).

One of the functions of age-related social and personal beliefs and expectations is the adaptive setting and pursuit of long-term goals (Heckhausen, 1999; Neugarten, Moore, & Lowe, 1965; Wrosch & Freund, 2001). Developmental goals provide an orientation for the development and selection of age-appropriate personal projects or goals. As developmental goals indicate age-dependent opportunity structures and the presence of resources, they also support the pursuit and maintenance of personal projects or goals (Freund & Baltes, 2005). The function of personal projects or goals for development is addressed in the next section.

The importance of adjusting personal projects or goals to match the social expectations and demands of a life context is stressed in the research by Salmela-Aro and Nurmi (1997). Using Little's (1983) personal project analysis (PPA), they found that young adults' personal projects predicted later actual transitions in the respective life domain (e.g., family-related personal projects predicted marriage or having a child). More interesting in this context, personal projects that referred to age-related developmental tasks (e.g., founding a family) predicted subjective well-being. Similarly, Salmela-Aro, Nurmi, Saisto, and Halmesmäki (2001) showed that an increase in family-related personal projects during pregnancy and after the birth of the child predicted a decline in depressive symptoms over time, whereas an increase in self-focused personal projects predicted an increase in depressive symptoms. In line with gender-related social expectations in the transition to parenthood, changes in the men's personal projects were less substantial than changes in women's personal projects (Salmela-Aro, Nurmi, Saisto, & Halmesmäki, 2000).

The influence of social expectations is not restricted to the content of personal projects or goals; it extends to the processes of goal selection and goal pursuit. In research on naive theory or folk psychology, proverbs are viewed as a body of folk knowledge or social expectations about human life. Proverbs are short statements summarizing advice on how to deal effectively or in morally correct ways with situations of everyday life (e.g., Mieder, 1993). If social expectations about processes of goal selection and pursuit as fundamental processes of development exist, it should be possible to identify proverbs reflecting such processes. Consistent with this expectation, Freund and Baltes (2002a) found that a substantial number of proverbs contain statements about behaviors reflecting goal processes. An example of a proverb reflecting the importance of goal pursuit for achieving higher levels of performance is "practice makes perfect," whereas an alternative proverb doubting any active role on the part of a person in goal attainment is "everything comes to he who waits." Goal-related and alternative proverbs were matched on a number of dimensions such as familiarity and meaningfulness. Younger and older adults chose proverbs reflecting goal processes more often than proverbs reflecting alternative strategies of life management as adaptive.

Personal Projects or Goals (Level 2)[1]

Personal projects or goals influence development by organizing behavior over time and situations into larger action sequences. Beyond concrete behaviors, personal projects or goals influence development

---

[1]The term *personal projects or goals* is used here to denote that this level subsumes personal goals as representations of abstract or concrete future states (to be achieved, maintained, or avoided) as well as personal projects in the sense of activities and concerns. In German, the connotation of projects (*Projekte*) is more concrete and more related to plans and actions than personal goals (*persönliche Ziele*). In Heckhausen's (1989) phase model of motivation, personal projects would be located beyond the Rubicon and denote the formulation of action plans. Personal goals, in contrast, also refer to the setting of goals in the predecisional phase. Level 2 is conceptualized to include all of these motivational states, namely the development, setting, commitment, pursuit, and termination (disengagement) of future and current concern, plans, actions, and goals.

because they motivate the acquisition, refinement, and coordination of resources and skills. As Little (1998) put it, personal projects "provide a sense of structure to human lives, a source of continuing personal identity and a point of active interchange between people and their surrounding contexts" (p. 194). Little (1999) stressed that personal projects are strongly related to the social context and that their meaning, manageability, and support differs across the life span. The following section elaborates on this important conceptualization of personal projects or goals in a life-span context.

Personal goals are important for individual development because they contribute to the specialization of general potentials. For instance, musicality is a general potential that, through a goal such as becoming a violinist, is translated through deliberate practice under the supervision of a teacher into concrete musical skills (Ericsson, Krampe, & Tesch-Römer, 1993). Pursuing personal goals can also contribute to general abilities such as delay of gratification that are important for positive development (Mischel, Cantor, & Feldman, 1996). A central function of personal projects or goals is often seen in their self-regulation function (Carver & Scheier, 1999). At the same time, self-regulation processes play an important role with respect to which goals are selected, and how goal-related behavior is initiated, executed, and terminated (Freund, 2001).

Personal projects or goals are typically conceived of as desired (or dreaded) states to which a person consciously and deliberatively commits. Speaking of nonconscious goals seems, at first glance, a contradiction in itself. During the past 15 years, however, Bargh (1990; Bargh & Ferguson, 2000) has theoretically elaborated and empirically investigated a model of how personal goals can become automatized and nonconscious. According to Bargh's automotive model, the repeated activation of a goal in a certain situation leads to an association of the respective goal and situational cues. Such situational features can then automatically trigger a goal and activate goal-relevant actions. In this model, goal-related behavior does not necessarily require conscious activation of the respective goal or conscious intention to engage in goal-relevant behavior (see e.g., Fitzsimons & Bargh, 2003, for a demonstration of how social partners can serve as stimuli activating goal-relevant behavior without intervening consciousness of the related goal). For instance, the personal project or goal to be more productive might be triggered automatically by seeing one's computer. The activation of this goal, in turn, might lead to the behavior of sitting down and working on revising a manuscript—without being consciously aware of the personal project "I want to be more productive." As this example shows, the model does not assume that the behavior is not under conscious control (most of us would consider revising a manuscript as an action that requires effortful and conscious mental activities). Instead, the automotive model proposes that the goal does not need to be conscious at every point in time to guide the relevant behavior.

Nonconscious goals are not the same as implicit (nonconscious) motives. Brunstein (2003) defined implicit motives as affective preferences for certain classes of stimuli that are acquired very early in life. Motives such as achievement, power, or affiliation are typically not consciously represented reasons for doing something. As Brunstein pointed out, motives and personal projects or goals do not necessarily overlap in content. For instance, achievement motivation might in one person be expressed in the personal project or goal to excel in the athletic domain, and in another person in the project or goal to start a new business. In this sense, then, motives can be seen as underlying projects or goals that are, at some point in time, conscious representations of relatively specific end states and that are informed by more basic motives. Schultheiss and Brunstein (1999) showed that conscious representations of projects or goals might serve a mediating role between motives and actual behavior. They found that goal imagery (i.e., the perception-like mental representation of the pursuit and attainment of a goal) increased the congruence between implicit motives and the commitment to and attainment of related goals. The next section takes a closer look at goals and self-regulation.

Personal Projects or Goals and Self-Regulation.   Since the cognitive revolution in psychology and in particular the research by Mischel (1968) on delay of gratification, a large number of psychological models have concerned themselves with processes of self-regulation. As research by investigators such as Mischel (1968) and Bandura (1969) exemplified, human behavior is only partly determined by external stimuli. An adequate description and prediction of behavior, the argumentation goes, has to refer to regulatory processes that lie within the individual. Central to the internal aspects that contribute to self-regulation are goals and standards (Freund & Baltes, 2000).

Baumeister and Heatherton (1996) defined self-regulation as "the extent to which people influence, modify, or control their own behavior" (p. 1). Following a feedback loop model (e.g., Carver & Scheier, 1999), self-regulation can be viewed as comprising three relevant aspects.

1. *Setting goals or standards.* If there is no goal (standard, desired state) to be achieved or maintained, each and every state is acceptable. Goals motivate behavior (toward the desired state) and give a direction to behavior. One aspect of the motivational process that is often overlooked by motivation theories is the question of which goals a person selects at a certain point in his or her life. Age-related expectations (Level 1) might serve as an important guideline for the selection of goals and standards.

2 *Testing phase.* Monitoring whether one is on the right track for achieving one's standards involves continually comparing the actual and desired state and using the resulting discrepancy to determine whether the means for achieving one's goal are appropriate or need to be changed (quantitatively and qualitatively). Monitoring can occur consciously or outside of conscious awareness.

3. *Operating phase.* This aspect refers to the investment of goal-relevant means to minimize the actual–ideal discrepancy. The central questions pertain to the initiation, maintenance, and termination of goal-relevant actions.

The coordination of these action phases is particularly complex when long-term and superordinate goals are involved. The pursuit of such goals entails the repeated initiation of actions, persistence, and often the overcoming of obstacles and setbacks. To complicate matters, once committed to a certain goal, there are a number of factors influencing the decision to give up trying to achieve or maintain it. One factor is known as *sunk cost* (Arkes & Ayton, 1999). The more a person has invested in achieving a goal (e.g., time, money, closing other doors), the more difficult it becomes to ignore these costs as sunk even if it is highly unlikely that the goal will be attained. Instead people are likely to try repairing and investing even more resources into achieving the goal. Distancing oneself from goals might hence become as important a matter as setting goals.

PERSONAL PROJECTS OR GOALS IN A LIFE-SPAN PERSPECTIVE: THE MODEL OF SELECTION, OPTIMIZATION, AND COMPENSATION

On the basis of the broad model of behavior regulation outlined earlier and adopting a life-span developmental perspective, Paul Baltes and I have developed over the past years an action-theoretical model of goal selection and pursuit. Based on a metamodel of selection, optimization, and compensation (SOC model; Baltes & Baltes, 1990), we propose to integrate the motivation-theoretical distinction of setting and pursuing goals (Atkinson, 1957; Heckhausen, 1989) into the life-span theoretical assumption of multidirectionality. Multidirectionality denotes that development comprises not only trajectories of growth but also trajectories of decline (Baltes, 1987; Labouvie-Vief, 1981). This integration of motivational and life-span theoretical distinctions leads to the identification of the four goal processes presented in Figure 9.2.

Applying the SOC model to personal goals, we (Freund & Baltes, 2000) argued that developing and committing to a hierarchy of personal goals (i.e., elective selection) and engaging in goal-directed actions and means (i.e., optimization) are essential for achieving higher levels of functioning. To maintain a given level of functioning in the face of loss and decline in goal-relevant means, we postulate that people need to invest in compensatory means (e.g., substitution for means that are no longer available). When the costs for goal achievement or maintenance outweigh their expected gains, it is adaptive to reconstruct one's goal hierarchy by focusing exclusively on the most important goals, developing new goals, or adapting goal standards (i.e., loss-based selection). Thus, the SOC model conceptualizes processes promoting gains (elective selection, optimization) but also processes to counteract losses that inevitably occur in life (compensation, loss-based selection). Selection, optimization, and compensation are proposed to advance

	Goal Setting	Goal pursuit
Gain orientation	Elective Selection	Optimization
Loss orientation	Loss-based Selection	Compensation

Figure 9.2. Distinction of goal processes on the basis of motivational and life-span developmental theory. (See Freund, Li, & Baltes, 1999)

positive development across the life span. The following sections provide a more detailed description of the three processes and their relation t motivation and positive development.

Selection

Throughout the life span, biological, social, and individual opportunities and constraints specify a range of alternative options (e.g., profession, city to live in, etc.). Within this great variety of options that is usually larger than the amount of resources available to the individual, people actively and passively, consciously and nonconsciously select goal domains in which to focus their resources and efforts. Selection of goals functions as a precondition for specialization and the further acquisition of resources. The general function of selection (i.e., developing, elaborating, and committing to goals), is that it directs development.

There are various taxonomies of goals (e.g., Carver & Scheier, 1999; Emmons, 1996). One important distinction that has its roots in early conceptions of motivation, relates to the focus of goals; that is, if a goal specifies an outcome that is to be approached or to be avoided (see Elliot & Friedman, chap. 3, this volume, for a discussion of approach and avoidance goals). It has been repeatedly shown in cognitive research on judgment and decision making (e.g., Kahneman & Tversky, 1979) as well as in the motivational literature (e.g., Emmons, 1996; Higgins, 1997) that it is important to distinguish between a gain and a loss focus when investigating goal-related processes. Impending or actual losses seem to affect people more strongly than gains (Hobfoll, 1989). In addition, the goal literature shows that the pursuit of avoidance rather than approach goals is detrimental for both well-being and actual attainment of goals (e.g., Coats, Janoff-Bulman, & Alpert, 1996; Elliot & Sheldon, 1997; Elliot, Sheldon, & Church, 1997).

The fundamental distinction between a gain focus and a loss focus is captured in the SOC model by distinguishing between two modes of selection, *elective selection* and *loss-based selection*. Loss-based selection involves changes in goals or the goal system such as reconstructing one's goal hierarchy, focusing on the most important goal(s), adapting standards, or searching for new goals (cf. assimilative coping, Brandtstädter & Wentura, 1995; compensatory secondary control, Heckhausen, 1999).

To hold and feel committed to goals contributes to feeling that one's life has a purpose and thereby gives meaning to life (e.g., Klinger, 1977;

Little, 1989). Moreover, goals reduce the complexity of any given situation as they guide attention and behavior. In other words, goals can also be seen as permanently available decision rules (an "implemental mind-set"; Gollwitzer, 1994) for directing attention (which of the numerous stimuli are, or what of the available information is goal relevant?) and for behavior selection (which of the many behavioral options in this situation are goal relevant?).

Empirical evidence supports the important function of prioritization for directing development. In a study with a sample of adults between 25 and 35 years old, Wiese and Freund (2001) found that, compared to young adults who pursue multiple goals at the same time, those who set priorities in one life domain over another (here, the work and the family domain) feel less conflicted about their goals and are more satisfied with their lives in general and with their domain-specific development. Moreover, attention is directed toward the prioritized goal (i.e., faster recognition of and preference for information relevant for the prioritized goal). Directing attention to goal-relevant information might enhance knowledge helping to achieve a given goal and might also alert to good opportunities to act on a goal, and thereby foster positive development.

Optimization

Achieving desired outcomes in the domains selected necessitates the acquisition, application, and refinement of goal-relevant means. Which means are best suited for achieving one's goals varies according to the specific goal domain (e.g., academic vs. social domain), personal characteristics (e.g., gender), and the sociocultural context (e.g., availability of institutional support systems). Social norms and expectations as well as explicit teaching typically provide information about which means are related to a given goal. On a general level, practice appears to be a key factor for the acquisition and refinement of goal-related means (Ericsson et al., 1993). Repeated practice also leads to the automatization of skills that thereby become less resource demanding and that free resources that can be devoted to other goal-related means.

Compensation

Compensation occurs in response to a loss in means. Some losses in means are due to a redirection of attention, others to more or less permanent losses in biological capacity. In contrast to loss-based selection, compensation refers to the investment of alternative means when maintaining the goal threatened by losses. From a life-span developmental perspective, the maintenance of functioning by compensation is as important for positive developmental regulation as a growth focus (optimization). As losses increase with age, there is presumably an increasing need to invest more and more resources into maintenance of functioning rather than into optimization (Staudinger, Marsiske, & Baltes, 1995; Freund & Ebner, 2005). This hypothesis was supported in cognitive experimental work on dual-task allocations associated with sensorimotor and memory functioning in young and old age (Li, Lindenberger, Freund, & Baltes, 2001). This study showed that older adults make increasingly more use of compensatory aids as the system of performance is challenged.

EMPIRICAL EVIDENCE FOR THE IMPORTANCE OF GOAL PROCESSES FOR POSITIVE DEVELOPMENT

A number of studies using a self-report measure of SOC addressed the importance of goal processes for positive development across adulthood. In a carefully worded questionnaire (Baltes, Baltes, Freund, & Lang, 1999), participants indicate whether they engage in behaviors of goal selection and goal pursuit or in alternative behaviors. Such alternatives are, for instance, keeping one's options open rather than committing to a set of goals (selection), being content with results of first trials rather than trying to maximize one's performance (optimization), or waiting for solutions and betterment of a loss situation rather than engaging in substitutive behaviors (compensation). Using this questionnaire in samples ranging in age from 14 to over 100 years, a number of studies (Freund & Baltes, 1998, 2002b; Wiese, Freund, & Baltes, 2000, 2001) have found that adults who report engaging in selection, optimization, and compensation of personal goals also report higher well-being (e.g., frequency of experiencing positive emotions, having a purpose in life, life satisfaction). Committing to personal goals, pursuing these goals and investing in their maintenance in the face of losses all contribute to positive subjective states across adulthood. In line with developmental assumptions, these findings also show that it is during adulthood when participants express the strongest indication of use of SOC.

Evidence for the functional usefulness of SOC is also available for young adults who are arguably at their prime with regard to resources in many areas of life. Such individuals seem to profit from engaging in the life management strategies of SOC. In a longitudinal study by Wiese et al. (2001), young adults reprting SOC behaviors scored higher on multiple subjective indicators of well-being, positive emotions, and partnership as well as job-related success.

Table 9.1 summarizes correlational findings of self-reported SOC and indicators of positive development. These studies show that all three SOC-related processes contribute to various indicators of emotional and social well-being across adulthood. The pattern of correlations is stable across adulthood into old and very old age. Moreover, it is robust against controlling for a number of rival predictors of positive development such as personality (e.g., Big Five) and motivation contructs (e.g., tenacious goal pursuit and flexible goal adjustment). To simplify the findings, I aggregated SOC into one overall SOC score.

TABLE 9.1

Summary of Correlational Findings on Self-Reported SOC and Subjective Indicators of Positive Development

Positive Development (subjective indicators)	SOC (overall score)
Freund & Baltes, 2002b (N = 395; 14–89 years; combined samples of studies 1 and 2)	
Positive Emotions	.33**
Personal Growth	.37**
Meaning in Life	.44**
Wiese, Freund, & Baltes, 2000 (N = 206, 25–36 years)	
Life Satisfaction	.49**
Emotional Balance	.37**
Self-Acceptance	.21**
Freund & Baltes, 1998 (N = 200; 72–102 years)	
Satisfaction with Aging	.33**
Positive Emotions	.47**
Emotional Loneliness	-.30**

Note. ** $p < .01$

Table 9.1 focuses on cross-sectional findings. Wiese et al. (2001) also found evidence for cross-lagged relations of SOC and outcomes of positive development. Self-reported SOC predicted *change* in job satisfaction and emotional balance over a time period of 3 years. Again, this result was robust when statistically controlling for rival predictors such as the NEO.

Changes in Motivational Orientation in Adulthood

Development does not occur in a social vacuum. Instead, the changes a person goes through over the life span occur in constant interaction with his or her social and physical environment. When trying to understand how goals change with age, we need to identify age-related changes in the person and the environment, as well as their interaction. On a very general level, the clearest change is that age is associated with increasing losses. Such multiple sources as increasing morbidity, loss of social partners, decline in information processing speed, loss of sensory acuity, and loss of stamina all contribute to the general sense that aging is associated with losses (for a summary see Freund & Riediger, 2003). Moreover, there is high social consensus that old age signals the onset of a larger number of undesirable personality traits (e.g., rigidity) and loss of desirable ones (e.g., extraversion; Heckhausen, Dixon, & Baltes, 1989). For very old age, this negative view appears to be empirically supported (Baltes & Smith, 2003; Smith & Baltes, 1999). This is not to say that aging can be described as a uniformly negative, loss-ridden time in life. This is neither true in the stereotypes of older people (Brewer, Dull, & Lui, 1981) nor with regard to the empirical evidence in various domains of functioning. On the one hand, some of the changes that are viewed as losses by younger age groups might, in fact, be seen as value-neutral or even positive changes in the eyes of older adults (Carstensen & Freund, 1994). On the other hand, there are a number of functional domains such as vocabulary skills, wisdom, or emotion regulation that show stability or even increase into old age (for an overview see Baltes et al., 2006). As any other phase in life, then, old age comprises both gains and losses (Baltes, 1987; Brandtstädter & Renner, 1990; Labouvie-Vief, 1981). The ratio of gains to losses, however, becomes more and more negative with age (Baltes et al., 2006; Smith & Baltes, 1999).

From a motivational perspective, optimization might have more positive emotional and motivational consequences than compensation. A number of studies (Coats et al., 1996; Elliot & Sheldon, 1997;

Elliot et al., 1997; Emmons, 1996) have shown that trying to achieve gains or growth is associated with a higher degree of self-efficacy, leads to positive emotions and well-being, and to better performance, whereas trying to avoid losses or decline is related to negative emotions and distress.

A set of studies investigated age-differential effects of goal framing on persistence in goal pursuit (Freund, 2006). These studies supported one of the life-span predictions of SOC-related behavior. Younger adults proved to be more motivated (operationalized as persistence) to achieve higher levels of performance (i.e., optimization) than to maintain performance when confronted with a loss on the same experimental task. Conversely, older adults when faced with a loss situation (i.e., compensation) showed higher persistence than compared to the same task aiming at improving performance.

This study used a highly artificial sensorimotor task. In both the optimization and the compensation condition, participants were asked to adjust the color of the lower half of a circle to the upper one displayed on a computer screen with a lever. In the optimization condition, the instruction was to "become as good as possible." In the compensation condition, the lever only responded with a certain delay and the task was to "try to get back to the prior level of performance." Feedback about performance was displayed on the screen at an interval of about every 2 minutes. To ensure that the difficulty of the task did not drive the effect, a condition of framing the optimization task as easy and the compensation task as difficult was introduced. As predicted, in this case, the age differences disappeared.

This result has important educational implications: For young adults, learning goals need to be formulated in a way that stresses the potential for improvement. Moreover, these studies show that for younger adults, individualized feedback on the degree of improvement is important for persistence. Regarding learning, this implies that individualized feedback referring to progress over time should be preferred over feedback on the relative standing when compared to other learners. This might be of particular importance when young adults have to work on overcoming difficulties or shortcomings in a given study domain. In contrast, older adults might profit more if goals are seen as instrumental for maintaining functioning. The motivation for acquiring new skills might be higher if the potential usefulness of these skills as compensatory tools or strategies is stressed. For instance, when learning a mnemonic technique, older adults might be more motivated to invest time and effort when they believe that this technique will help them to counteract loss in memory. In contrast, younger adults might be more motivated if they believe that they can enhance their memory performance with a given technique. For them, loss avoidance might seem less relevant. As of yet, this hypothesis is speculative and awaits empirical investigation.

CONCLUSION

Revisiting the opening question of this chapter: Do goals matter in a person's life? I hope that the theoretical and empirical evidence, incomplete and sketchy as it still is in many places, has provided a cautiously positive answer: Goals do matter. Asking a job candidate about her personal goals regarding research and career is most likely predictive of her future work-related commitment and engagement. Furthermore, expectations of her immediate and more distal social environment about the number and quality of papers, research projects, mentoring, and teaching she should accomplish at what point in her life will influence her own beliefs and expectations as we all as her personal goals and projects. If routinely activated, these goals will be represented and operate without conscious awareness. This might seduce some to believe that explicit personal goals are a mere epiphenomenon. In contrast to this view, I endorse a more comprehensive conceptualization than is typically subsumed under the definition of goals as conscious personal goals and projects. A more comprehensive model of goals distinguishes between different levels of representation: age-related expectations (Level 1) and personal projects or goals (Level 2). Together, these two levels predict what kinds of projects people pursue in everyday life at different points in their lives and how they do so.

Empirical evidence supports the notion that cultural and social knowledge represents the importance of personal projects or goals for successful development (e.g., Freund & Baltes, 2002a). Using self-report methodology, a number of correlative studies show that processes of setting, pursuing, and maintaining goals, as specified in the model of SOC, are associated with indicators of positive development in adulthood. Age-related changes in motivational orientation suggest that compensation becomes more important with age. Considering the increasingly negative ratio of gains to losses with age, this might be an adaptive mechanism contributing to positive development in adulthood (Freund & Ebner, 2005).

Future research in this framework needs to address more directly the interaction of the different levels of goal representations and their changes across adulthood. Regarding the relative importance of the different levels of goals for development, one could, on the one hand, speculate that the relative importance of social and personal beliefs and expectations gains in importance for individual development across adulthood. On the other hand, one could argue that personal projects and goals become more important because, due to being activated more often, they are more likely to be automatized, leading to automatic situation–action links that are relatively immune to social expectations. According to this view, goals should be less likely to be conscious, which would make it particularly difficult to change them. According to such an automatization model (cf., Bargh & Gollwitzer, 1994), personal projects and goals would become less flexible with increasing age. This, in turn, might lead to a decrease in the match of personal projects and goals and individual abilities and available resources. According to Vallacher and Wegner (1985), goals are likely to become conscious when they are blocked and, therefore, goal pursuit is interrupted. Loss-based selection could, then, become a correction mechanism in old age to adapt automatized goals to changes in the environment or the person. As of yet, the interplay of conscious and nonconscious goal processes across adulthood is unexplored.

Taken together, the proposed framework of levels of goal representation attempts to integrate existing literature on life-span developmental psychology, motivation, and goals. At its current stage, however, it also raises a variety of open questions awaiting theoretical and empirical investigation.

REFERENCES

Arkes, H. R., & Ayton, P. (1999). The sunk cost and Concorde effects: Are humans less rational than lower animals? *Psychological Bulletin, 125,* 591–600.

Atkinson, J. W. (1957). Motivational determinants of risk-taking behavior. *Psychological Review, 64,* 359–372.

Baltes, P. B. (1987). Theoretical propositions of life-span developmental psychology: On the dynamics between growth and decline. *Developmental Psychology, 23,* 611–626.

Baltes, P. B., & Baltes, M. M. (1990). Psychological perspectives on successful aging: The model of selective optimization with compensation. In P. B. Baltes & M. M. Baltes (Eds.), *Successful aging: Perspectives from the behavioral sciences* (pp. 1–34). New York: Cambridge University Press.

Baltes, P. B., Baltes, M. M., Freund, A. M., & Lang, F. (1999). *The measurement of selection, optimization, and compensation (SOC) by self report* (Tech. Rep. No. 1999). Berlin: Max Planck Institute for Human Development.

Baltes, P. B., Lindenberger, U., & Staudinger, U. M. (2006). Life-span theory in developmental psychology. In R. M. Lerner (Ed.), *Handbook of child psychology. Vol. 1: Theoretical models of human development* (6th ed., pp. 569–664). New York: Wiley.

Baltes, P. B., & Smith, J. (2003). New frontiers in the future of aging: From successful aging of the young old to the dilemmas of the fourth age. *Gerontology, 49,* 123–135.

Bandura, A. (1969). *Principles of behavior modification.* New York: Holt, Rinehart, & Winston.

Bargh, J. A. (1990). Auto-motives: Preconscious determinants of social interaction. In E. T. Higgins & R. M. Sorrentino (Eds.), *Handbook of motivation and cognition: Foundations of social behavior* (Vol. 2, pp. 93–130). New York: Guilford.

Bargh, J. A., & Ferguson, M. J. (2000). Beyond behaviorism: On the automaticity of higher mental processes. *Psychological Bulletin, 126,* 925–945.

Bargh, J. A., & Gollwitzer, P. M. (1994). Environmental control of goal-directed action: Automatic and strategic contingencies between situations and behavior. *Nebraska Symposium on Motivation, 41,* 71–124.

Baumeister, R. F., & Heatherton, T. F. (1996). Self-regulation failure: An overview. *Psychological Inquiry, 7,* 1–15.

Brandtstädter, J. (1998). Action perspective on human development. In W. Damon (Series Ed.) & R. Lerner (Vol. Ed.), *Handbook of child psychology: Vol. 1. Theoretical models of human development* (5th ed., pp. 807–863). New York: Wiley.

Brandtstädter, J., & Renner, G. (1990). Tenacious goal pursuit and flexible goal adjustment: Explication and age-related analysis of assimilative and accommodative strategies of coping. *Psychology and Aging, 5,* 58–67.

Brandtstädter, J., & Wentura, D. (1995). Adjustment to shifting possibility frontiers in later life: Compensatory adaptive modes. In R. A. Dixon & L. Bäckman (Eds.), *Psychological compensation: Managing losses and promoting gains* (pp. 83–106). Hillsdale, NJ: Lawrence Erlbaum Associates.

Brewer, M. B., Dull, V., & Lui, L. (1981). Perceptions of the elderly: Stereotypes as prototypes. *Journal of Personality and Social Psychology, 41,* 656–670.

Brunstein, J. C. (2003). Implizite Motive versus motivationale Selbstbilder: Zwei Prädiktoren mit unterschiedlichen Gültigkeitsbereichen [Implicit motives versus motivational self-images: Two predictors with different realms of application]. In J. Stiensmeier-Pelster & F. Rheinberg (Eds.), *Diagnostik von Motivation und Selbstkonzept* (pp. 59–88). Göttingen, Germany: Hogrefe.

Cantor, N. (1994). Life task problem solving: Situational affordances and personal needs. *Personality and Social Psychology Bulletin, 20,* 235–243.

Carstensen, L. L., & Freund, A. M. (1994). The resilience of the aging self. *Developmental Review, 14,* 81–92.

Carver, C. S., & Scheier, M. F. (1999). Themes and issues in the self-regulation of behavior. In R. S. Wyer, Jr. (Ed.), *Perspectives on behavioral self-regulation* (pp. 1–105). Mahwah, NJ: Lawrence Erlbaum Associates.

Coats, E. J., Janoff-Bulman, R., & Alpert, N. (1996). Approach versus avoidance goals: Differences in self-evaluation and well-being. *Personality and Social Psychology Bulletin, 22,* 1057–1067.

Elliot, A. J., & Sheldon, K. M. (1997). Avoidance achievement motivation: A personal goals analysis. *Journal of Personality and Social Psychology, 73,* 171–185.

Elliot, A. J., Sheldon, K. M., & Church, M. A. (1997). Avoidance personal goals and subjective well-being. *Personality and Social Psychology Bulletin, 23*, 915–927.

Emmons, R. A. (1996). Striving and feeling: Personal goals and subjective well-being. In P. M. Gollwitzer & J. A. Bargh (Eds.), *The psychology of action: Linking cognition and motivation to behavior* (pp. 313–337). New York: Guilford.

Ericsson, K. A., Krampe, R. T., & Tesch-Römer, C. (1993). The role of deliberate practice in the acquisition of expert performance. *Psychological Review, 100*, 363–406.

Fitzsimons, G. M., & Bargh, J. A. (2003). Thinking of you: Nonconscious pursuit of interpersonal goals associated with relationship partners. *Journal of Personality and Social Psychology, 84*, 148–163.

Freund, A. M. (1997). Individuating age-salience: A psychological perspective on the salience of age in the life course. *Human Development, 40*, 287–292.

Freund, A. M. (2001). Developmental psychology of life-management. In N. J. Smelser & P. B. Baltes (Eds.), *International encyclopedia of the behavioral and social sciences* (Vol. 13, pp. 8827–8832). Oxford, UK: Elsevier Science.

Freund, A. M. (2003). Die Rolle von Zielen für die Entwicklung [The role of goals for development]. *Psychologische Rundschau, 54*, 233–242.

Freund, A. M. (2006). Differential motivational consequences of goal focus in younger and older adutls. *Psychology and Aging, 21*, 240–252.

Freund, A. M., & Baltes, P. B. (1998). Selection, optimization and compensation as strategies of life-management: Correlations with subjective indicators of successful aging. *Psychology and Aging, 13*, 531–543.

Freund, A. M., & Baltes, P. B. (2000). The orchestration of selection, optimization and compensation: An action-theoretical conceptualization of a theory of developmental regulation. In W. J. Perrig & A. Grob (Eds.), *Control of human behavior, mental processes, and consciousness: Essays in honor of the 60th birthday of August Flammer* (pp. 35–58). Mahwah, NJ: Lawrence Erlbaum Associates.

Freund, A. M., & Baltes, P. B. (2002a). The adaptiveness of selection, optimization, and compensation as strategies of life management: Evidence from a preference study on proverbs. *Journals of Gerontology: Psychological Sciences, 57*, P426–P434.

Freund, A. M., & Baltes, P. B. (2002b). Life-management strategies of selection, optimization, and compensation: Measurement by self-report and construct validity. *Journal of Personality and Social Psychology, 82*, 642–662.

Freund, A. M., & Baltes, P. B. (2005). Entwicklungsaufgaben als Organisationsstrukturen von Entwicklung und Entwicklungsoptimierung [Developmental tasks as organizing structures of optimal development]. In W. Scheider (Ed.), *Enzyklopädie für Psychologie. Serie V: Entwicklungspsychologie des mittleren und höheren Erwachsenenalters* (vol. 6., pp. 35–78). Göttingen, Germany: Hogrefe.

Freund, A. M., & Ebner, N. C. (2005). The aging self: Promoting gains and balancing losses: Goal orientation in old age. In W. Greve, D. Wentura, & K. Rothermund (Eds.), *The adaptive self: Personal continuity and intentional self-development* (pp. 185–202). Ashland, OH: Hogrefe & Huber.

Freund, A. M., Li, K. Z. H., & Baltes, P. B. (1999). Successful development and aging: The role of selection, optimization, and compensation. In J. Brandtstädter & R. M. Lerner (Eds.), *Action and self-development: Theory and research through the life span* (pp. 401–434). Thousand Oaks, CA: Sage.

Freund, A. M., & Riediger, M. (2003). Successful aging. In R. M. Lerner, M. A. Easterbrooks, & J. Mistry (Eds.), *Handbook of psychology: Vol. 6. Developmental psychology* (pp. 601–628). New York: Wiley.

Freund, A. M., & Smith, J. (1999). Content and function of the self-definition in old and very old age. *Journals of Gerontology: Psychological Science, 54,* P55–P67.

Gollwitzer, P. M. (1994). Goal achievement: The role of intentions. In W. Stroebe & M. Hewstone (Eds.), *European review of social psychology* (Vol. 4, pp. 141–185). London: Wiley.

Hagestad, G. O., & Neugarten, B. L. (1985). Age and the life course. In R. H. Binstock & E. Shanas (Eds.), *Handbook of aging and the social sciences* (2nd ed., pp. 35–61). New York: Van Nostrand Reinhold.

Heckhausen, H. (1989). *Motivation und Handeln* [Motivation and Action]. Berlin: Springer.

Heckhausen, J. (1999). *Developmental regulation in adulthood: Age-normative and sociostructural constraints as adaptive challenges.* New York: Cambridge University Press.

Heckhausen, J., Dixon, R. A., & Baltes, P. B. (1989). Gains and losses in development throughout adulthood as perceived by different adult age groups. *Developmental Psychology, 25,* 109–121.

Higgins, E. T. (1997). Beyond pleasure and pain. *American Psychologist, 52,* 1280–1300.

Hobfoll, S. E. (1989). Conservation of resources: A new attempt at conceptualizing stress. *American Psychologist, 44,* 513–524.

Kahneman, D., & Tversky, A. (1979). Prospect theory: An analysis of decision under risk. *Econometrica, 47,* 263–291.

Klinger, E. (1977). *Meaning and void: Inner experience and the incentives in people's lives.* Minneapolis: University of Minnesota Press.

Labouvie-Vief, G. (1981). Proactive and reactive aspects of constructivism: Growth and aging in life-span perspective. In R. M. Lerner & N. A. Busch-Rossnagel (Eds.), *Individuals as producers of their development: A life-span perspective* (pp. 197–230). New York: Academic.

Lerner, R. M., & Busch-Rossnagel, N. A. (Eds.). (1981). *Individuals as producers of their development: A life-span perspective.* New York: Academic.

Li, K. Z. H., Lindenberger, U., Freund, A. M., & Baltes, P. B. (2001). Walking while memorizing: Age-related differences in compensatory behavior. *Psychological Science, 12,* 230–237.

Little, B. R. (1983). Personal projects: A rationale and method for investigation. *Environment and Behavior, 15,* 273–309.

Little, B. R. (1996). Free traits, personal projects and ideo-tapes: Three tiers for personality psychology. *Psychological Inquiry, 7,* 340–344.

Little, B. R. (1989). Personal projects analysis: Trivial pursuits, magnificent obsessions, and the search for coherence. In D. M. Buss & N. Cantor (Eds.), *Personality psychology: Recent trends and emerging directions* (pp. 15–31). New York: Springer-Verlag.

Little, B. R. (1998). Personal project pursuit: Dimensions and dynamics of personal meaning. In P. T. P. Wong & P. S. Fry (Eds.), *The human quest for meaning: A handbook of psychological research and clinical applications* (pp. 193–212). Mahwah, NJ: Lawrence Erlbaum Associates.

Little, B. R. (1999). Personal projects and social ecology: Themes and variations across the life span. In J. Brandtstädter & R. M. Lerner (Eds.), *Action and self-development: Theory and research through the life span* (pp. 197–221). Thousand Oaks, CA: Sage.

Mayer, K. U. (1986). Structural constraints on the life course. *Human Development, 29,* 163–170.

McAdams, D. P. (1995). What do we know when we know a person? *Journal of Personality, 63,* 365–396.

Mieder, W. (1993). *Proverbs are never out of season: Popular wisdom in the modern age.* New York: Oxford University Press.

Mischel, W. (1968). *Personality and assessment.* New York: Wiley.

Mischel, W., Cantor, N., & Feldman, S. (1996). Principles of self-regulation: The nature of willpower and self-control. In E. T. Higgins & A. W. Kruglanski (Eds.), *Social psychology: Handbook of basic principles* (pp. 329–360). New York: Guilford.

Neugarten, B. L. (1968). Adult personality: Toward a psychology of the life cycle. In B. L. Neugarten (Ed.), *Middle age and aging: A reader in social psychology* (pp. 137–147). Chicago: University of Chicago Press.

Neugarten, B. L., Moore, J. W., & Lowe, J. C. (1965). Age norms, age constraints, and adult socialization. *American Journal of Sociology, 70,* 710–717.

Nurmi, J.-E. (1992). Age differences in adult life goals, concerns, and their temporal extension: A life course approach to future-oriented motivation. *International Journal of Behavioral Development, 15,* 487–508.

Salmela-Aro, K., & Nurmi, J.-E. (1997). Goal contents, well-being, and life context during transition to university: A longitudinal study. *International Journal of Behavioral Development, 20,* 471–491.

Salmela-Aro, K., Nurmi, J.-E., Saisto, T., & Halmesmäki, E. (2000). Women's and men's personal goals during the transition to parenthood. *Journal of Family Psychology, 14,* 171–186.

Salmela-Aro, K., Nurmi, J.-E., Saisto, T., & Halmesmäki, E. (2001). Goal reconstruction and depressive symptoms during the transition to motherhood: Evidence from two cross-lagged longitudinal studies. *Journal of Personality and Social Psychology, 81,* 1144–1159.

Schultheiss, O. C., & Brunstein, J. C. (1999). Goal imagery: Bridging the gap between implicit motives and explicit goals. *Journal of Personality, 67,* 1–38.

Settersten, R. A., & Hagestad, G. O. (1996a). What's the latest? Cultural age deadlines for educational and work transitions. *The Gerontologist, 36,* 602–613.

Settersten, R. A., & Hagestad, G. O. (1996b). What's the latest? Cultural age deadlines for family transitions. *The Gerontologist, 36,* 178–188.

Smith, J., & Baltes, P. B. (1999). Trends and profiles of psychological functioning in very old age. In P. B. Baltes & K. U. Mayer (Eds.), *The Berlin aging study: Aging from 70 to 100* (pp. 197–226). New York: Cambridge University Press.

Staudinger, U. M., Freund, A., Linden, M., & Maas, I. (1996). Selbst, Persönlichkeit und Lebensgestaltung: Psychologische Widerstandsfähigkeit und Vulnerabilität [Self, personality and life-management: Psychological resilience and vulnerability]. In K. U. Mayer & P. B. Baltes (Eds.), *Die Berliner Altersstudie* [The Berlin Aging Study] (pp. 321–350). Berlin: Akademie Verlag.

Staudinger, U. M., Marsiske, M., & Baltes, P. B. (1995). Resilience and reserve capacity in later adulthood: Potentials and limits of development across the life span. In D. Cicchetti & D. Cohen (Eds.), *Developmental psychopathology: Vol. 2. Risk, disorder, and adaptation* (pp. 801–847). New York: Wiley.

Vallacher, R. R., & Wegner, D. M. (1985). *A theory of action identification.* Hillsdale, NJ: Lawrence Erlbaum Associates.

Wegner, D. M. (2002). *The illusion of conscious will.* Cambridge, MA: MIT Press.

Wiese, B. S., & Freund, A. M. (2001). Zum Einfluss persönlicher Prioritätensetzungen auf Maße der Stimuluspröferenz [The impact of personal priorities on stimulus preference]. *Zeitschrift für Experimentelle Psychologie, 48,* 57–73.

Wiese, B. S., Freund, A. M., & Baltes, P. B. (2000). Selection, optimization, and compensation: An action-related approach to work and partnership. *Journal of Vocational Behavior, 57,* 273–300.

Wiese, B. S., Freund, A. M., & Baltes, P. B. (2001). Longitudinal predictions of selection, optimization, and compensation. *Journal of Vocational Behavior, 59,* 1–15.

Wood, J. V., & Taylor, K. L. (1991). Serving self-relevant goals through social comparison. In J. Suls & T. A. Willis (Eds.), *Social comparison—contemporary theory and research* (pp. 23–49). Hillsdale, NJ: Lawrence Erlbaum Associates.

Wrosch, C., & Freund, A. M. (2001). Self-regulation of normative and non-normative developmental challenges. *Human Development, 44,* 264–283.

Wrosch, C., & Heckhausen, J. (1999). Control processes before and after passing a developmental deadline: Activation and deactivation of intimate relationship goals. *Journal of Personality and Social Psychology, 77,* 415–427.

10

Personal Persistence and Personal Projects: Creating Personal and Cultural Continuity

Monika Brandstätter and Christopher E. Lalonde

The overall goal of our contribution to this volume—our own personal project—is to showcase the ways in which personal projects analysis can be used to explore variation in the construction and understanding of the meaning of self. More than that, we mean to use personal projects analysis as a vehicle for examining this variation across both individuals and whole cultures. We realize, of course, that studies of self and culture are contentious within the social sciences. We recognize, too, that announcing our plan to link the personal and the cultural in the pages that follow amounts to uttering what some would consider fighting words. However, the kernel idea that we offer up as a way of avoiding fisticuffs, is this: Professional and cultural differences aside, in our everyday experience, both selves and cultures are commonly understood to both change and yet remain the same. That is, whatever else divides us, we routinely experience ourselves and others as temporally stable or continuous, yet we also expect people to change—and often strive to bring about change in ourselves and others. In much the same fashion, we understand that cultures must change and yet, if they are to survive pressures of assimilation, or colonization, or conquest, must somehow remain "the same." Some hope for resolving this apparent paradox of sameness and change—and of bridging the gulf between studies of individual persons and of entire cultures—can be found, we argue, in notions of personal and cultural continuity that are capable of preserving identity (both personal identity and cultural identity) across time and through change.

The obvious first step in our personal project, if we are to convince you that an accounting of our own attempts to resolve this paradox is worthy of your sustained attention, is to provide some working definition of just what we mean by personal persistence or cultural continuity. In addition, we need to demonstrate why, against tradition, we seem intent on casually collapsing all those usual levels of analysis that routinely separate studies of persons from studies of the cultures they inhabit. Getting all of this straight occupies the first part of the chapter and, after some meandering through the philosophical literature, brings us to the second part, in which we present reasons for believing that such notions actually apply to real instances of both persons and cultures. The third part concerns the fact that failures in continuity hold real and dire consequences that can be measured in elevated suicide risk for individuals and in the suicide rates of entire cultural communities. Next, we come to the real heart of the matter by introducing new evidence in support of the view that personal projects analysis (PPA) offers a novel way to understand how the everyday plans and routine personal strivings of young adults can function to maintain and modify more deep-seated and culture-bound conceptions of self and personhood. In the closing section of the chapter, we outline our future research plans and discuss the feasibility of adding a new dimension to PPA that quantifies the extent to which personal projects intersect with communal and cultural experience to define (and redefine) the meaning of self within different cultural contexts.

All of that seems a tall order—and of course it is—so let us begin by asking a seemingly simple question: How is it that you are still the same person you used to be? Think about it. What connects the person that you once were to the person you take yourself to be today or the person you are en route to becoming? What argumentative strategy would you adopt to warrant the claim that, despite having changed in perhaps dramatic fashion over the years, you are still importantly the same person? Before summarizing what some 600 young persons have told us about their own sense of self-continuity and before presenting our scheme for categorizing these attempts to resolve the paradox of personal persistence, we begin, as promised, with a brief discussion of what philosophers have had to say on the topic.

SELF-CONTINUITY AND THE PARADOX
OF PERSONAL PERSISTENCE

Our ordinary understanding of the concept of person or self includes, it is said, two seemingly contradictory features: Selves are commonly taken to "embody both change and permanence simultaneously" (Fraisse, 1963, p. 10). On the one hand, we appreciate that persons change—often dramatically so—over the course of their development. Yet, on the other, persons must somehow persist as continuous or numerically identical individuals, and remain, as Locke (1694/1956) famously put it, "as the same thinking thing in different times and places" (p. 335). If persons were not understood to persist from one moment to the next, and to somehow own their own pasts, then no one could be held accountable for their actions and our concepts of moral responsibility would be emptied of meaning (Rorty, 1973), just as planning for an anticipated future would be fundamentally nonsensical. Our everyday meaning of self, then, creates a paradox: How can persons both change and yet remain the same? How is it, for example, that you are still the same person that you were 10, 20, or 30 years ago? If pondering this question is new to you, and if answers fail to come readily to mind, then all is as we had hoped. Take heart: Not only have whole generations of philosophers puzzled over the problem of numerical identity, but so too (as we show in a later section) does every new generation of young persons.

References to this paradox of change and stability can be found in the writings of Aristotle, who held that "animals differ from what is not naturally constituted in that each of these [living] things has within it a principle of change and of staying unchanged" (cited in Wiggins , 1980, pp. 88–89), as well as in the works of Locke (1694/1956) and James (1910), and on into the modern era. Cassirer (1923), for example, spoke of "temporal unity"; Chisholm (1971) of "intact persistence"; and Strawson (1999) of "diachronic singleness." Solutions to the problem, however, are not quite so common.

The most frequent solution offered by philosophers concerns not connections to a previously experienced past, but rather to an anticipated and not yet realized future. Selves, in MacIntyre's (1984) words, are on a perpetual quest. Persons are made, according to Bakhtin (1986), not only out of "remnants of the past, but also from rudiments and tendencies of the future" (p. 26), rudiments that give "a sense to one's life as having a direction toward what one not yet is" (Taylor, 1988, p. 298). What holds our past, present, and future together in time is, as Flanagan (1996) put it, the fact that, "As beings in time, we are navigators. We care how our lives go" (p. 67).

Psychologists have taken up this same forward-looking notion in various guises, most notably in Markus's work on possible selves (e.g., Markus & Nurius, 1986; Markus & Ruvolo, 1989). For Markus and Nurius (1986), possible selves are the mechanisms of change for the self-concept. Whereas traditional instruments assessing the "now-self" provide ratings that are highly stable across periods as long as 35 years, possible selves—representing the "context of possibility that surrounds and embeds these self-views—may have undergone substantial changes during this period" (p. 965). Whether hoped for or feared, possible selves, like Cantor's (1990) life tasks and Markus's (1983) self-schemas, "focus more globally on what individuals hope to accomplish with their lives and what kind of people they would like to become as the significant elements of motivation" (Markus & Nurius, 1986, pp. 956–957).

Few would argue that people ordinarily fail to see themselves and others as temporally continuous, or indeed, that we fail to care how our lives go. That we hold selves to be continuous or persistent is not really at issue—it is a definitional part of the term *person*. What the philosophical literature does not, and perhaps cannot, tell us, however, is whether people routinely feel the need to resolve this paradox within the confines of their own lives, and, if they do, how is it accomplished? The answer to this last question can only be found by asking people how it is that they are still the same person despite the obvious ways in which they seem to have changed over time. The following section is devoted to summarizing the results of a series of studies designed to put this question to persons of various ages and cultural backgrounds. Our purpose in rehearsing these empirical findings, the details of which can be found in other publications, is to show that questions of personal persistence are matters of real concern to real young persons, and that the solution strategies they entertain are not only shaped by their own developmental station, but also by their cultural environment.

ACCESSING AND ASSESSING THOUGHTS ABOUT PERSONAL PERSISTENCE

Getting young people of differing ages and cultural groups to offer up their best thoughts about the paradox of sameness and change turns out to be more difficult than simply asking them how it is that they manage to both change and yet remain the same. At least this was our experience. In hindsight, the blank stares that attended this first-off, dead-simple assessment technique are perfectly understandable because (a) no one is born with clear thoughts about how it is that selves persist across time and there must be some developmental process that lies behind whatever grown-up mode of thinking might eventually emerge, and (b) there is no reason to assume (and every reason to doubt) that even the most articulate and self-aware among us would have a ready answer to this rather odd question, especially when it is lobbed in cold from somewhere out in left field. Some more roundabout way was needed, we soon discovered, of warming young people to the prospect of discussing this rather heady matter of their own persistence through time. The assessment strategy that we eventually adopted involved introducing the topic more gradually and by way of example by presenting fictional case histories of personal change over time and then soliciting comments on the continuity of the person in question before more gently turning attention to the participant's thoughts about continuity in his or her own life.

The procedure as it has come to be standardized in our studies involves presenting participants with a condensed comic-book version of the life story of a character (e.g., Victor Hugo's Jean Valjean in *Les Misérables*) who is said to undergo radical personal change over the course of the narrative. A set of probe questions are then used to elicit the participant's best thoughts as to why the protagonist, as described at the outset, should still be considered "the same person" at the end of the story. Following a pair of such stories, participants are then asked to describe themselves both as they perceive themselves in the present moment and at some point in their own distant past. Similar probe questions are then used to draw out the participants' views on the issue of their own self-continuity. This semistructured interview procedure has been employed, in various forms, to study reasoning about personal persistence in childhood (Chandler, Boyes, Ball, & Hala, 1987), adolescence (Chandler & Ball, 1990; Ferris, 2001), and adulthood (Brandstätter &

Lalonde, 2003), as well as in different cultural contexts (Chandler, Lalonde, Sokol, & Hallett, 2003). A more detailed accounting of the procedural means of conducting this interview can be found in these other sources, but for the moment, the point to be made is that there are practical ways in which to query persons of different ages about what have previously been seen as matters of interest only to professional philosophers. More important, here is what these studies have found.

First, on the basis of interviews conducted with more than 600 young persons to date, there appears to be a natural developmental progression to thoughts about personal persistence. Children, in their middle-school years, claim that persistence is found in any and all things that remain constant across time: pointing to one's name, favored activities, or physical appearance is seen to be sufficient. Change, if it is acknowledged at all, is seen as peripheral: "I am still the same because I still play soccer." In time, children begin to offer more substantial reasons that become increasingly abstract with advancing age. The hidden forces of unchanging personality traits often come to form the focus of arguments offered by preteens: "I'm still the same because I'm still aggressive: I used to get in fights at school, now I'm only aggressive on the soccer field where it's OK to be like that." For adolescents, the reasons lie deeper still: "I am the ship that sails through the troubled waters of my life." Making sense of these arguments is sometimes difficult, but a clear age-graded pattern in terms of increasing conceptual sophistication has been documented (Chandler et al., 2003).

The second general finding from these earlier studies is that these arguments in favor of continuity can be effectively sorted into one of two general kinds. One way of winning the argument that you are still the same person is to claim that you have not really changed at all, and to work to discount or trivialize anything that looks like evidence of change while clinging to all of those things about you that have managed to somehow withstand the ravages of time. Claiming, for example, that the basic structure of your personality has remained the same despite the differing ways in which it might be expressed over time, is just such a change-defeating, or *essentialist* argument. A second, and quite different *narrative* strategy involves first granting that real change has, in fact, occurred and then placing all hope of persistence on the existence of some narrative or plotlike way of seeing all of the different ways one has been in the past as connected through a series of storied and coherent cause-and-effect chains to the person one currently takes oneself to be. Brief descriptions and examples of these alternative essentialist and narrative self-continuity warranting strategies and the five-level sequence of reasoning types are presented in Table 10.1.

TABLE 10.1
Summary of Personal Persistence Warranting Strategies

Essentialist Strategies	Narrative Strategies
Level 1: Simple Inclusion Arguments The self is understood to be a simple assemblage of parts without internal structure. Continuity is maintained by finding any aspect of the self, no matter how trivial, that has managed to remain intact: one remains the same because, for example, their fingerprints or hair color has not changed.	*Level 1: Episodic Arguments* What passes for permanence here is a simple chronological listing out of events without providing any true plot structure. The mere contingency of events in time is thought to vouchsafe personal persistence across changes of any and all sorts.
Level 2: Topological Arguments Anything seemingly novel is argued to have already been present from the beginning, although perhaps temporarily obscured (e.g. "It looks to you like I've changed, but that's just because you've never seen this side of me before"). Change is discounted as a matter of mere appearance.	*Level 2: Picaresque Arguments* Respondents at this level construct somewhat more complex narratives, according to which, what passes for a plot is simply a listing out of episodes in which the hero acts in ways that confirm their true character. Within such stories, circumstances change, but persons do not.
Level 3: Epigenetic Arguments Change is seen as the result of an unfolding epigenetic plan that includes anticipated periods of immaturity that can create an illusion of discontinuity in those lacking an understanding of how life normally unfolds (e.g. "I know I seem different, but I always had it in me to be just the way I am right now").	*Level 3: Foundational Arguments* Past and present lives are seen as cause and effect— the "person" one has become is the inevitable consequence of antecedent events which have set his/her life on an unwavering and fatalistic course. The plot of such narratives concerns the sequence and impact of these cause and effect chains.
Level 4: Entity Arguments Change can be written off as mere phenotypic variations, while, beneath this changing surface structure, there remains a core of essential sameness capable of paraphrasing itself in endless superficial variations (e.g., "I have always been competitive—as a child I wanted to win races, now I want to get the best grades").	*Level 4: Embodiment Arguments* Selves are embodied agents" who share responsibility for the eventual shape of their own biographies. Arguments of this sort are true bildungsroman, or stories of character development governed by a real discoverable plot that is seen to reveal the precise reasons that things turned out as they did.

(continued)

TABLE 10.1   *(continued)*

Level 5: Theory Based Arguments	Level 5: Interpretive Arguments
While self is still a kind of "entity," permanence and change are now seen to exist simultaneously, forming a dynamic equilibrium. Accounts of self are provisional, or theory-like, and seen as being in need of active and continual revision.	The current narrative is seen to be only the latest in a perhaps endless series of attempts to interpretively re-read the past in light of the present. Continuity arises only out of the abstract pattern of one's efforts to make ongoing sense of oneself.

As might be expected, the list of variables associated with individual differences in performance on this 5-point scale includes the usual suspects of chronological age and level of cognitive development, a finding that is now supported by both cross-sectional and longitudinal data (Chandler et al., 2003). Explaining why it is that individual young people appear to prefer one of these solution strategies over the other, as they evidently do according to our data, and typically cling through thick and thin to that style of argumentation across this developmental progression is another matter. However, our data show just this sort of calculated loyalty: Although most can appreciate and even offer up arguments that belong to the other camp, their usual default strategy is unambiguously either essentialist or narrative. A partial answer to this question seems to reside in the cultural background of our interviewees. Among the "culturally mainstream" Canadian youth we have interviewed to date, more than 80% have employed essentialist strategies, whereas more than 70% of the Canadian Aboriginal (or First Nations) youth in our studies make use of narrative strategies. It is through these cross-cultural studies that personal and cultural continuity begin to connect.[1]

The intuition behind these cross-cultural comparisons was that young persons construct a sense of self—an identity—from materials made available to them by their cultural surroundings and that cultural groups differ in the kinds of materials that are ready to hand (see also

[1]Readers interested in possible relations between our essentialist–narrativist distinction and the work of Dweck (2000) may be interested to know that her Implicit Theories of Personality Scale was included in an earlier study in our research program. In a sample of Aboriginal youth who completed both our interview procedure and Dweck's (2000) 6-item inventory, essentialists were more likely to endorse an entity view of personality, whereas their narrativist peers took an altogether more process view.

Freund, chap. 9, this volume, for a discussion of societal levels of goals). For mainstream Canadian youth, growing up as they do within a European American intellectual tradition that places special value on what Polkinghorne (1988) called a "metaphysics of substance," according to which truth and beauty and virtue are always to be found at a depth beneath a shifting surface layer of mere appearance, essentialism is all but bred in the bone. By contrast, indigenous groups are said to promote a "metaphysics of potentiality and actuality" (Polkinghorne, 1988) that is consistent with their interpretive and oral traditions and their more thorough-going "ecocentric" approach to matters of knowledge and identity (Kirmayer, Brass, & Tait, 2000), so they favor a narrative stance. Seen in this light, the sharp differences that are apparent in the ways that Aboriginal and non-Aboriginal youth reason about personal persistence are entirely consistent with the cultural traditions within which they develop.

All of the foregoing was intended to make four key points. First, the issue of self-continuity or personal persistence is nothing new under the sun: Philosophers and psychologists and others have long wrestled with the paradox of sameness and change. Second, when the topic is presented in a suitable manner, as it is in our interview procedure, even middle-school children can be counted on to carefully consider the problem and are able to offer up reasons in favor of their own persistence in time. Third, there is a developmental progression in the sophistication of the reasoning used: Across the period of their teen years, the typical participants in our studies can be expected to pass from Level 1 to Level 5 of our coding scheme. Fourth and finally, there are clear differences in the argumentative strategies that young persons from different cultural backgrounds adopt. Aboriginal youth generally admit that real and transformative change has occurred in their lives, but work to construct a coherent narrative that weaves together the separate time slices of their experience. Non-Aboriginal youth, by contrast, typically labor to trivialize or deny change in favor of a hidden and unchanging essence that endures despite changes to the visible surface structure of the self.

All of that, we hope, has proven interesting enough, but wait (as they say), there is more. The "more" does not concern the normative process of development but rather the effect of certain kinds of failures or challenges faced in moving along this developmental sequence. As noted earlier, the consequences of such failures are found in elevated suicide risk for individual persons and whole communities.

ON THE PERSONAL AND CULTURAL
CONSEQUENCES OF FAILURES OF CONTINUITY

The theoretically driven nature of our work on identity formation led us to suppose that the stepwise function of increasing sophistication in reasoning about continuity we had observed would also leave room for a certain class of structural failures that attend any putative developmental sequence. In this particular case, we wondered about the consequences of transitional failures—of failing to step smoothly from one phase or stage in this normative sequence to the next. What would it mean, for example, if you were midway in your journey up this developmental staircase and found yourself suddenly off-balance by having abandoned your previous working notion of personal persistence as childish or naive, all before having any more fully formed or adequate alternative firmly in place? What if you fully lost—even for a brief developmental moment—that otherwise concrete sense of continuity in time that effectively binds together your own past, present, and future? Caught in that awkward transitional moment, with both feet temporarily off the ground and bereft of your usual and certain commitment to your own future, what would keep you from acting on those fleeting self-destructive impulses that occasionally haunt us all? What if, in the usual course of events, you were expected to ascend the full flight of this precarious set of stairs in your tumultuous teen years?

If failures to maintain a sense of personal persistence were as dangerous as we supposed, then young persons who are known to be actively suicidal, we reasoned, should also be marked by an inability to resolve the paradox of sameness and change as presented in our interview procedure. Studies of young people housed in psychiatric settings (Ball & Chandler, 1989; Ferris, 2001) have confirmed this suspicion. Unlike their nonhospitalized peers and unlike their wardmates who are hospitalized for reasons other than suicidality, over 80% of those known to be suicidal at the time of their interview were also unable to mount any kind of argument whatsoever as to why they themselves, or any story characters we presented, should be understood to persist through time. Of course, even controlling as we did for obvious third-variable candidates such as depression, we could still be reading the causal relation in the wrong direction: Perhaps being suicidal robs you of your sense of self-continuity. Perhaps, but that would still leave us all to wonder why suicide is most often attempted and committed by the young, and why it is that once past early adulthood, one's risk for suicide diminishes rather than grows.

If failures of personal persistence are associated with individual acts of suicide and if such failures are most likely to occur in the teen years when the pace of change is at its height, then perhaps we have the beginnings of an explanation for the sudden and dramatic spiking in suicidal behavior that occurs during adolescence and early adulthood. This at least has been the guiding assumption behind our continued work in this area.

If the usual forces of development regularly put young people in harm's way during their adolescent years, then why are suicide rates so much higher still among Aboriginal youth? Available evidence suggests that Aboriginal youth in Canada are three to five times more likely to die by their own hand than non-Aboriginal youth (Lalonde, 2001). Indeed, the Aboriginal population of Canada is said to suffer the highest suicide rate of any culturally identifiable group in the world (Kirmayer, 1994). Usual explanations for this dramatic difference in suicide rates invoke demographic differences in poverty or transience, or point toward higher rates of mental illness in the Aboriginal population. By focusing as they do on population-level variables, such explanations gloss over the diversity that exists within Aboriginal groups and promote the mistaken notion that there is an epidemic of suicide sweeping through the Aboriginal population. In fact, although it is true that suicide rates are extremely high in some Aboriginal communities, our research has shown that in British Columbia, in over half of all First Nations communities no suicides were recorded in a 14-year period from 1987 to 2001 (Chandler & Lalonde, 1998; Lalonde, 2001). Apparently, some communities have effectively "solved" the suicide problem. Within the remaining communities, rates range from well below the provincial average to 50 times higher. This is a rather selective epidemic.

The question that immediately leaps to mind, of course, is just what separates the high-suicide communities from those in which suicide is remarkably rare or entirely absent? The answer—or at least some part of an answer—is to be found in mechanisms that work to maintain continuity, not of individual persons but of cultural communities. Just as conceptions of self-continuity work on the individual level to extend the self both forward and backward in time by keeping us committed to an anticipated future and responsible for our own past, and so provide a hedge against suicide risk, so also do conceptions of cultural continuity, but this time on a much larger scale. Communities that have been especially successful in protecting their youth from suicide risk, at least according to our research, are also marked by efforts to preserve and promote their cultural heritage, assert direct local control over key aspects of civic life, reacquire and maintain access to their traditional territories, and secure political self-determination. That is, those communities that effectively own their own past and control their own future have the lowest suicide rates (Chandler & Lalonde, 1998; Lalonde, 2001).

Once again, however, we could be reading this epidemiological relation in the wrong direction. It could be that individual acts of suicide rob a community of a sense of cultural continuity. Perhaps, and although no one would doubt that a suicide—particularly the suicide of a young person—can have a devastating effect within a small community, that would again leave us to wonder why the presence of these same factors is associated with higher rates of school completion and lower rates of unintentional injuries. Cultural continuity appears to be associated with many measures of healthy youth development. Our own more hopeful reading of this growing data set is that youth who develop within communities that actively promote their cultural heritage and have been successful in achieving a measure of self-government tend to care about their own personal and cultural future.

PERSONAL PERSISTENCE AND PERSONAL PROJECTS

What, you might wonder, does all of this talk of suicide have to do with personal projects? It illustrates the importance and utility of personal self-constructions and the key role that the cultural environment can play to support or undercut such constructions. What all of the research reported thus far cannot tell us, however, is how these essentialist or narrative views are formed, maintained, or reconstructed over time. What actions or activities—personal or cultural—function to prop up particular conceptions of the self? What impels young people to abandon one way of thinking in favor of another? In other words, how are differing conceptions of the self expressed in everyday life? Some large measure of our own hopes for answering just these sorts of questions has come to rest on personal projects analysis. Our reasons are as follows.

If our personal projects are predictive of general well-being (Little, 1985, 1988, 1989, 1998, 2000) and if failures in personal persistence are associated with acts of suicide, then we might predict a relation between the two measures, at least at the extremes. That is, the personal projects of suicidal persons should be markedly different than those of more rank-and-file young persons. Indeed, evidence from personal project research involving students seeking psychological counseling (Salmela-Aro, 1992) as well as clinically depressed populations (Röhrle, Hedke, & Leibold, 1994) supports this hypothesis. However, beyond these extraordinary or tragic cases, there are other reasons to suppose that personal projects hold the potential to tell us something of value about the self-conceptions of their authors. First, personal projects are more than an arbitrary assemblage of mundane tasks or running "to-do" lists. Rather, our personal tasks and goals represent a personal project *system*—an organized and focused set of plans that orient us toward an anticipated and valued future. As such, they can be seen to embody the person we take ourselves to be en route to becoming. If that is so, if personal projects are an expression of our ability to envision our own future and to work toward bringing it about, then an analysis of such project systems should provide a window onto conceptions of the self. Viewed in the opposite direction, it should be the case that conceptions of selfhood play an important role in the inception, construction, and execution of personal projects.

Personal projects represent concrete efforts to manipulate the environment and to engineer our own experience in ways that create the future we envision for ourselves. Our beliefs about the true or authentic self—the self that endures despite the changes that our own efforts are designed to bring about—are the yardsticks against which the success of personal projects is measured. If Flanagan (1996) was right, that is, if "we are navigators" and really do "care how our lives go," then combining the study of self-continuity with the conceptualization of personal projects as "conative units of analysis" pertaining to motivation (Little, 1999) and self (Little, 1993) may help us better understand how and why we plot the particular life course that we work to follow. In short, then, here are the twin working hypotheses that prompted this research: Personal projects propel our ongoing construction and reconstruction of self, and conceptions of personal persistence provide a rudder and a compass.

The sea swell of contemporary interest in studying the meaning of selfhood is sustained by the availability of tools (e.g., PPA and the personal persistence interview) that claim to capture both idiographic and nomothetic dimensions of the self. Moving between these levels of analysis is, of course, an inherently risky business. The real end of our work, however, is not simply the private thoughts of individuals about the routine business of managing their lives (their personal projects), nor even their deeply held notions of personhood (self-continuity). Rather, it is the conjunction of these two—how the ways in which we understand and navigate our own lives work to create the self. By applying both tools to the problem at hand, we would seem to have a better chance of capturing Bruner's "self in use" or McAdams's (1996c) "selfing" or the elusive connection between self and culture:

> The Self, then, like any other aspect of human nature, stands both as guardian of permanence and as a barometer responding to the local cultural weather. The culture, as well, provides us with guides and stratagems for finding a niche between stability and change: it exhorts, forbids, lures, denies, rewards the commitments that the Self undertakes. And the Self, using its capacities for reflection and for envisaging alternatives, escapes or embraces or reevaluates and reformulates what the culture has on offer. (Bruner, 1990, p. 110)

The joint assessment of personal projects and conceptions of personal persistence would, we reasoned, tell us something of value about the public and private ways in which our participants attempt to influence the course of their own development by identifying the ways in which they quite literally preserve, alter, enhance, and re-create themselves as they navigate through time. To this end, we collected personal projects questionnaires from close to 400 undergraduate students, and interviewed a subsample of 75 participants to collect their thoughts about their own and others' continuity in time. Among the many questions that we sought to answer with this large and rich data set, two are especially relevant to the purpose here. First, because of our particular interest in selves in time, we wanted to know whether personal projects are targeted at the temporal aspects of the self. That is, do projects differently address one's past, present, and anticipated future? Second, we wanted to examine the personal projects of essentialists and narrativists as classified in our self-continuity interview. Do the groups differ in terms of the kinds of personal projects they pursue? Do they differ in terms of the functions that these projects are understood to serve with reference to their conceptions of self?

Do Personal Projects Target Temporal Aspects of the Self?

The modular nature of PPA made it possible to add to the 17 core dimensions established by Little (1998) a total of 12 ad hoc dimensions that, among other things, address the temporal aspects of the self. The standard set was complemented by 2 previously tested dimensions, distractibility and commitment (Brandstätter & Baumann, 2003), as well as 10 ad hoc dimensions developed for this study. Nine of these ad hoc dimensions were added to capture specific ways in which projects might function in relation to the maintenance and change of a person's self-conceptions. (For a complete listing and description of the additional dimensions, see Table 10.2.) These self-related dimensions were hypothesized to align according to their temporal orientation to past self, present self, and future self (see Figure 10.1). Finally, a community/culture dimension was added to capture the relatedness to one's community or cultural group that might be gained by involvement in a project. (For a comparison of the traditional factor structure with the derived factors from this expanded set, see Table 10.3.)

The hypothesized structure of these self-related dimensions appears in Figure 10.1. As can be seen in this figure, our nine self-related dimensions were hypothesized to reflect the manner in which personal pro-

TABLE 10.2
Dimensions added to Personal Projects Analysis

Dimension	Description
Community/ Culture:	how much this personal project conveys or reflects a sense of connection to your community or culture
Self-related dimensions	
Centrality:	how central this personal project is to your sense of self
Expression:	to what extent this personal project highlights or showcases an aspect of the self that already exists—a part of you that has not reached the surface but already exists
Enhancement:	to what extent this personal project aims at improving upon an existing positive aspect of the self
Experimentation:	to what extent this personal project reflects trying new ways of being
Exploration:	to what extent this project examines aspects of the self
Extension:	to what extent this project reflects an existing part of the self that is pushed or applied to new settings or displayed in a new manner
Preservation:	to what extent this project prevents changes to existing aspects of the self by taking actions that strengthen the current self
Improvement:	to what extent this personal project serves the improvement of an existing (negative) aspect of the self
Re-establishment:	to what extent this personal project serves to reconnect to or regain an earlier aspect of the self

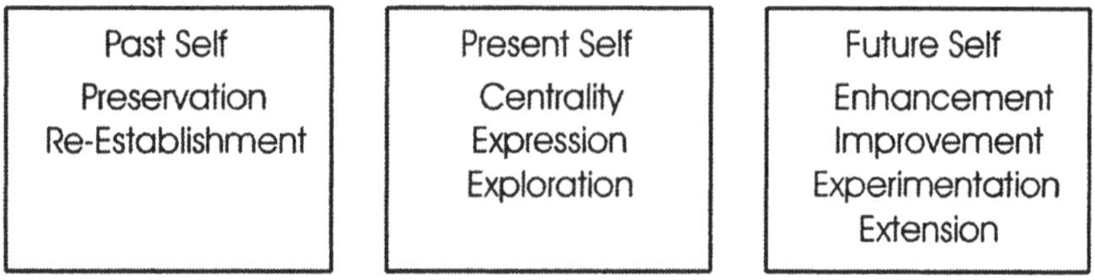

Past Self	Present Self	Future Self
Preservation Re-Establishment	Centrality Expression Exploration	Enhancement Improvement Experimentation Extension

Figure 10.1. Hypothesized structure of self-related dimensions.

jects are used to express central aspects of the current self (present: centrality, expression, exploration) to bring about changes to the self (future: experimentation, extension, improvement, enhancement), and to preserve or regain valued aspects of self (past: preservation, reestablishment). An evaluation of this hypothesis using exploratory factor analyses, however, revealed that all of the self-related dimensions are highly intercorrelated, resulting in a one-factor solution. This suggests that projects that are generally experienced as "closer to home" relate fairly consistently to all of these factors. In other words, whereas some projects may not be relevant to any of these self-functions, others simultaneously serve present, past, and future self-functions. Interestingly, however, eliciting two-, three-, and four-factor solutions yielded support for the more finely grained structure of our hypothesized temporal alignment with two noteworthy exceptions.

First, exploration, which we had imagined would constitute a function of the present self, relates instead to the future-oriented factors. Our working definition of exploration included processes of reflecting on one's personality or self—a sort of stock-taking exercise—although our participants clearly conceived it as an activity closer to experimentation: It seems to have been understood as more external than internal and as having to do with where they imagine themselves going rather than where they have been. Second, our hypothesized future-related dimensions generated two factors rather than one: Improvement and enhancement turn out to be all about attempts to (as the old song goes) "accentuate the positive, eliminate the negative,"or, in short, about becoming a better self (i.e., future-better). Experimentation, extension, and exploration build a separate factor capturing self functions that are more oriented toward becoming a different self (i.e., future-other). These findings are illustrated in Figure 10.2.

The high intercorrelations among self-functions indicate that both projects and project systems typically serve all four of the self-functions, although usually with differing degrees of emphasis on any one func-

TABLE 10.3
Traditional and Derived Factor Structure

Traditional Factory	Dimension	Derived Factor
	Community/Culture[a]	
Meaning	Value congruency	Identity/Culture
	Self-identity	
	Enjoyment	
	Importance	
	Absorption	
	Distractibility[a]	Efficacious involvement
	Commitment[a]	
Efficacy	Project state	
	Progress	
	Outcome	
Structure	Control	Structure
	Initiation	
	Negative impact	
Stress	Stress	Stress
	Difficulty	
	Challenge	
Community	Support	Community
	Others' view of importance	
	Visibility	

[a]New dimension.

tion. That is, at the microlevel (project-level analyses), a project may emphasize the future-better self-function, at the same time maintaining some minimal threshold level of focus on the other self functions. Similarly, at the macrolevel (project system-level analyses), the project sys-

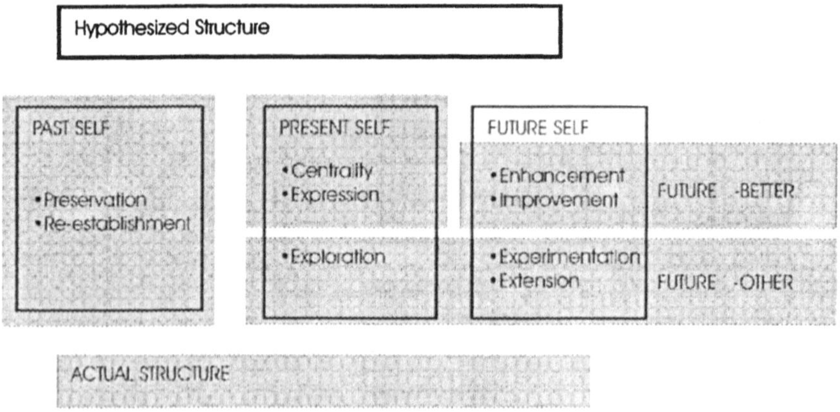

Figure 10.2.   Hypothesized and actual structure of self-related dimensions. The hypothesized structure is overlapped by the actual structure (gray boxes).

tem of a given person also comprises all four self-functions and aims to achieve a balance among them. Hence, people seem to achieve coherence both within and across their projects, rather than dedicating part of their project system toward change and other parts toward sameness. Sameness and change, it seems, are relentlessly on the agenda for everybody, in every project, and within the whole project system at any given point in time.

Do the Personal Projects of Essentialists and Narrativists Differ?

Among the 75 participants who completed both the PPA and the self-continuity interview, 48 were classified as essentialist and 27 as narrativist (see Table 10.4 for the distribution of these participants across levels and tracks). The groups did not differ in the level of reasoning used (a measure of argumentative sophistication), nor on other demographic variables that might be of interest (e.g., age, gender). More centrally, however, and in ways that we initially found discouraging, the groups also did not differ with regard to their overall ratings on the personal project dimensions or on the higher level project factors (as shown in Table 10.3, the factors derived through exploratory factor analysis were stress, efficacious involvement, identity/culture, community, and structure, as well as the self-related factors of future-other self,

TABLE 10.4

Number of participants by track and level of self-continuity strategy

Track	Level					Total
	I	II	III	IV	V	
Essentialist	1	11	18	14	4	48
Narrative	2	1	6	14	4	27
Total	3	12	24	28	8	75

present self, future-better self, and past self). At first blush, then, there seemed little to choose between them: For essentialists and narrativists alike, personal projects are, just as Little intended, used to manage the minutiae of everyday life.

On reflection, however, this absence of overall or global differences should have come as no surprise. There are no good reasons to imagine, for example, that essentialists should rate their projects as any more or less important or central than narrativists, nor to think that one group would necessarily experience higher levels of stress or lower levels of structure. Differences did appear, however, when we probed more deeply and examined the kinds of projects that essentialists and narrativists were engaged in, and the ways in which they negotiated the meaning–manageability trade-off (Little, 1998) in the service of over-arching needs for self-expression, preservation, enhancement, and ex-tension. As we argue later, these differences are reflective of their divergent conceptions of selfhood.

Projects were categorized in the usual manner into one of six content categories: academic or occupational, health or appearance, interper-sonal, intrapersonal or value concerns, leisure, and administrative or maintenance. A series of group differences emerged with respect to cer-tain kinds of projects but for the sake of brevity, the results of the long series of analyses we carried out on these project content categories can be summarized in just two claims about overall differences between essentialists and narrativists. Both claims are consistent with the self-continuity strategies of these groups: It appears that narrativists have a more distributed sense of self (distributed across both people and pro-jects) and tend to engage in projects that emphasize meaning over man-ageability. Essentialists appear to be resistant to change and tend to engage in projects that are more manageable rather than meaningful.

Distributed Self and Meaning. The claim that narrativists have a more distributed sense of self is evident in both the greater frequency with which they engage in interpersonal projects (more distributed across people) and in the fact that they show higher ratings of self-identity for administrative tasks. These higher levels of self-identity associated with administrative projects—with the nitty-gritty of our lives—seem to indicate that narrativists invest a substantial amount of self even into seemingly mundane tasks such as searching for an apartment, filling out job applications, or cleaning the house. Perhaps because these projects are extensions of the self, they are also stressful: Narrativists deem their administrative projects only slightly less stressful than their academic ones, whereas essentialists experience much lower stress in conjunction with their administrative projects than with academic ones. For narrativists, administrative projects are more relevant to their sense of self than their academic or their health projects. For essentialists, on the other hand, these other project categories are more reflective of their true self than administrative undertakings.

Change Resistance and Manageability. The claim that essentialists are resistant to change arises mainly from our analysis of their intrapersonal and health projects. Intrapersonal projects are particularly theoretically interesting, as they reflect "an individual's own motivation, personal characteristics, and sense of identity" (Little, 1993, p. 173). In the context of our study, they were expected to be particularly revealing with regard to possible differences between essentialists and narrativists. Indeed, when we conducted discriminant function analyses using the combination of the 29 project rating dimensions averaged across intrapersonal projects, essentialists and narrativists could be reliably distinguished on the basis of their intrapersonal project ratings alone. Essentialists' intrapersonal projects were more visible, value-congruent, self-explorative, and self-extending but lower in initiation than those of narrativists. However, intrapersonal projects also tend to be stressful and onerous (Little, 1993; Salmela-Aro, 1992), and essentialists seem to avoid such projects whenever possible. When essentialists do engage in these projects, they are likely to be initiated (or coinitiated) by other people. It is interesting to note that although essentialists are less likely to initiate intrapersonal projects, they do not report fewer of these projects. Furthermore, essentialists tend to use their intrapersonal projects to a larger extent to achieve future-other self functions (exploration and extension). A similar tendency is observed for health-related projects, suggesting that when essentialists experience personal change it is either a result of projects that were pressed on them by others or else occurs incidentally through projects that are undertaken for reasons other than personal change.

Body and Soul Projects. Health projects appear to have a particularly important role in achieving self-continuity for essentialists. In being highly relevant to both their preservation needs (preservation, past self) and their need for change (future-other: exploration, extension, experimentation), health projects may be a main vehicle of self-continuity for essentialists—extending from the past via the present to the future. In effect, this may represent the embodiment idea that is the *essence* in essentialist: defining their body as a core aspect of what they count as self over time, or what they use to achieve an enduring sense of self—a body that needs to be taken care of, exercised, fed well, and given a haircut now and then.

For narrativists, intrapersonal projects are the more likely candidates to fulfill such self-preservation or self-continuity functions, as expressed in higher preservation ratings (and as a trend in higher past self factor ratings) of projects in this category as compared to health projects. Unlike health projects that target physical aspects of the self, intrapersonal projects are aimed at bringing about psychological change. As such, our findings suggest that narrativists—in accord with our conceptualization of their self-continuity reasoning strategy—are looking for stability or continuity not in essences but in psychological constructs, and in the construction and reconstruction of personal narratives as suggested by McAdams (1995, 1996a, 1996b), Sarbin (1997), and other life story theorists (e.g., Bruner, 2001; Ezzy, 1998). In summary, intrapersonal projects are highly relevant to the two future-related self functions and present self for both groups, and for past self foremost for narrativists.

Meaning and Manageability. The meaning–manageability tradeoff—the need to "jointly optimize the manageability and the meaningfulness of projects" (Little, 1989, p. 21)—is essentially a question of project *phrasing level*. Little (1988) suggested that the level at which a project is phrased can be determined "simply by reference to its abstraction level, its syntactical or linguistic complexity, and the scope and span of activities entailed" (p. 44). In Little's example, the meaning–manageability trade-off consists of the need to choose between or balance molecular-level projects such as "return the ladder to my neighbour" and highly molar-level superordinate activities such as "challenge the rise of Australian realist philosophy" (Little, 1989, p. 21). Our own claim that essentialists favor more manageable projects whereas narrativists emphasize meaning is supported not only by the fact that essentialists report fewer interpersonal projects (just over half of essentialists [54%] report such projects, compared with 85% of narrativists), but that these projects appear to be more concrete and more "doable." This is reflected in the project stage ratings: Essentialists deem their interpersonal projects as being closer to completion and, therefore, as possibly having more defined and concrete beginnings and endings rather than as representative of more extended and overarching personal strivings.

Essentialists not only rate their interpersonal projects as higher in progress than narrativists rate theirs, they also rate them as more progressed compared to their own academic and leisure projects (and narrativists rate projects in each of these categories to be at similar stages). This indicates that, if essentialists do construe their interpersonal projects at lower phrasing levels (Emmons, 1992; Little, 1988, 1989), then this is a content-specific phenomenon, which does not generalize to the categories of academic and leisure projects. If project stage does, in fact, signify a proxy measure of project phrasing level, then essentialists seem to tip the balance toward more manageable and narrativists may tend to choose the meaningful.

Personal Persistence and Subjective Well-Being

Essentialists and narrativists also differed in terms of their subjective well-being (for a discussion of the facets of well-being, see Wiese, chap. 11, this volume). For essentialists, positive affect is particularly—and only—associated with past self aspects, indicating that they experience positive affect when personal projects provide self-preservation and reestablishment, rather than any of the other self-functions. For narrativists, positive affect relationships are more evenly distributed across the self-functions. Among narrativists, the extent to which projects reflect a sense of personal identity as well as a sense of belonging to their community or culture was strongly reflected in their affective experience. Higher identity and culture ratings are associated with high positive and low negative affect. For essentialists, these relationships are completely absent. For this group, it is the more tangible aspects of community, such as support and others' view of importance, that are more relevant to the experience of positive affect as well as affect balance.

This latter result is particularly interesting in view of the inverse relation between cultural continuity and suicide rates in Aboriginal communities. The extent to which personal projects reflect both a personal sense of agency and a sense of belonging to one's community plays an important role in the well-being of individuals preferring a narrative approach to self-continuity, although having little effect for essentialists. This finding, combined with the fact that Aboriginal youth prefer narrativist strategies by a margin of four to one, provides (indirect) evidence of the differential importance that cultural connectedness can have for different cultural groups. Cultural continuity may be particularly important to communities (e.g., Aboriginal communities) in which a narrativist approach to self-continuity is the preferred or predominant strategy.

CONCLUSION AND FUTURE DIRECTIONS: BOOSTING OUR OWN FUTURE-BETTER RATINGS

Our work is predicated on the notion that we construct and reconstruct and invent and reinvent ourselves in ways that bear the marks of both social and personal construction. Who we are, the persons we take ourselves to be, the persons we hope to become or fondly recall having been, are neither fully determined by our cultural surround nor wholly matters of personal invention. The aim of the new research outlined here was to empirically demonstrate that the process of "selfing" connects our deep-seated, enduring, and implicit conceptions of self with the more routine, changeable, and explicit actions we undertake in our workaday personal and social worlds.

By necessity, we have painted the research in very broad strokes, leaving out great swaths of detail concerning our procedures and statistical analyses, but hope to have persuaded you that there is general merit in this approach and, more specifically, that narrativists and essentialists use personal projects in ways that are consistent with their conceptions of personal change. Narrativists emphasize the relational and interpersonal aspects of change whereas essentialists, although less likely to actively seek change, maintain continuity by structuring their project systems in ways that shore up their own more embodied view of self. For essentialists and narrativists alike, personal projects can, and evidently do, work to propel the self through time by providing the necessary connective tissue that binds past, present, and future aspects of the self.

The success of this initial effort to connect self-continuity and personal projects—and so to connect the personal and the cultural—rests on the effectiveness of the new dimensions we introduced to the personal projects procedure. Our intent was to focus the attention of our respondents on two previously underexplored aspects of personal project systems. First, we wanted them to comment on the temporal aspects of their projects—on the ways that projects might specifically target their own past, present, and future. We did this by creating a set of self-related dimensions that eventuated in our past self, present self, future-other, and future-better factors.

Second, we asked our respondents about the extent to which each project "conveys or reflects a sense of connection to your community or culture." This community/culture dimension did not load on the traditional community factor but instead helped create a new factor (identity/culture) constructed out of the core dimensions of the traditional meaning factor (value-congruency, self-identity, enjoyment). This new factor appears to capture those aspects of the personal project system that operate to connect personal identity and meaning with a sense of communal identity and cultural belonging.

Interestingly, the identity/culture factor is the only one that related to all four of the self factors (past self, present self, future-other, and future-better) indicating that participants who rate their projects as high on identity/culture have projects that serve all self-functions, be they past-, present-, or future-self related. The relation between identity/culture and future-other is in many ways the most informative from a theoretical point of view. How can something that is not yet realized be invested with such a heavy load of personal and cultural meaning? We believe this points to the importance of *potential*—of a sense of identity that is projected through a realm of possibilities and possible selves. These are the projects that involve the highest degrees of uncertainty and risk. Future-other projects involve stepping away from the roots of the current and past self into new and unknown territory. The association with identity/culture shows that such tasks are only undertaken when they are close to the heart and offer the possibility of strengthening a sense of cultural belonging.

Here we arrive at our last point. To borrow Flanagan's language again, if both persons and whole cultures can be understood as "beings in time" and "navigators" that care how their lives go, then understanding how personal and cultural activities work to preserve continuity in the face of change, and ultimately, how such activities or projects operate to bring about a better future—a personal future and collective future—should be high on our list of research priorities. Within the Aboriginal communities that have collaborated in our work on youth suicide, finding ways to preserve culture and to promote a strong sense of cultural belonging among youth consistently tops the list of community goals. Our research suggests that these efforts to strengthen cultural continuity are likely to pay particularly large dividends in terms of lowering suicide rates given the preponderance of the narrative strategy among Aboriginal youth. Relative to essentialists, whose sense of self-continuity is largely self-contained, narrativists derive strength from the interleaving of shared personal histories. For youth who adopt narrativist strategies, the effect of threats to culture or of positive community actions on a sense of personal persistence will be magnified. When your own sense of personal persistence is dependent on the persistence of your culture, the need for strategies that maintain self- and cultural continuity is more vital.

Aboriginal communities do not, of course, need to be told—especially by ivory tower academics—that maintaining their culture is important or that threats to their culture bring dangers that are disproportionately visited on their youth. However, community leaders are open to new methods of assessing the impact that their own efforts to promote self-determination can have on youth development, and we believe that a suitably refined version of the self-continuity and personal projects methodology we employed could be especially valuable in supporting these efforts. The usual methods of program evaluation—those that focus on changes in the attitudes or behaviors of persons exposed to this or that particular form of intervention—are particularly ill-suited to the task of evaluating the effect of multilevel community-based efforts to promote culture. Consider, for example, the fact that Aboriginal communities in British Columbia that have succeeded in gaining control over local police and fire services have lower rates of suicide than communities without control. Any evaluation strategy that focused on youth attitudes toward the acquisition of fire-fighting equipment or a local constabulary would clearly miss the point. What we really want to know is why youth who come of age in communities that acquire such services are so much better off. What we want, then, is a means of connecting personal identity with a sense of cultural identity. This is the promise offered by our methodology.

REFERENCES

Bakhtin, M. (1986). *Speech genres and other late essays.* Austin: University of Texas Press.

Ball, L., & Chandler, M. J. (1989). Identity formation in suicidal and non-suicidal youth: The role of self-continuity. *Development and Psychopathology, 1,* 257–275.

Brandstätter, M., & Baumann, U. (2003, June). Personal projects in Austrian students: Project stability and relationship to subjective well-being. In J. J. Van Bavel (Chair), *A symposium on the role of context in acculturation, identity and meaning.* Symposium conducted at the annual convention of the Canadian Psychological Association, Hamilton, ON, June 12–14.

Brandstätter, M., & Lalonde, C. E. (2003, June). *Self-continuity and personal projects: Abstract reasoning and everyday undertakings as functions of the self.* Paper presented at the annual meeting of the Jean Piaget Society, Chicago.

Bruner, J. (1990). *Acts of meaning.* Cambridge, MA: Harvard University Press.

Bruner, J. (2001). Self-making and world-making. In J. Brockmeier & D. Carbaugh (Eds.), *Narrative and identity: Studies in autobiography, self and culture* (pp. 25–37). Amsterdam: John Benjamins.

Cantor, N. (1990). From thought to behavior: "Having" and "doing" in the study of personality and cognition. *American Psychologist, 45,* 735–750.

Cassirer, E. (1923). *Substance and function.* Chicago: Open Court.

Chandler, M. J., & Ball, L. (1990). Continuity and commitment: A developmental analysis of the identity formation process in suicidal and non-suicidal youth. In H. Bosma & S. Jackson (Eds.), *Coping and self-concept in adolescence* (pp. 149–166). New York: Springer-Verlag.

Chandler, M. J., Boyes, M., Ball, L., & Hala, S. (1987). The conservation of selfhood: A developmental analysis of children's changing conceptions of self-continuity. In T. Honess & K. Yardley (Eds.), *Self and identity: Perspectives across the life-span* (pp. 108–120). London: Routledge & Kegan Paul.

Chandler, M. J., & Lalonde, C. (1998). Cultural continuity as a hedge against suicide in Canada's First Nations. *Transcultural Psychiatry, 35,* 191–219.

Chandler, M. J., Lalonde, C. E., Sokol, B. W., & Hallett, D. (2003). Personal persistence, identity development, and suicide: A study of Native and non-Native North American adolescents. *Monographs of the Society for Research in Child Development, 68*(2).

Chisholm, R. M. (1971). On the logic of intentional action. In R. Binkley, R. Bronaugh, & A. Marras (Eds.), *Agent, action, and reason* (pp. 38–80). Toronto: University of Toronto Press.

Dweck, C. S. (2000). *Self-theories: Their role in motivation, personality, and development.* Philadelphia: Psychology Press.

Emmons, R. A. (1992). Abstract versus concrete goals: Personal striving levels, physical illness, and psychological well-being. *Journal of Personality and Social Psychology, 62,* 292–300.

Ezzy, D. (1998). Theorizing narrative identity: Symbolic interactionism and hermeneutics. *Sociological Quarterly, 39,* 239–252.

Ferris, J. M. (2001). *Reasoning about self-continuity and self-unity among psychiatrically ill adolescents.* Unpublished bachelor's thesis, University of Victoria, Victoria, BC, Canada.

Flanagan, O. (1996). *Self-expressions: Mind, morals and the meaning of life.* New York: Oxford University Press.

Fraisse, P. (1963). *The psychology of time.* New York: Harper & Row.

James, W. (1910). *Psychology: The briefer course.* New York: Holt.

Kirmayer, L. (1994). Suicide among Canadian aboriginal people. *Transcultural Psychiatric Research Review, 31,* 3–57.

Kirmayer, L. J., Brass, G. M., & Tait, C. L. (2000). The mental health of Aboriginal peoples: Transformations of identity and community. *Canadian Journal of Psychiatry, 45,* 607–616.

Lalonde, C. E. (2001). *Suicide rates among First Nations persons in British Columbia (1993–2000).* Victoria: British Columbia Ministry of Health and Ministry Responsible for Seniors.

Little, B. R. (1985). *Personal projects and social ecology: Exploring the determinants of human well-being.* Ottawa, ON, Canada: Carleton University, Social Ecology Laboratory, Department of Psychology.

Little, B. R. (1988). *Personal projects analysis: Theory, method and research.* Ottawa, ON, Canada: Social Sciences and Humanities Research Council of Canada.

Little, B. R. (1989). Personal projects analysis: Trivial pursuits, magnificent obsessions, and the search for coherence. In D. M. Buss & N. Cantor (Eds.), *Personality psychology: Recent trends and emerging directions* (pp. 15–31). New York: Springer-Verlag.

Little, B. R. (1993). Personal projects and the distributed self: Aspects of a conative psychology. In J. M. Suls (Ed.), *The self in social perspective: Psychological perspectives on the self* (Vol. 4, pp. 157–185). Hillsdale, NJ: Lawrence Erlbaum Associates.

Little, B. R. (1998). Personal project pursuit: Dimensions and dynamics of personal meaning. In P. T. P. Wong & P. S. Fry (Eds.), *The human quest for meaning: A handbook of psychological research and clinical applications* (pp. 193–212). Mahwah, NJ: Lawrence Erlbaum Associates.

Little, B. R. (1999). Personality and motivation: Personal action and the conative evolution. In L. A. Pervin & O. P. John (Eds.), *Handbook of personality: Theory and research* (2nd ed., pp. 501–524). New York: Guilford.

Little, B. R. (2000). Free traits and personal contexts: Expanding a social ecological model of well-being. In W. B. Walsh, K. H. Craik, & R. H. Price (Eds.), *Person–environment psychology: New directions and perspectives* (2nd ed., pp. 87–116). Mahwah, NJ: Lawrence Erlbaum Associates.

Locke, J. (1956). *Essay concerning human understanding.* Oxford, UK: Clarendon. (Original work published 1694)

MacIntyre, A. (1984). *After virtue: A study in moral theory.* Notre Dame, IN: University of Notre Dame Press.

Markus, H. (1983). Self-knowledge: An expanded view. *Journal of Personality, 51,* 543–565.

Markus, H., & Nurius, P. (1986). Possible selves. *American Psychologist, 41,* 954–969.

Markus, H., & Ruvolo, A. (1989). Possible selves: Personalized representations of goals. In L. A. Pervin (Ed.), *Goal concepts in personality and social psychology* (pp. 211–241). Hillsdale, NJ: Lawrence Erlbaum Associates.

McAdams, D. P. (1995). What do we know when we know a person? *Journal of Personality, 63,* 365–396.

McAdams, D. P. (1996a). Alternative futures for the study of human individuality. *Journal of Research in Personality, 30,* 374–388.

McAdams, D. P. (1996b). Personality, modernity, and the storied self: A contemporary framework for studying persons. *Psychological Inquiry, 7,* 295–321.

McAdams, D. P. (1996c). What this framework can and cannot do. *Psychological Inquiry, 7,* 378–386.

Polkinghorne, C. (1988). *Narrative knowing and the human sciences.* Albany: State University of New York Press.

Röhrle, B., Hedke, J., & Leibold, S. (1994). Persönliche Projekte zur Herstellung und Pflege sozialer Beziehungen bei depressiven und nicht depressiven Personen [Social relationships as personal projects in depressives and nondepressives]. *Zeitschrift für Klinische Psychologie, 23,* 43–51.

Rorty, A. O. (1973). The transformations of persons. *Philosophy, 48,* 261–275.

Salmela-Aro, K. (1992). Struggling with self: The personal projects of students seeking psychological counselling. *Scandinavian Journal of Psychology, 33,* 330–338.

Sarbin, T. R. (1997). The poetics of identity. *Theory and Psychology, 7,* 67–82.

Strawson, G. (1999). Self and body: Self, body, and experience. *Supplement to the Proceedings of Aristotelian-Society, 73,* 307–332.

Taylor, C. (1988). The moral topography of the self. In S. B. Messer, L. A. Sass, & R. L. Woolfolk (Eds.), *Hermeneutics and psychological theory: Interpretive perspectives on personality, psychotherapy, and psychopathology* (pp. 298–320). New Brunswick, NJ: Rutgers University Press.

Wiggins, D. (1980). *Sameness and substance.* Cambridge, MA: MIT Press.

IV

Projects, Goals, and the Varieties of Well-Being

11

Successful Pursuit of Personal Goals and Subjective Well-Being

Bettina S. Wiese

Does achieving our goals make us happy? Is it achieving our goals or successfully pursuing them that matters? What do we mean by successful goal pursuit? Although the answers to these questions might intuitively seem simple, recent research reveals that the relation between personal goal achievement and subjective well-being is more complex.

Personal goals[1] and subjective well-being have often been linked (e.g., Brunstein, 1993; Emmons, 1986). Within the framework of personal goal constructs, it has been repeatedly stated that striving toward personal goals provides a person's life with structure and meaning (e.g., Klinger, 1977; Little, 1989), and empirical evidence has shown that people who are involved in the pursuit of subjectively important personal goals indicate higher subjective well-being than individuals who lack a sense of goal directedness (e.g., Emmons, 1986; Freund & Baltes,

---

[1]In this chapter, the term *personal goals* is used as a generic, inclusive equivalent for concepts focusing on self-set action-related endeavors such as personal projects, personal strivings, current concerns, and so on (see Little, 1999, for similarities and differences among these concepts).

2002). It seems plausible that if being committed to and acting on meaningful personal goals has positive consequences for well-being (e.g., Emmons, 1986), then making progress or attaining this goal should also have a positive effect (or have an even more pronounced effect). Hence, it is not surprising that a basic assumption of the personal goal literature is that the successful pursuit of meaningful goals plays an important role in the development and maintenance of psychological well-being (see Brunstein, 1993). This chapter summarizes theoretical and empirical approaches concerning the effects of successful goal pursuit on different facets of well-being. Before reviewing and integrating respective empirical research, however, the concepts of progress and attainment, as well as the multifaceted construct of subjective well-being, are introduced briefly.

DIFFERENTIATING BETWEEN GOAL PROGRESS AND GOAL ATTAINMENT

The term *successful goal pursuit* is not very precise because it might embrace both a phase of goal progress and the state of goal attainment. In theories of action regulation, however, it is common to differentiate between goal progress and goal attainment (Heckhausen & Kuhl, 1985).

At first sight, this differentiation appears to be an easy task. In a straightforward conceptualization, goal *progress* denotes all successful steps that help to attain a goal, whereas goal *attainment* refers to a prescribed end state of the goal-striving process. A deeper conceptual analysis, however, reveals a much more complex picture because not all goals are necessarily represented as approach goals with predefined end states (see Chambers, chap. 5, this volume; Elliot & Friedman, chap. 3, this volume). As summarized by Emmons (1996), personal goals denote what a person wants to attain (e.g., "I plan to marry"), to maintain (e.g., "I want to preserve marital happiness") or to avoid (e.g., "I do not want to argue with my wife"). For maintenance goals, at least the desired state is clear because it equals the status quo. However, with such a goal the process of goal pursuit never ends (or ends only if a person decides to disengage from the goal). Avoidance goals are especially difficult to describe in terms of goal attainment because it is difficult, if not impossible, to detect goal progress or attainment success (see Elliot & Friedman, chap. 3, this volume). As for maintenance goals, no final attainment is to be expected.

Whether or not attainment is a meaningful outcome criterion is not only a logical concomitant feature of the verbal representation of a personal goal, but also a matter of the systemic level and standing of the specific goal under consideration. Emmons (1989), for instance, posited that a goal such as "make life easier for my parents" can be an enduring striving that is not associated with a clear final attainment (see also the concept of core projects; Little, 2005; Little & Chambers, 2004) but rather with progress in or attainment of related subgoals (e.g., "save money," "get along with my brother"). Hence, a person would consider herself or himself successful in goal pursuit of enduring personal strivings whenever subgoals that serve this striving are realized.

FACETS OF SUBJECTIVE WELL-BEING

Subjective well-being is a multifaceted psychological construct embracing emotional and cognitive components (e.g., Andrews & McKennell, 1980). The first component is often measured as positive and negative affect and the second component as explicit satisfaction judgments. In addition, subjective well-being can refer to life in general or to specific life domains and tasks (Diener, Suh, Lucas, & Smith, 1999). Finally, one can differentiate between short-lived patterns of experienced states and more enduring experiences of well-being (Watson, Clark, & Tellegen, 1988; trait affect: Watson & Walker, 1996; trait cognitive well-being: Pavot & Diener, 1993; state cognitive well-being: Oishi & Diener, 2001). Therefore, it makes sense to distinguish trait-like and state-like components. Referring to the possible combinations of the aforementioned well-being criteria—(a) affective versus cognitive, (b) domain-general versus domain-specific, and (c) short-term, midterm, and long-term—one can roughly differentiate among 12 variants of subjective well-being (see Table 11.1).

To some degree, these different facets of well-being are expected to interrelate. It has been shown, for instance, that cognitive and affective well-being are distinct lower order constructs, but that they also load onto a single higher order factor of well-being (Lucas, Diener, & Suh, 1996). In addition, trait-based well-being might influence midterm well-being experiences and actual well-being states because some proportion of long-term, midterm, and short-term well-being might be equally influenced by a genetically determined predisposition for well-being. Finally, one might speculate that cognitive and affective well-being are functionally interrelated. It has been posited, for instance, that

TABLE 11.1

Facets of Well-Being: Content Focus and Time Perspective

	Well-Being Content Focus	
Well-Being Time Perspective	Cognitive	Affective
Short-term (state-like)	General Domain vs Specific	General Domain vs Specific
Mid-term	General Domain vs Specific	General Domain vs Specific
Long-term (trait-like)	General Domain vs Specific	General Domain vs Specific

cognitive well-being can buffer the impact of negative events on mood states, probably because of differences in interpreting these events (Robinson, 2000). Concerning the link between domain-general and domain-specific well-being, both top-down and bottom-up relations have been found (see Diener et al., 1999).

THEORETICAL LINKS BETWEEN SUCCESSFUL GOAL PURSUIT AND SUBJECTIVE WELL-BEING

Successful goal pursuit has been linked to cognitive as well as affective components of well-being. On a conceptual level, these links have been drawn in both models of well-being and goal-theoretical approaches.

Concepts of cognitive well-being often display a clear telic character by proposing that the fulfilment of needs, goals, and desires is crucial for experiencing happiness and life satisfaction (Diener, 1984). Andrews and McKennell (1980), for instance, postulated that satisfaction "requires some kind of comparison—either explicit or implicit—between a level of achievement and some standard (e.g., what one expects or aspires to) and hence involves the kind of judgmental thinking and knowledge that is the hallmark of cognition" (p. 135). In other words, satisfaction indicates a match between goals and their achievement. In Ryff's (1989) dimensional conceptualization of well-being, positive psychological functioning comprises six key components: self-acceptance, positive relations with others, autonomy, environmental mastery, purpose in life, and personal growth. One of these dimensions, purpose in life, makes direct reference to having meaningful personal goals, and two other dimensions of her well-being approach, namely environmental mastery and personal growth, have progress and attainment-related foci by stressing the importance of self-efficacy experiences and feelings of continued self-development.

With regard to affective well-being, functional links to goal-related behavior and experiences have been drawn by a number of scholars (e.g., Bagozzi, Baumgartner, & Pieters, 1998; Carver & Scheier, 1990). Within Bagozzi et al.'s (1998) model of goal-directed emotions, anticipatory as well as goal-outcome emotions are considered. Anticipatory emotions are elicited by the prospects of goal success or failure (e.g., "If I succeed in achieving my goal of decreasing my bodyweight, I will feel happy"). They have the potential to motivate goal-directed volitional processes and behavior that are necessary for goal attainment, which, in turn, causes goal-outcome emotions (e.g., "Because I achieved my bodyweight goal, I feel happy"). In their communicative theory of emotions, Oatley and Johnson-Laird (1996) proposed that positive emotions are associated with the attainment of subgoals and usually lead to a decision to continue with one's current plans, whereas negative emotions result from problems with the current goal pursuit.

Goal theories, such as the one put forth by Carver and Scheier (1990), also draw a direct link between goal progress and emotional well-being. Here, emotions are seen as indicators of distance-reducing processes between the actual and the desired states. From the perspective of self-regulation, positive emotions during goal pursuit indicate a diminishing discrepancy between the actual and the desired state. In this sense then, goal progress can be seen as representing a proximate cause of emotional well-being (mainly in terms of affective states). In addition, goal success is hypothesized to increase self-efficacy beliefs that, in turn, are related to well-being. However, even on the microlevel of self-regulatory processes, the relation between goal progress and affect seems to be more complex. For instance, Carver and Scheier (1990) postulated that positive affect results only when goal attainment is realized faster than expected (see later).

In their dual-function model of personal projects, McGregor and Little (1998) suggested that personal projects serve both an instrumental function via the experience of efficacy and a symbolic function via feelings of integrity. Both experiences are expected to relate to well-being, although to different facets: Efficacy is expected to relate to happiness (i.e., life satisfaction, positive affect, absence of negative affect), whereas integrity is expected to relate to meaningfulness (i.e., feelings of connectedness, purpose, and growth). Although McGregor and Little (1998) did not explicitly elaborate on goal progress, their concept of goal efficacy as doing well obviously embraces a progress component. Hence, one could infer that (a) goal progress evinces a direct link to subjective well-being in terms of happiness, more or less regardless of goal content, and that (b) working on and progressing toward goals that are consistent with important aspects of one's self-identity could additionally foster well-being in terms of meaningfulness.

One should note, however, that there are also researchers who are more skeptical about the beneficial role of successful goal pursuit for well-being. McIntosh and Martin (1992), for instance, argued that the positive well-being effects of goal attainment are short-lived. With reference to Helson's (1964) adaption-level theory, McIntosh and Martin (1992) posited that one reason for this failure of goal attainment to foster long-term well-being is that people's assessments of outcomes shift with their experiences. Therefore, McIntosh and Martin doubted that goal attainment can add to the long-term prediction of well-being. They proposed, however, that nonattainment might increase negative affect and dissatisfaction, especially among those individuals who believe that goal attainment is a prerequisite for their happiness. In the case of nonattainment, these "linkers" would ruminate about failure. This rumination, in turn, would lead to negative moods and unhappiness.

Are Goal Pursuit and Attainment Differentially Related to Well-Being?

The process of moving toward goals may provide individuals with many small satisfying experiences that cumulate to influence general well-being (see the bottom-up model of well-being; Diener et al., 1999). Goal attainment, however, might result in well-being changes via a top-down route, at least if attainment is associated with clear positive changes in one's self-perception and life circumstances (see Sheldon, Kasser, Smith, & Shore, 2002).

The idea that goal pursuit and progress themselves might be beneficial to well-being has been rooted in philosophy since Aristotle and is still advocated nowadays by various scholars (e.g., Csikszentmihalyi, 1990; Little, 2005; Omodei & Wearing, 1990). Recently, Little (2005; Little & Chambers, 2004) posited that positive psychological functioning is contingent on the sustainable pursuit of core personal projects. Although Little (2005) did not specify whether sustainable goal pursuit is bound to experiences of successful goal pursuit, one might speculate that personal goals that are pursued without the experience of any kind of progress will hardly have the potential of supporting sustainable proactive self-development.

Austin and Vancouver (1996) suggested that there might be qualitatively different well-being experiences between goal progress and attainment. They argued that "flow"-like (Csikszentmihalyi, 1990) experiences are to be expected only during the ongoing phase of goal progress. Assumptions concerning distinct emotional experiences during goal pursuit and following goal attainment have also been formulated in brain research. For example, Davidson (1994; Davidson, Pizzagalli, Nitschke, & Kalin, 2003) posited that an approach-related form of positive affect (i.e., a form of affect that is generated in the context of planning goal-directed action and moving toward a desired goal) is associated with an activation of the left side of the dorsolateral prefrontal cortex, whereas postattainment affect is qualitatively different (phenomenologically experienced as contentment) and is expected to occur when the prefrontal cortex goes offline.

In sum, there is a broad conceptual foundation, both in the well-being and in the goal-related literature, for assuming positive links between goal progress and subjective well-being, as well as between the attainment of personal goals and well-being. From the viewpoint of personality psychology, most conceptual approaches to personal goals are in the middle range between fixed traits and motivational dispositions and the more ephemeral states of functioning (e.g., specific action units; see Emmons, 1989). At first sight, this might predispose goal-related success experiences to be linked mainly to midterm well-being indicators (see Table 11.1). However, particularly within the day-to-day process of goal pursuit, short-term effects on state well-being are also likely to occur.

EMPIRICAL FINDINGS ON THE LINK BETWEEN SUCCESSFUL GOAL PURSUIT AND WELL-BEING

In the first meta-analysis of the relation between goal progress and well-being, based on nine published studies, Koestner, Lekes, Powers, and Chicoine (2002) reported a significant overall effect of $d = .61$. A clear strength of the included studies is that, with one exception (King, Richards, & Stemmerich, 1998), they were based on longitudinal data. However, all of the studies were built on samples that were exclusively comprised of university students (for a critical discussion of systematic biases in student populations, see Sears, 1986). Of course, this restricts generalizability.

The Appendix gives a more recent overview of 30 longitudinal studies on the link between successful goal pursuit and well-being that, overall, provides clear evidence of a positive relation.[2] With few exceptions, main effects in the expected direction were found in student samples as well as in diverse adult samples. However, in Affleck et al.'s (1998) study that is based on a sample of women diagnosed with primary fibromyalgia syndrome, only daily goal progress toward social-interpersonal goals, but not goal progress in the area of health, predicted improvements in positive mood. Many of these health-related goals have perhaps been formulated as avoidance goals (here, goals focusing on avoiding pain) that are difficult to be judged in terms of goal progress, but this was not analyzed by the authors. Interestingly, in their study on bodyweight-related goals, Bagozzi et al. (1998) showed that for respondents who wanted to lose weight the link between goal attainment and positive outcome emotions was stronger than for those who wanted to maintain their weight. This gives further evidence that it might be fruitful to distinguish among approach, maintenance, and avoidance goals (see also Elliot & Friedman, chap. 3, this volume).[3]

---

[2]With regard to the samples, 20 studies were conducted with college and university students, one study with high school students (Lüdtke, 2004), 9 studies with adult samples (7 with working adults [Brown et al., 1997; Harris et al., 2003; Kehr, 2003; Maier & Brunstein, 2001; Wiese, 2004; Wiese & Freund, 2005; Wiese & Heimann, 2006], 1 with a clinical sample [Affleck et al., 1998], and 1 with an adult sample where the professional status was not explicitly described [Bagozzi et al., 1998]). With the exception of 4 studies (Bagozzi et al., 1998; Brown et al., 1997; Elliot & Sheldon, 1997; Harris et al., 2003), all studies were based on goal assessment techniques in which participants were asked to freely list their goals (for details on different elicitation techniques see Little & Gee, chap. 2, this volume). Within some of the free-listing instructions, however, participants had to concentrate on specific goal domains such as work, interpersonal relationships, or health (e.g., Affleck et al., 1998; Elliot & Church, 2002; Maier & Brunstein, 2001; Wiese & Freund, 2005). As we had to be selective, we refrained from including in this analysis findings from cross-sectional research (e.g., Christiansen, Backman, Little, & Nguyen, 1999; Emmons, 1986; King et al., 1998; Salmela-Aro, 1992), studies that focused solely on physical symptoms (e.g., Elliot & Sheldon, 1998), studies in which ratings of goal progress were summed up with other goal appraisals (e.g., stressfulness of goal pursuit, knowledge about how to accomplish a project, etc. [e.g., Salmela-Aro & Nurmi, 1996, 1997b]), studies for which it was not specified whether the goals under consideration were actually self-set personal goals or rather assigned tasks (e.g., Alliger & William, 1993), and studies in which goal assessment was restricted to the indication of an aspiration level with regard to a predefined goal (preferred and acceptable college grades [Mone & Baker, 1992; Thomas & Mathieu, 1994]).

[3]There were other important differences from the overall pattern of a positive linkage. Brunstein et al. (1998), for example, found significant raw correlations between goal progress and well-being but no significant well-being changes due to goal progress; significant changes were found only when motive-congruent goals were pursued. Sheldon and Elliot (2000) failed to find a significant effect of the attainment of friendship goals on friendship-related satisfaction, and Wiese & Heimann (2006, Study 1) failed to find a significant increase in satisfaction with university studies due to study-related goal progress. Finally, Sheldon et al. (2002) demonstrated that goal progress is associated with significant increases in affective well-being and vital judgments, but only marginally with psychosocial well-being indicated by an aggregate score based on the Ryff (1989) subscales.

So far, a clear differentiation between well-being experiences related to goal progress versus well-being experiences related to goal attainment has not been the focus of empirical research. Most studies included either a progress measure or a measure where it was rather difficult to differentiate between progress and attainment. Some authors subsumed their goal success measure under the heading of goal attainment although asking for progress. Harris, Daniels, and Briner (2003) explicitly elaborated on the differentiation between progress and attainment. However, as they measured only goal attainment, empirical comparisons were not possible. In sum, it seems that there is a lack of empirical research that includes clear measures of progress and attainment that would help to disentangle differential effects of these phases of the goal cycle.

With regard to the different forms of well-being, a broad range of variables have been measured, including both the more cognitively oriented and the more emotionally oriented concepts. However, there is some dominance of domain-general well-being criteria (e.g., generalized positive affect, life satisfaction) that might be due to the common method of aggregating goal-related assessments across goals from different life domains (for a critique concerning this method see Sheldon & Elliot, 2000). Concerning the different qualitative facets of emotional well-being (i.e., positive and negative affect), there is clear evidence that goal progress is related to positive affect. Those studies that differentiated between positive and negative affect mostly showed a comparatively lower or no effect of successful goal pursuit on negative affect (e.g., Affleck et al., 1998; Bagozzi et al., 1998; Sheldon & Kasser, 1998; Wiese & Freund, 2005; Wiese & Heimann, 2006, Studies 1 & 2), thereby reinforcing the well-known two-factor model of emotional experiences (Watson et al., 1988).

In addition, so far, there is mixed evidence concerning the question whether progress is more strongly related to domain-general or to domain-specific well-being (Wiese & Heimann, 2006, Study 1—stronger link to domain-general well-being, Study 2—links of similar size). Brunstein (1999) reported that the positive well-being effects for goal progress were similar for affective and cognitive well-being measures (both measured as states). Although not the focus of this chapter, one should also note that prior well-being predicts goal progress (e.g., Brunstein, 1993; Wiese & Heimann, 2006), which is probably at least partly due to the potential of positive affect to motivate goal-related behavior (e.g., Bagozzi et al., 1998; Brown, Cron, & Slocum, 1997).

It is rather surprising that, so far, studies on successful pursuit of personal goals and well-being have paid little attention to the fact that a fair number of personal goals are formulated as "well-being goals" in the first place (e.g., to reach and maintain marital happiness, to be satisfied with one's life, to feel balanced; see Wiese, 2000). These kind of goals make it difficult (if not impossible) to disentangle goal progress from well-being outcome criteria and might therefore inflate the overall relation between successful goal pursuit and well-being. Future studies might pay attention to this issue.

Are Success-Related Well-Being Increases Only Ephemeral?

Given the positive overall effect of successful goal pursuit, Sheldon and Houser-Marko (2001) raised a further challenging research question: Can we maintain an increased level of well-being or can our well-being continue to grow due to ongoing successful goal pursuit experiences? Two studies conducted by Sheldon and Houser-Marko showed that one can at least maintain well-being, if not magnify it by continuous success in goal pursuit. However, if one fails to be continuously successful, one's sense of well-being regresses. Sheldon and Houser-Marko's approach implies the possibility of unlimited growth of well-being given that an individual is continuously successful in goal pursuit. One might argue, however, that genetic influences set limits to the possible range of increases in well-being. This would support a less restrictive conceptualization of a well-being baseline as was proposed, for instance, by Heady and Wearing (1989), who assumed that any change in the individual's unique baseline level will only be temporary. Baseline levels can be expected to change under specific circumstances, but only within predetermined limits.

MODERATORS OF THE LINK BETWEEN SUCCESSFUL GOAL PURSUIT AND WELL-BEING

Do the characteristics of the goal-pursuit process, as well as characteristics of goals and goal systems themselves, have an influence on the degree to which successful goal pursuit predicts subjective well-being? To shed light on this question, the following section deals with (a) the rate of goal progress, (b) the subjective importance and difficulty of goals, (c) causal attributions of goal-related success, (d) the "organismic congruence" of goals, (e) the sociocultural appropriateness of goals, and (f) the influence of success and failure in multiple goal systems as possible moderators of the link between successful goal pursuit and subjective well-being.

Goal Progress Dynamics: The Role of Velocity

As mentioned in the preceding section, a main assumption of Carver and Scheier's control-theoretical approach is that the rate of progress toward one's goals is crucial for predicting positive and negative affect. They stated, "If the rate is below the criterion, negative affect arises. If the rate is at the criterion, the person is affect-free. If the rate exceeds the criterion, positive affect arises" (Carver, Sutton, & Scheier, 2000, p. 744). In addition, negative affect is expected to result when no progress toward a goal is realized (Carver, Lawrence, & Scheier, 1996).

So far, empirical evidence in favor of the assumption that unexpectedly fast progress is a prerequisite for a positive effect of successful goal pursuit on well-being is sparse. Carver and Scheier (2000) themselves cited only one unpublished study (Lawrence, Carver, & Scheier, 1999) from their own research group that supports its validity. The cited experiment, however, did not include progress toward self-set personal goals but toward an assigned task, and progress was not caused by individuals' behavior but was manipulated via faked feedback. Another experiment sometimes cited to document the velocity hypothesis was conducted by Hsee and Abelson (1991). This experiment did provide evidence that satisfaction is positively related to the rate of progress toward desired outcomes. Again, Hsee and Abelson (1991) did not test their assumption with regard to self-set personal goals but only with fictitious and assigned tasks. In addition and contrary to Carver and Scheier's (1990) position (i.e., velocity as the primary determinant of affect), Hsee and Abelson (1991) not only found a velocity effect but also an effect on the actual absolute level of task fulfillment.

In sum, although there is a broad array of intended applications (Carver & Scheier, 1990), we still do not know whether and what role velocity plays in the link between successful pursuit of personal goals and well-being. Obviously, a logical precondition for the applicability of the velocity assumption is that a person has a clear expectation concerning the time he or she assumes to be necessary for successful goal pursuit. Even if such time-related expectations exist, however, the importance of velocity might depend on specific characteristics of the goals or the project domains under consideration. In fact, Carver and Scheier (1990) themselves conceded that there might be goals for which pacing matters little. One might imagine that a person is happy on reaching an important personal goal (e.g., founding a family, getting tenure), even if it took him or her longer than he or she had expected.

Goal Importance and Goal Difficulty

It has been posited that domain-specific psychological involvement strengthens the link between goal progress in the respective domain and well-being (Alliger & Williams, 1993; Wiese & Freund, 2005). Someone who feels highly involved and invested in his or her job, for instance, should respond more strongly to being successful in job-related goals. Nevertheless, in a diary study, Alliger and Williams (1993) failed to demonstrate a significant interaction effect between job involvement and work-related goal progress on affective well-being. It was not clearly outlined, however, whether the goals under consideration were self-set or assigned work tasks. In a 3-year longitudinal study concerning the job-related personal goals of working adults, Wiese and Freund (2005) found some evidence that the subjective importance of the work domain (in terms of one's current work involvement) induced progress-dependent increases in well-being. The moderating effect of subjective importance was even more convincingly demonstrated in a diary study conducted by Harris et al. (2003), who showed that the interaction between the subjective importance of personal work goals and goal attainment predicted positive change in pleasurable affect. With reference to Little's (2005) concept of core personal projects (that, by definition, are of high personal importance), one might assume that it is particularly the successful pursuit of these core projects (or the successful pursuit of subgoals related to these goals) that has high potential for promoting subjective well-being.

Another appraisal dimension that has been proposed to be related to the potentially beneficial effects of successful goal pursuit on well-being is goal difficulty (Wiese & Freund, 2005). Especially in work and organizational psychology, difficulty is one of the most prominent goal characteristics focused in empirical research. The strong interest in goal difficulty mainly stems from Locke and Latham's (1990) influential goal setting theory, which, it should be noted, was originally formulated mainly with reference to assigned goals. Numerous studies have supported the validity of Locke and Latham's (1990) proposition that difficult goals lead to higher achievement than ill-defined do-your-best goals (for a review, see also Locke, Shaw, Saari, & Latham, 1981). Within the present context, however, it is not the positive impact on performance that is central but the question of whether progressing toward or attaining difficult goals has a higher impact on well-being than progressing toward or attaining comparatively easier goals. In fact, in the aforementioned longitudinal study conducted by Wiese and Freund (2005), difficulty was identified as the most powerful moderating goal characteristic in terms of strengthening the affective response to a positive evaluation of one's goal success in the work domain (see Figure 11.1). Hence, it seems that setting difficult goals not only fosters performance but also leads to stronger positive emotional responses when goal progress is experienced.

Goal Success Attribution

From the viewpoint of attribution theory, one might postulate that whether the reasons for goal-related success are perceived as internal or external is important. Mone and Baker (1992), as well as Thomas and Mathieu (1994), conducted studies that explicitly focused on goal-related success, attribution styles, and well-being. Mone and Baker (1992) reported that internal attributions were significantly more likely to lead to positive affective responses than external attributions of success. In Thomas and Mathieu's (1994) study, however, a moderating effect of internal attributions was found solely for the beginning of university studies.

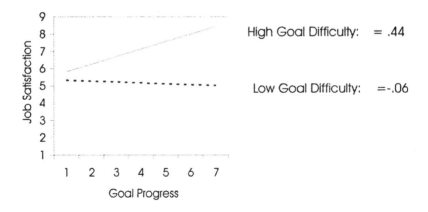

Figure 11.1. Interaction between goal difficulty and progress for job satisfaction. (From Wiese & Freund, 2005)

Two further studies (one with university students, one with working adults) on goal-related success, causal attributions, and well-being were conducted by Wiese and Heimann (2006). In contrast to Mone and Baker (1992) and Thomas and Mathieu (1994), who restricted the personal goal assessment to measuring individual indications of preferred or acceptable college grades, Wiese and Heimann (2006) used a combined idiographic-nomothetic approach in which each participant was allowed to freely generate goals that he or she pursued in the academic or work domain. Half a year later, each participant was asked to indicate for each individual goal how much progress he or she had made toward that goal. Wiese and Heimann's approach also differed with regard to the operationalization of internal success attribution. Whereas the studies by Mone and Baker (1992) and Thomas and Mathieu (1994) restricted the measurement of internal causes to asking whether the cause was something about the person herself or himself (see Russell, 1982), Wiese and Heimann (2006) presented a set of possible internal causes. They postulated that attributions to one's own proactvity (i.e., attributions to action or volitional strategies such as effort, persistence, adequate time management, etc.) should especially strengthen the well-being effects of successful goal pursuit. In their two half-year longitudinal studies, however, they did not find evidence for the postulated moderation. One reason for the missing positive moderation might be that, conceptually, attributions are of prime importance when individuals find themselves in situations where they have an acute need for an explanation (see Skinner, 1995). Weiner (1985) posited that people primarily ask themselves for causal explanations when something negative or unexpected happens. Progressing toward self-set goals, however, is neither negative nor unexpected. Nevertheless, Wiese and Heimann (2006) found that proactivity attributions of goal success predicted subjective well-being and self-efficacy.

Organismic Congruence of Goals

In personality psychology, it has repeatedly been stated that, for positive psychological functioning, it is crucial to select self-appropriate personal goals; that is, goals that serve basic needs (e.g., autonomy, competence, and relatedness; Deci & Ryan, 2000) and that converge with underlying motives (e.g., affiliation), stable personality traits (e.g., extraversion), and individual talents (Sheldon, 2002; see also Sheldon, chap. 13, this volume). For a person with a high communion motive, for instance, a congruent personal goal might be "to plan to volunteer in a nursing home." For a highly extraverted person, personal goals such as "organizing a birthday party for my husband" or "spending my holidays on a cruise ship" might be highly self-congruent. During the last decade, several researchers have started to investigate whether the degree to which self-set goals are self-compatible is predictive of subjective well-being (e.g., Brunstein, Schultheiss, & Grässman, 1998; Sheldon & Elliot, 1998).

In their goal-achievement-motive-satisfaction hypothesis Brunstein et al. (1998) suggested that individuals feel happiest when they succeed in the pursuit of goals that converge with their implicit motives. Motive congruency in Brunstein et al.'s study referred to the degree of convergence between two motives (i.e., communion, agency) and self-generated personal goals. In fact, in their study with university students, goal progress itself did not predict positive change in emotional well-being, whereas progress toward motive-congruent goals did predict positive change (Brunstein et al., 1998, Study 1).

With reference to humanistic theories of motivation (e.g., Deci & Ryan, 1985; Rogers, 1963), it has been assumed that goal progress best promotes well-being when goals display high organismic congruence (Sheldon & Kasser, 1995, 1998) in terms of both the reasons for goal pursuit (the "why") and the content (the "what") of the goals pursued. Although in a nominal sense, personal goals are self-set, these goals do not always feel self-determined (see Sheldon & Kasser, 2001). Individuals who pursue personal goals for autonomous reasons are expected to experience a high degree of well-being in the case of successful goal pursuit. With regard to the content of goals, it has been assumed that goals aiming at self-acceptance, affiliation, community feelings, and health—subsumed under the heading of intrinsic goals—are most beneficial to well-being (Kasser & Ryan, 1996; note, however, that the content-focused operationalization of the intrinsic or extrinsic value of goals is not without problems; Carver & Baird, 1998). On the contrary, extrinsic goals—goals that focus on rewards and on other people's opinions and expectations (e.g., goals related to financial success, physical attraction, social recognition)—are expected to bear risks for well-being, at least when they dominate over intrinsic goals, because an excessive concentration on external rewards can distract people from intrinsic endeavors that are important for supporting one's well-being (Deci & Ryan, 1985; Kasser & Ryan, 1993, 1996).

Following Sheldon and Kasser's (2001) considerations on organismic congruence, one might assume that individuals experience the strongest increases in well-being when they successfully pursue goals that they have chosen for self-determined reasons and that are coherent in terms of helping to bring about higher level goals of intrinsic value. Sheldon and Kasser (1998) tested this assumption based on short-term (5 days) and long-term (semester) data collected from a university sample. As expected, participants showed the largest increase in well-being when they progressed toward goals that displayed high degrees of organismic congruence. More precisely, Sheldon and Kasser (1998) found positive moderator effects of the self-determination and the intrinsic value of projects (in terms of reference to self-acceptance, intimacy, or societal contribution) on combined measures of well-being. They reported that making short-term progress in either self-determined or intrinsic goals predicted greater short-term and long-term overall well-being. In addition, Sheldon and Kasser (1998) found that merely pursuing projects for self-determined reasons or pursuing intrinsic goals does not lead to increases in well-being unless one experiences success in goal pursuit. Sheldon and Elliot (1999) showed that for university students, positive change in well-being is mainly due to the need for satisfying experiences, which is especially pronounced among those individuals who attained self-concordant goals.

As outlined by Sheldon and Kasser (2001), findings from personal goal research show that striving toward goals for authentic, self-concordant reasons facilitates goal progress and attainment, which, in turn, predict positive change in well-being. This well-being effect probably has at least two sources: Referring to humanistic as well as to social-cognitive theoretical approaches, Sheldon, Ryan, and Reis (1996) showed that both the experience of autonomy (a central well-being prerequisite in humanistic theories; e.g., Deci & Ryan, 1985) and the experience of efficacy (a central prerequisite in social-cognitive approaches but also associated with the basic need for competence in humanistic approaches; see Bandura, 1977, and Deci & Ryan, 2000, respectively) add to the prediction of daily well-being. This also converges with McGregor and Little's (1998) argument that acting efficaciously and with integrity are important predictors of well-being, as noted earlier. Overall, the self-efficacy-triggered effect on well-being seems not to be content related. However, Kasser and Ryan (1993) argued that individuals who concentrate on contingent, external goals (e.g., financial success) tend to experience only superficial and fleeting satisfaction because their success experiences are unrelated to their inherent needs. This is an intriguing assumption that clearly warrants testing in future research.

Life-Span Contextualization of Goals

In life-span psychology, the predominant culture (e.g., individualistic vs. collectivistic value systems) as well as biological constraints (e.g., females' fertility-based deadlines for founding a family) build a meaningful background for adaptive goal selection. These cultural and biological influences are often reflected in social norms and age-related expectations (see Freund, chap. 9, this volume). A number of scholars have stated that it is desirable to choose personal goals that not only converge with personal motives, interests, and capacities, but also with age-related societal demands (Baltes & Baltes, 1990; Cantor, 1994; Heckhausen, 1999; Nurmi, 1992; Salmela-Aro & Nurmi, 1997a). In fact, setting personal goals in accordance with normative age-related expectations (e.g., setting goals in the work domain in late adolescence and young adulthood) may help to take advantage of available resources, thereby increasing the likelihood of successful goal pursuit, and also to ensure later access to resources (e.g., to attain further promotions; see Freund, chap. 9, this volume). Recent work in personality psychology also acknowledges the necessity to focus not only on the match between personal goals and individual needs, motives, and traits, but also on the match between personal goals and the dominant culture (see Little, 2005; Sheldon, chap. 13, this volume).

The importance of culture is illustrated by Oishi and Diener (2001), who posited that the positive effects of intrinsically motivated goals might depend on the cultural context. They conducted a series of studies with university students from different cultural contexts to explore the role of culture for the beneficial well-being effects (in terms of life satisfaction) of attaining independent versus interdependent goals. They found that for European Americans, the positive well-being change was especially large when they attained goals that were pursued for independent reasons. However, this did not hold true for Asian Americans and Japanese college students. On the contrary, the Asian Americans and Japanese tended to experience positive well-being changes when successfully striving for interdependent goals.

The life-span aspects are evidenced in the work of Nurmi and Salmela-Aro (2002; Salmela-Aro & Nurmi, 1997a; Salmela-Aro, Nurmi, Saisto, & Halmesmäki, 2001), which stresses the importance of adjusting personal goals to match age-related social expectations and an individual's actual life situation. These studies demonstrated that personal projects that fit age-related developmental tasks (e.g., founding a family in young adulthood) predicted well-being (Salmela-Aro & Nurmi, 1997a; Salmela-Aro et al., 2001). In two cross-lagged panel studies on the transition to motherhood, for instance, Salmela-Aro et al. (2001) found that an increase in family-related goals during pregnancy and after childbirth predicted a decline in women's depressive symptoms. However, this does not necessarily imply that one has to be "on the clock" to enhance well-being; on the contrary, achieving personal goals at an "inappropriate" age may still have the potential to increase well-being. Imagine, for instance, a middle-aged man in his 40s having his first child. Although later than socially expected, this father might be very happy that he finally succeeded in realizing his personal goal of founding a family.

Success Relations of Multiple Goals

Goal progress and attainment in one's life domain may be judged not only with reference to intradomain standards (e.g., goal difficulty), but also with reference to personal development and circumstances in other life domains. Indeed, as pointed out by Austin and Vancouver (1996), multiple goal striving appears to be the rule (see also Riediger, chap. 4, this volume). Therefore, in their study with working adults, Wiese and Freund (2005) investigated goal progress in the work domain and simultaneous goal progress in the partnership and family domains. One might argue that affective reactions to attainment or nonattainment of goals in one life domain might be influenced by the experience of being successful or unsuccessful in other important domains of functioning. Kruglanski (1996), for instance, postulated that individuals who are pursuing numerous goals may invest less in each goal and hence may react less intensely to attainment or nonattainment than individuals with fewer goals (see also Linville, 1985). From a socionormative perspective, however, high attainment in different domains (e.g., work and family) seems desirable for successful adult development. Therefore, one might also argue that nonattainment in the family domain could have a negative effect on personal evaluations of attainments in the occupational domain if one recognizes that work-related goal-attainment (e.g., getting promoted) was realized only at the expense of partnership-related goals (e.g., having not been successful in goals such as preserving marital stability or having another child).

Wiese and Freund's (2005) results showed that individuals who indicated little progress in the partnership and family domain were characterized by a steeper increase in satisfaction with their professional development following work-related goal progress than those who indicated huge goal progress in the partnership and family domain. For job satisfaction and global emotional well-being, the moderator effect of goal progress in the partnership and family domain failed to attain significance. However, the result pattern was similar. One could interpret this finding as indicating that individuals with little success in the partnership domain exhibit some sort of compensatory switching to concentrate their emotion regulation on positive experiences in the work domain. Note, however, that the measurement of general well-being was limited to a selected subset of self-reported emotions. In future studies, well-being assessment should be broadened to also include criteria such as meaningfulness, which might depend on other goal-progress constellations (e.g., simultaneous progress in both the family and work domains). It is also important to note that, at least with reference to the central life domains of work and family, a substantial number of adults indicate the integration of work-related and family-related goals as central personal goals in themselves (Hoff & Ewers, 2003). Given such integration goals, we might expect a stronger interrelatedness of the well-being effects of goal progress in different life domains.

CONCLUSION

In this chapter, I summarized theoretical and empirical approaches concerning the effects of successful goal pursuit on different facets of well-being. There is growing evidence of the positive effect of successful goal pursuit on well-being and on conditions that determine how pronounced this well-being effect is. In a number of research programs, the question was raised as to whether goal progress for all kinds of goals is equally beneficial to well-being. With reference to possible moderators of the relation between successful goal pursuit and subjective well-being, empirical research has repeatedly shown that striving toward self-concordant goals strengthens the link between goal progress and well-being. The predominant reliance on student populations sets limits on the generalizability of the respective findings, however. Attributing goal progress to one's own efforts did not turn out to moderate the link between goal progress and well-being. However, there is indirect evidence that personal investments strengthen the link between goal progress and well-being because individuals who indicate high goal difficulty experience greater well-being increases when progressing toward their goals than individuals with comparatively easier goals.

Overall, there seems to be a lack of systematization in empirical research when it comes to the differentiation between progress-related and attainment-related well-being effects, as well as a lack of research that explicitly compares the effects of successful goal pursuit on different forms of subjective well-being. In addition, from a life-span perspective, one might also advocate that research not focus solely on the immediate effects of goal progress and attainment on well-being. The question of whether or not one has succeeded in realizing meaningful personal goals might also be important in the context of individual life reviews. Finally, successful goal pursuit can be analyzed not only from the individual perspective but also on the dyadic and group levels. It would be interesting to see, for instance, whether a partner's reaction to one's goal success in the occupational domain influences well-being.

Of course, any attempts to study and track goal pursuit and its correlates is challenging because the dynamic nature of goals implies that their content and relative importance might change. This complexity increases when one takes into account that individuals have multiple goals and that successful life management is often as much an individual as it is a socially interdependent enterprise. Throwing light on these issues, however, would be an intriguing goal for future research.

REFERENCES

Affleck, G., Tennen, H., Urrows, S., Higgins, P., Abeles, M., Hall, C., et al. (1998). Fibromyalgia and women's pursuit of personal goals: A daily process analysis. *Health Psychology, 17,* 40–47.

Alliger, G. M., & Williams, K. J. (1993). Using signal-contingent experience sampling methodology to study work in the field: A discussion and illustration examining task perception and mood. *Personnel Psychology, 46,* 525–549.

Andrews, F. M., & McKennell, A. C. (1980). Measures of self-reported well-being: Their affective, cognitive, and other components. *Social Indicators Research, 8,* 127–155.

Austin, J. T., & Vancouver, J. B. (1996). Goal constructs in psychology: Structure, process, and content. *Psychological Bulletin, 120,* 338–375.

Bagozzi, R. P., Baumgartner, H., & Pieters, R. (1998). Goal-directed emotions. *Cognition and Emotion, 12,* 1–26.

Baltes, P. B., & Baltes, M. M. (1990). Psychological perspectives on successful aging: The model of selective optimization with compensation. In P. B. Baltes & M. M.

Baltes (Eds.), *Successful aging: Perspectives from the behavioral sciences* (pp. 1–34). New York: Cambridge University Press.

Bandura, A. (1977). Self-efficacy: Toward a unifying theory of behavioral change. *Psychological Review, 84,* 191–215.

Brown, S. P., Cron, W. L., & Slocum, J. W. (1997). Effects of goal-directed emotions on salesperson volitions, behavior, and performance: A longitudinal study. *Journal of Marketing, 61,* 39–50.

Brunstein, J. C. (1993). Personal goals and subjective well-being: A longitudinal study. *Journal of Personality and Social Psychology, 65,* 1061–1070.

Brunstein, J. C., Schultheiss, O. C., & Grässman, R. (1998). Personal goals and emotional well-being: The moderating role of motive dispositions. *Journal of Personality and Social Psychology, 75,* 494–508.

Cantor, N. (1994). Life task problem solving: Situational affordances and personal needs. *Personality and Social Psychology Bulletin, 20,* 235–243.

Carver, C. S., & Baird, E. (1998). The American dream revisited: Is it what you want or why you want it that matters? *Psychological Science, 9,* 289–292.

Carver, C. S., Lawrence, J. W., & Scheier, M. F. (1996). A control-process perspective on the origins of affect. In L. L. Martin & A. Tesser (Eds.), *Striving and feeling: Interactions among goals, affect, and self-regulation* (pp. 11–52). Hillsdale, NJ: Lawrence Erlbaum Associates.

Carver, C. S., & Scheier, M. F. (1990). Origins and functions of positive and negative affect: A control-process view. *Psychological Review, 97,* 19–35.

Carver, C. S., & Scheier, M. F. (2000). On the structure of behavioral self-regulation. In M. Boekaerts, P. P. Pintrich, & M. Zeidner (Eds.), *Handbook of self-regulation* (pp. 41–84). San Diego, CA: Academic.

Carver, C. S., Sutton, S. K., & Scheier, M. F. (2000). Action, emotion, and personality: Emerging conceptual integration. *Personality and Social Psychology Bulletin, 26,* 741–751.

Christiansen, C. H., Backman, C., Little, B. R., & Nguyen, A. (1999). Occupations and well-being: A study of personal projects. *American Journal of Occupational Therapy, 53,* 91–100.

Csikszentmihalyi, M. (1990). *Flow: The psychology of optimal experience.* New York: Harper & Row.

Davidson, R. J. (1994). Asymmetric brain function, affective style, and psychopathology: The role of early experience and plasticity. *Development and Psychopathology, 6,* 741–758.

Davidson, R. J., Pizzagalli, D., Nitschke, J. B., & Kalin, N. H. (2003). Parsing the subcomponents of emotions and disorders of emotions: Perspectives from affective neuroscience. In R. J. Davidson, H. H. Goldsmith, & K. Scherer (Eds.), *Handbook of affective science* (pp. 8–24). New York: Oxford University Press.

Deci, E. L., & Ryan, R. M. (1985). *Intrinsic motivation and self-determination in human behavior.* New York: Plenum.

Deci, E. L., & Ryan, R. M. (2000). The "what" and "why" of goal pursuits: Human needs and the self-determination of behavior. *Psychological Inquiry, 11,* 227–268.

Diener, E. (1984). Subjective well-being. *Psychological Bulletin, 95,* 542–575.

Diener, E., Suh, E. M., Lucas, R. E., & Smith, H. L. (1999). Subjective well-being: Three decades of progress. *Psychological Bulletin, 125,* 276–302.

Elliot, A. J., & Church, M. A. (2002). Client articulated avoidance goals in the therapy context. *Journal of Counseling Psychology, 49,* 243–254.

Elliot, A. J., & Sheldon, K. M. (1997). Avoidance achievement motivation: A personal goals analysis. *Journal of Personality and Social Psychology, 73,* 171–185.

Elliot, A. J., & Sheldon, K. M. (1998). Avoidance personal goals and the personality–illness relationship. *Journal of Personality and Social Psychology, 75,* 1282–1299.

Elliot, A. J., Sheldon, K. M., & Church, M. A. (1997). Avoidance personal goals and subjective well-being. *Personality and Social Psychology Bulletin, 23,* 915–927.

Emmons, R. A. (1986). Personal strivings: An approach to personality and subjective well-being. *Journal of Personality and Social Psychology, 51,* 1058–1068.

Emmons, R. A. (1989). The personal strivings approach to personality. In L. A. Pervin (Ed.), *Goal concepts in personality and social psychology* (pp. 87–126). Hillsdale, NJ: Lawrence Erlbaum Associates.

Emmons, R. A. (1996). Striving and feeling: Personal goals and subjective well-being. In P. M. Gollwitzer & J. A. Bargh (Eds.), *The psychology of action: Linking cognition and motivation to behavior* (pp. 313–337). New York: Guilford.

Freund, A. M., & Baltes, P. B. (2002). Life-management strategies of selection, optimization and compensation: Measurement by self-report and construct validity. *Journal of Personality and Social Psychology, 82,* 642–662.

Harris, C., Daniels, K., & Briner, R. (2003). A daily diary study of goals and affective well-being at work. *Journal of Occupational and Organizational Psychology, 76,* 401–410.

Heady, B., & Wearing, A. (1989). Personality, life events, and subjective well-being: Toward a dynamic equilibrium model. *Journal of Personality and Social Psychology, 57,* 731–739.

Heckhausen, H., & Kuhl, J. (1985). From wishes to actions: The dead ends and short cuts on the long way to action. In M. Frese & J. Sabini (Eds.), *Goal-directed behavior: The concept of action in psychology* (pp. 134–159). Hillsdale, NJ: Lawrence Erlbaum Associates.

Heckhausen, J. (1999). *Developmental regulation in adulthood: Age-normative and sociostructural constraints as adaptive challenges.* New York: Cambridge University Press.

Helson, H. (1964). *Adaption level theory.* New York: Harper & Row.

Hoff, E. H., & Ewers, E. (2003). Zielkonflikte und Zielbalance: Berufliche und private Lebensgestaltung von Frauen, Männern und Paaren [Goal conflicts and balance: Professional and private life management of women, men, and couples]. In A. E. Abele, E. H. Hoff, & H. U. Hohner (Eds.), *Frauen und Männer in akademischen Professionen* (pp. 131–156). Heidelberg, Germany: Asanger.

Hsee, C. K., & Abelson, R. P. (1991). Velocity relation: Satisfaction as a function of the first derivative of outcome over time. *Journal of Personality and Social Psychology, 60,* 341–347.

Kasser, T., & Ryan, R. M. (1993). A dark side of the American dream: Correlates of financial success as a central life aspiration. *Journal of Personality and Social Psychology, 65,* 410–422.

Kasser, T., & Ryan, R. M. (1996). Further examining the American dream: Well-being correlates of intrinsic and extrinsic goals. *Personality and Social Psychology Bulletin, 22,* 281–288.

Kehr, H. M. (2003). Goal conflicts, attainment of new goals, and well-being among managers. *Journal of Occupational Health Psychology, 8,* 195–208.

King, L. A., Richards, J. H., & Stemmerich, E. (1998). Daily goals, life goals, and worst fears: Means, ends, and subjective well-being. *Journal of Personality, 66,* 713–744.

Klinger, E. (1977). *Meaning and void: Inner experience and the incentives in people's lives.* Minneapolis: University of Minnesota Press.

Koestner, R., Lekes, N., Powers, T. A., & Chicoine, E. (2002). Attaining personal goals: Self-concordance plus implementation intentions equals success. *Journal of Personality and Social Psychology, 83,* 231–244.

Kruglanski, A. W. (1996). Goals as knowledge structures. In P. M. Gollwitzer & J. A. Bargh (Eds.), *The psychology of action: Linking cognition and motivation to behavior* (pp. 599–618). New York: Guilford.

Lawrence, J. W., Carver, C. S., & Scheier, M. F. (1999). *Velocity and affect in immediate personal experience.* Unpublished manuscript.

Linville, P. W. (1985). Self-complexity and affective extremity: Don't put all of your eggs in one cognitive basket. *Social Cognition, 3,* 94–120.

Little, B. R. (1989). Personal projects analysis: Trivial pursuits, magnificent obsessions, and the search for coherence. In D. M. Buss & N. Cantor (Eds.), *Personality psychology: Recent trends and emerging directions* (pp. 15–31). New York: Springer.

Little, B. R. (1999). Personality and motivation: Personal action and the conative evolution. In L. A. Pervin & O. P. John (Eds.), *Handbook of personality: Theory and research* (2nd ed., pp. 501–524). New York: Guilford.

Little, B. R. (2005). Personality science and personal projects: Six impossible things before breakfast. *Journal of Research in Personality, 39,* 4–21.

Little, B. R., & Chambers, N. C. (2004). Personal project pursuit: On human doings and well beings. In W. M. Cox & E. Klinger (Eds.), *Handbook of motivational counseling: Concepts, approaches, and assessment* (pp. 65–82). Chichester, UK: Wiley.

Locke, E. A., & Latham, G. P. (1990). *A theory of goal setting and task performance.* Englewood Cliffs, NJ: Prentice-Hall.

Locke, E. A., Shaw, K. N., Saari, L. M., & Latham, G. P. (1981). Goal setting and task performance: 1969–1980. *Psychological Bulletin, 90,* 125–152.

Lucas, R. E., Diener, E., & Suh, E. (1996). Discriminant validity of well-being measures. *Journal of Personality and Social Psychology, 71,* 616–628.

Lüdtke, O. (2004). Persönliche Ziele im jungen Erwachsenenalter [Personal goals in early adulthood]. Unpublished dissertation, Free University, Berlin.

Maier, G. W., & Brunstein, J. C. (2001). The role of personal work goals in newcomers' job satisfaction and organizational commitment: A longitudinal analysis. *Journal of Applied Psychology, 86,* 1034–1042.

McGregor, I., & Little, B. R. (1998). Personal projects, happiness, and meaning: On doing well and being yourself. *Journal of Personality and Social Psychology, 74,* 494–512.

McIntosh, W. D., & Martin, L. L. (1992). The cybernetics of happiness: The relation of goal attainment, rumination, and affect. *Review of Personality and Social Psychology, 49,* 222–246.

Mone, M. A., & Baker, D. D. (1992). A social-cognitive, attributional model of personal goals: An empirical evaluation. *Motivation and Emotion, 16,* 297–321.

Nurmi, J.-E. (1992). Age differences in adult life goals, concerns, and their temporal extension: A life course approach to future-oriented motivation. *International Journal of Behavioral Development, 15,* 487–508.

Nurmi, J.-E., & Salmela-Aro, K. (2002). Goal construction, reconstruction and depressive symptoms in a life-span context: The transition from school to work. *Journal of Personality, 70,* 385–420.

Oatley, K., & Johnson-Laird, P. N. (1996). The communicative theory of emotions: Empirical tests, mental models, and implications for social interaction. In L. L. Martin & A. Tesser (Eds.), *Striving and feeling: Interactions among goals, affect, and self-regulation* (pp. 363–393). Hillsdale, NJ: Lawrence Erlbaum Associates.

Oishi, S., & Diener, E. (2001). Goals, culture, and subjective well-being. *Personality and Social Psychology Bulletin, 27,* 1674–1682.

Omodei, M. M., & Wearing, A. J. (1990). Need satisfaction and involvement in personal projects: Toward an integrative model of subjective well-being. *Journal of Personality and Social Psychology, 59,* 762–769.

Pavot, W., & Diener, E. (1993). Review of the Satisfaction with Life Scale. *Psychological Assessment, 5,* 164–172.

Robinson, M. D. (2000). The reactive and prospective functions of mood: Its role in linking daily experiences and cognitive well-being. *Cognition and Emotion, 14,* 145–176.

Rogers, C. (1963). The actualizing tendency in relation to "motives" and to consciousness. In M. R. Jones (Ed.), *Nebraska symposium on motivation* (Vol. 11, pp. 1–24). Lincoln: University of Nebraska Press.

Russell, D. W. (1982). The causal dimension scale: A measure of how individuals perceive causes. *Journal of Personality and Social Psychology, 42,* 1137–1145.

Ryff, C. D. (1989). Happiness is everything, or is it? Explorations on the meaning of psychological well-being. *Journal of Personality and Social Psychology, 57,* 1069–1081.

Salmela-Aro, K. (1992). Struggling with self: The personal projects of students seeking psychological counselling. *Scandinavian Journal of Psychology, 33,* 330–338.

Salmela-Aro, K., & Nurmi, J.-E. (1996). Depressive symptoms and personal project appraisals: A cross-lagged longitudinal study. *Personality and Individual Differences, 21,* 373–381.

Salmela-Aro, K., & Nurmi, J.-E. (1997a). Goal contents, well-being, and life context during transition to university: A longitudinal study. *International Journal of Behavioral Development, 20,* 471–491.

Salmela-Aro, K., & Nurmi, J.-E. (1997b). Personal project appraisals, academic achievement and related satisfaction: A prospective study. *European Journal of Psychology of Education, 12,* 77–88.

Salmela-Aro, K., Nurmi, J.-E., Saisto, T., & Halmesmäki, E. (2001). Goal reconstruction and depressive symptoms during the transition to motherhood: Evidence from two cross-lagged longitudinal studies. *Journal of Personality and Social Psychology, 81,* 1144–1159.

Sears, D. O. (1986). College sophomores in the laboratory: Influences of a narrow data base on social psychology's view of human nature. *Journal of Personality and Social Psychology, 51,* 515–530.

Sheldon, K. M. (2002). The self-concordance model of healthy goal-striving: When personal goals correctly represent the person. In E. L. Deci & R. M. Ryan (Eds.), *Handbook of self-determination research* (pp. 65–86). Rochester, NY: University of Rochester Press.

Sheldon, K. M., & Elliot, A. J. (1998). Not all personal goals are personal: Comparing autonomous and controlled reasons for goals as predictors of effort and attainment. *Personality and Social Psychology Bulletin, 24,* 546–557.

Sheldon, K. M., & Elliot, A. J. (1999). Goal striving, need satisfaction, and longitudinal well-being: The self-concordance model. *Journal of Personality and Social Psychology, 76,* 482–497.

Sheldon, K. M., & Elliot, A. J. (2000). Personal goals in social roles: Divergences and convergences across roles and levels of analysis. *Journal of Personality, 68,* 51–84.

Sheldon, K. M., & Houser-Marko, L. (2001). Self-concordance, goal attainment, and the pursuit of happiness: Can there be an upward spiral? *Journal of Personality and Social Psychology, 80,* 152–165.

Sheldon, K. M., & Kasser, T. (1995). Coherence and congruence: Two aspects of personality integration. *Journal of Personality and Social Psychology, 68,* 531–543.

Sheldon, K. M., & Kasser, T. (1998). Pursuing personal goals: Skills enable progress, but not all progress is beneficial. *Personality and Social Psychology Bulletin, 24,* 1319–1331.

Sheldon, K. M., & Kasser, T. (2001). Goals, congruence, and positive well-being: New empirical support for humanistic theories. *Journal of Humanistic Psychology, 41,* 30–50.

Sheldon, K. M., Kasser, T., Smith, K., & Shore, T. (2002). Personal goals and psychological growth: Testing an intervention to enhance goal attainment and personality integration. *Journal of Personality, 70,* 5–31.

Sheldon, K. M., Ryan, R., & Reis, H. T. (1996). What makes for a good day? Competence and autonomy in the day and in the person. *Personality and Social Psychology Bulletin, 22,* 1270–1279.

Skinner, E. A. (1995). *Perceived control, motivation, and coping.* Thousand Oaks, CA: Sage.

Thomas, K. M., & Mathieu, J. E. (1994). Role of causal attributions in dynamic self-regulation and goal processes. *Journal of Applied Psychology, 79,* 812–818.

Watson, D., Clark, L. A., & Tellegen, A. (1988). Development and validation of brief measures of positive and negative affect: The PANAS scales. *Journal of Personality and Social Psychology, 54,* 1063–1070.

Watson, D., & Walker, L. M. (1996). The long-term stability and predictive validity of trait measures of affect. *Journal of Personality and Social Psychology, 70,* 567–577.

Weiner, B. (1985). "Spontaneous" causal thinking. *Psychological Bulletin, 97,* 74–84.

Wiese, B. S. (2000). *Berufliche und familiäre Zielstrukturen* [Work and family goal structures]. Münster, Germany: Waxmann.

Wiese, B. S. (2004). Konflikte zwischen Beruf und Familie im Alltagserleben erwerbstätiger Paare: Querschnittliche und prozessuale Analysen [Work–family conflicts of dual-earner couples: Cross-sectional and process analyses]. *Zeitschrift für Sozialpsychologie, 35,* 45–58.

Wiese, B. S., & Freund, A. M. (2005). Goal progress makes one happy, or does it? Longitudinal findings from the work domain. *Journal of Occupational and Organizational Psychology, 78,* 287–304.

Wiese, B. S., & Heimann, M. (2006). *Goal progress in the academic and work domains: The role of affect, self-efficacy, and internal success attributions.* Manuscript submitted for publication.

APPENDIX

Selected Longitudinal/Process Studies on Successful Goal Pursuit and Well-Being

Author(s)	Sample	Time Interval	Dependent Measure(s): Content Focus of Well-Being
Affleck et al. (1998)	N = 50 Adult Sample Nationality: American	Thirty days (with sixty measurements)	Affective Well-Being: • Positive Affect • Negative Affect
Bagozzi et al. (1998)	N = 406 Adult sample Nationality: Dutch	Four weeks (with two measurements)	Affective Well-Being: • Positive Affect • Negative Affect
Brown et al. (1997)	N = 122 Adult sample Nationality: American	Three months (with two measurements)	Affective Well-Being: • Positive Affect • Negative Affect
Brunstein (1993)	N = 88 University Students Nationality: German	14 weeks (with four measurements)	Combined Well-Being Scale (Positive Affect, Negative Affect, Satisfaction with Life)
Brunstein et al. (1998)	Study 1: N = 98 University Students Nationality: German Study 2: N = 127 University Students Nationality: German	Study 1: Two weeks (with thirteen measurements) Study 2: Four months (with four measurements)	Study 1: Affective Well-Being: • Positive Affect minus Negative Affect Study 2: Affective Well-Being: • Positive Affect minus Negative Affect
Elliot & Church (2002)	N = 53 University Students (seeking psycho-therapy services) Nationality: American	Twelve weeks (with two measurements)	Combined Well-Being Scale (Positive Affect, Negative Affect, Satisfaction with Life)
Harris et al. (2003)	N = 22 Adult Sample Nationality: British	Twelve days (with 24 measurements)	Affective Well-Being: • Pleasurable Affect • Activated Affect
Kehr (2003)	N = 99 Adult Sample Nationality: German	Five months (with three measurements)	Affective Well-Being: • Positive Affect Negative Affect
Koestner et al. (2002)	Study 1: N = 106 University Students Nationality: Canadian Study 2: N = 59 University Students Nationality: Canadian	Study 1: Weekend (with two measurements) Study 2: Six weeks (with three measurements)	Study 1: Affective Well-Being: • Positive Affect minus Negative Affect Study 2: Affective Well-Being: • Positive Affect minus Negative Affect

Lüdtke (2004)	$N = 84$ High School Students Nationality: German	Six weeks (with five measurements)	Affective Well-Being: • Positive Affect minus Negative Affect Cognitive Well-Being: • Satisfaction with School
Maier & Brunstein (2001)	$N = 81$ Adult Sample Nationality: German	Eight months (with three measurements)	Cognitive Well-Being: • Job Satisfaction
Oishi & Diener (2001)	Study 1: $N = 106$ University Students Nationality: American (87 Europ. Amer.; 19 Asian Amer.)	Study 1: One month (with two measurements)	Study 1: Cognitive Well-Being: • Life Satisfaction
	Study 2: $N = 131$ University Students Nationality: American (67 Europ. Amer.; 64 Asian Amer.)	Study 2: One week (with two measurements)	Study 2: Cognitive Well-Being: • Life Satisfaction
	Study 3: $N = 70$ College Students Nationality: Japanese	Study 3: One week (with two measurements)	Study 3: Cognitive Well-Being: • Life Satisfaction
Sheldon & Elliot (1999)	Study 1: $N = 169$ University Students Nationality: American	Study 1: One semester (with five measurements)	Study 1: Combined Well-Being Scale (Positive Affect, Negative Affect, Satisfaction with Life)
	Study 3: $N = 73$ University Students Nationality: American	Study 3: One semester (with ten measurements)	Study 3: Combined Well-Being Scale (Positive Affect, Negative Affect, Satisfaction with Life)

Sheldon &
Elliot (2000)
	Study 2:
	$N = 82$
	University Students
	Nationality: American
		Study 2:
		15 weeks
		(with four
		measurements)
			Study 2:
			Cognitive Well-Being:
			• Life Satisfaction
			• Satisfaction with …
			  Child Role
			  Employee Role
			  Romance Role
			  Student Role
			  Friendship Role

Sheldon & Houser-Marko (2001)	Study 1: $N = 114$ University Students Nationality: American	Study 1: About two semesters (with five measurements)	Study 1: Cognitive Well-Being: • Adjustment to College
	Study 2: $N = 94$ University Students Nationality: American	Study 2: Two weeks (with three measurements)	Study 2: Cognitive Well-Being: • Sense of Growth

Sheldon & Kasser (1998)	$N = 90$ University Students Nationality: American	Two months (with seven measurements)	Combined Well-Being Scale (Positive Affect, Negative Affect, Satisfaction with Life, Depression; partly separated for analyses)
Sheldon et al. (2002)	$N = 78$ University Students Nationality: American	About one semester (with three measurements)	Cognitive Well-Being: • Psychosocial Well-Being • Psychological Vitality Affective Well-Being: • Positive Affect minus Negative Affect
Wiese (2004)	$N = 70$ Adult Sample Nationality: German	Two weeks (fourteen measurements)	• Positive Affect
Wiese & Freund (2005)	$N = 82$ Adult Sample Nationality: German	Three years (two measurements)	Cognitive Well-Being: • Job Satisfaction • Satisfaction with Professional Development Affective Well-Being: • Positive Affect • Negative Affect
Wiese & Heimann (2006)	Study 1: $N = 34$ University Students Nationality: German	Study 1: Six months (two measurements)	Study 1: Cognitive Well-Being: • Satisfaction with University Studies Affective Well-Being: • Positive Affect • Negative Affect
	Study 2: $N = 53$ Adult Sample Nationality: German	Study 2: Six months (two measurements)	Study 2: Cognitive Well-Being: • Job Satisfaction Affective Well-Being: • Positive Affect • Negative Affect

12

Personal Projects
in Health and Illness

Amy H. Peterman and Len Lecci

I t is 8:00 a.m. Monday morning and several patients are sitting in the outer office of a medical clinic waiting for their names to be called. Nearest to the reception desk is Bryan, a 45-year-old writer and father of two children who recently separated from his wife after a 14-year marriage. He is no stranger to the clinic, frequenting its waiting room for countless visits, and his days are filled with numerous illness-related projects. Yet this is by no means a routine experience from an emotional standpoint. In fact, he is particularly apprehensive about today's appointment. Although Bryan has been reasonably healthy his entire life, he cannot seem to shake the belief that there is something seriously wrong with him. This morning, he is scheduled to see Dr. Watkinson to get the results of a prostate exam. This is his third exam, with the two previous tests resulting in no unusual findings. Earlier this year, Bryan was convinced that he had a cancerous tumor in his brain, and was heard commenting frequently that it was so large that he could feel it when he blinked. That too proved to be a false alarm. The nurses, who know him by name, assure him that today will be like all other days, and the end result will be fine.

Seated across from Bryan is Emily, who looks calm despite the fact that she, too, is dealing with serious concerns about her health. A 41-year-old woman, Emily also has an appointment to discuss the results of some recent tests. She had an MRI of her brain and a thorough neurological exam to determine the cause of the blurry vision and balance problems that seemed to have come out of nowhere within the past month or so. Most worrisome to her, though, was something that happened yesterday: She had been having a conversation with her husband when she lost consciousness for about a minute. Her husband had driven her to the emergency room where a physician accessed the MRI results, refused to give her any information about them, and told her to see her own doctor as soon as possible. Emily was able to get an appointment with Dr. Jenkins the very next day. She was worried, but also annoyed because it interfered with two of her most important personal projects: To attend the appointment, she had to cancel an important meeting at work and find someone to pick up her two children from school. However, she was alert enough to know that she might be getting some bad news. This was worrisome, but she resolved not to become too upset before she found out what the doctor had to say.

There are a wide range of contexts within which one's physical health can be conceptualized, and the meaning attributed to one's physical health is central to how it is experienced and how it effects day-to-day functioning. One avenue for conceptualizing physical health, as well as any concerns about one's health, is motivation. Motivation can be broadly defined as the processes that direct a person's selection, initiation, maintenance, change, and termination of personal projects, as well as the processes that influence the intensity of action and the schematic organization of personal projects (e.g., Little, 1983; Little & Chambers, 2004; see also Bandura, 1988). Consequently, changes in an individual's personal projects can provide a particularly meaningful and sensitive measure of the overall impact of disease, both real and imagined, as well as any treatments or interventions, as experienced from the patient's perspective.

In this chapter we review the literature that has examined the manifestation of personal projects, the processes that govern them, and their relation to both physical health and beliefs regarding health and illness. We also present new data on the personal projects of cancer patients. It is important to note that, although there is a more expansive literature examining the link between health and goal units broadly defined (e.g., Chen, Matthews, Salomon, & Ewart, 2002; Emmons & King, 1988;

Karoly & Lecci, 1997), we focus our discussion here on research utilizing the personal projects methodology.

THE INCIDENCE OF HEALTH PROJECTS

Although most research involving personal projects has concentrated on the affective and cognitive appraisal of projects, some researchers have also considered their content. As a result, there are examples in the literature of content coding schemes that are used by researchers to define participants' projects after the fact (e.g., Lawton, Moss, Winter, & Hoffman, 2002), as well as procedures where the participants themselves categorize their personal projects (e.g., Karoly & Lecci, 1993). Both of these content scoring schemes include a category referring to health projects, where health projects could be broadly defined as any activities involving the individual's appearance, health, health improvement, or fitness (see Little, 1987). Common examples of health projects have included "lose weight," "quit smoking," and "see my doctor," as well as direct references to participants' health (for a detailed description of the methodology behind personal projects analysis [PPA], see Little & Gee, chap. 2, this volume).

When considering either the participant- or experimenter-assessed content analysis, it appears that approximately 14% of personal projects generated can be categorized as having a health focus. Indeed, there is a surprising degree of convergence with respect to the percentage of projects that are defined as health projects, as these findings emerge despite substantial differences in the total number of personal projects elicited, as well as differences in the ages and life circumstances of the participants (e.g., these figures have emerged in samples ranging from female college students to community residents over the age of 70; see Karoly & Lecci, 1993; Lawton et al., 2002). Thus, this supports the idea that health projects are present for a wide range of individuals. Despite the fact that researchers have documented the robust presence of health projects, a more detailed analysis of these projects has not been undertaken. Do content distinctions among health projects reflect developmental, generational, or cultural differences in health beliefs?

Research has examined whether individual differences in health beliefs affect the rate of endorsement of health-related personal projects. For example, participants who scored high on a measure of health preoccupation and fear generated more health projects, or were more likely to endorse health projects from a prearranged list, and were more likely to define their health projects as their "most important projects" (see Karoly & Lecci, 1993; Lecci, Karoly, Ruehlman, & Lanyon, 1996). The fact that individuals who are concerned about health engage in more health projects is important because these individuals will, by definition, have fewer (or fewer resources for) projects in other domains. As a result, when considering the domain of health projects, problems for those with a disproportionate number of health concerns might be relevant in domains other than health, as reflected by insufficient time to deal with other normative pursuits. It is also possible that individual differences in illness beliefs can affect how health projects are construed.

HEALTH PROJECT CONSTRUAL AND ILLNESS BELIEFS

Most individuals in the normal population are biased toward believing that they are healthy unless confronted with overwhelming evidence to the contrary. Weinstein (1984, 1987), for example, showed that most people assess their risk for illness as lower than average. When "normal" individuals have a health fear activated, they avoid actions that may facilitate the detection of a health threat, and are temporarily unwilling to undertake protective acts (e.g., Leventhal & Watts, 1966; Millar & Millar, 1995). Only when an individual adopts an illness schema that is perceived to be serious will he or she report more symptoms, desire additional information about his or her health, and seek out medical information specific to the medical problem (Jemmot, Ditto, & Croyle, 1986; Leventhal, 1970). Thus, when such individuals have a health fear activated, the outcome is an avoidance of actions that move one toward detecting a threat and a temporary undermining of a willingness to undertake a protective act if minor discomfort or pain is involved (Leventhal & Watts, 1966; see also Miller & Miller, 1995).

This response is in direct contrast to the response exhibited by individuals evidencing a subclinical level of preoccupation and fear of illness; something that has been termed *hypochondriacal tendencies* (see Barsky, Cleary, Sarnie, & Klerman, 1993). As would be the case with Bryan, such individuals evidence a strong bias toward believing they are unhealthy, seek out medical information, and may undergo uncomfortable procedures to validate their beliefs (Kellner, 1986). They, along with those evidencing negative affectivity, show a heightened incidence of self-reported illness (e.g., Ellington &

Wiebe, 1999; Feldman, Cohen, Doyle, Skoner, & Gwaltney, 1999; Pennebaker, 1982; Watson & Pennebaker, 1989). Because the nonclinical population is best described as having a continuum of illness beliefs (Pilowsky, 1978), ranging from those having an aversion to believing that they are ill to those evidencing hypochondriacal tendencies (see also Lecci, 2004), then an assessment of individual differences in illness belief acquisition is important when considering an individual's personal projects.

Kuhl and his colleagues have accumulated substantial evidence suggesting that motivation or volition is critical for the long-term maintenance of cognitive, behavioral, and affective states, even when such states are maladaptive (e.g., Kuhl, 1985; Kuhl & Helle, 1986). A well-established means of operationalizing the broad concepts of volition and motivation is via the sampling of personal projects (e.g., Cantor & Zirkel, 1990; Pervin, 1989). Personal projects prompt information seeking, guide coping efforts, and can serve as an endpoint in a self-regulatory framework (e.g., Klinger, Barta, & Maxeiner, 1981; Leventhal, Meyer, & Nerenz, 1980; Posner, 1988; Simon, 1994). Although the theoretical link between psychopathology and personal project (i.e., goal) functioning is not new to the field of psychology (e.g., Adler, 1927; Karoly, 1999; Little, 1987), it should be acknowledged that there is a dearth of empirical investigations of goal functioning relative to nonnormative health beliefs (e.g., hypochondriacal tendencies). In fact, there have been only two such published studies.

In the first of these studies, the Minnesota Multiphasic Personality Inventory (MMPI) Hypochondriasis (*Hs*) scale was administered to 1,541 undergraduate students, and participants scoring in the clinical range and those scoring below the mean (but well within the normal range) were recalled for further testing (Karoly & Lecci, 1993). Participants were then retested with the MMPI *Hs* scale, and only those showing consistency in their MMPI *Hs* scores were retained for further analysis. Participants were given PPA (Little, 1983), which required them to identify and rate their 10 most important projects using a series of appraisal dimensions (e.g., stress, enjoyment, progress to date, etc.). Participants also categorized their projects using a content scoring system and, as previously mentioned, those evidencing a preoccupation and fear of illness listed significantly more health projects and were more likely to identify their health projects as most important relative to those not evidencing a preoccupation and fear of illness. Two other findings also emerged:

1. When examining the ratings for the health projects, MMPI *Hs* scores were associated with generally aversive cognitive evaluations (e.g., stress, difficulty, less enjoyment, and less progress). For nonhealth projects, MMPI *Hs* scores did not show this pattern of aversive cognitive evaluations. Instead, MMPI *Hs* scores were associated with the inability to progress on, control, and have sufficient time to work on nonhealth projects.

2. For those individuals with higher MMPI *Hs* scores, the content of their most important health projects was benign and similar to the health projects nominated by normal individuals (e.g., lose 10 pounds, stop smoking, exercise more). However, when examining the projects not considered among the most important, more medically oriented projects emerged for those with high MMPI *Hs* scores (e.g., see all my doctors, lower blood pressure, keep illness under control, see new psychiatrists, keep myself unsick, etc.). These results may highlight the distinction between illness prevention projects and more normative health promotion projects. If these qualitative (health promotion vs. illness prevention) differences are robust, then differences in strategic tendencies might also exist (see also Elliot & Sheldon, 1998; Ogilvie & Rose, 1995).

In a follow-up study (Lecci et al., 1996) based on a sample of adults representatively selected from across the United States, the previously mentioned findings were confirmed and extended. Specifically, goal ratings associated with hypochondriacal tendencies were found to be distinct from those associated with depression, pure symptom endorsements, and the self-reported diagnosis of physical illness. This suggests that the relation between the construal of personal projects and hypochondriacal tendencies is independent of other related (traditionally comorbid) conditions. Second, with regard to goal (i.e., project) content, hypochondriacal tendencies were positively associated with the endorsement of illness-type health pursuits, but were unrelated to the endorsement of more normative health promotion projects. Third, hypochondriacal tendencies showed no relation to assessments of project value and self-efficacy.

Based on the results from these two studies, it appears that the connection between health project pursuit and hypochondriacal tendencies occurs at both the level of project content and in the cognitive and affective elaborations associated with the pursuit of one's health projects. Moreover, these associations appear to follow a developmental trend. Specifically, with regard to content, it has been shown that, whereas nonhypochondriacal individuals normatively engage in health promotion pursuits, hypochondriacal tendencies are associated with illness prevention projects. These types of projects appear to become increasingly important as those evidencing hypochondriacal tendencies get older (see also chapters in this volume examining developmental project construal; e.g., Freund, chap. 9, this volume). Thus, avoiding negative health outcomes rather than achieving positive health outcomes may be an important feature for those evidencing hypochondriacal tendencies. This conclusion is consistent with the principle of behavioral activation versus inhibition and its relation to mental health (e.g., Gray, 1987). Specifically, by focusing on the avoidance of negative outcomes (illness prevention) rather than the approach of positive outcomes (health promotion), the individual's cognitive experience is decidedly more negative (see also the distinction between disease detection and health promotion discussed by Millar & Millar, 1995).

It can also be hypothesized that through the process of specialization, young individuals with hypochondriacal tendencies may eventually focus their maladaptive project construals in the health domain (e.g., a generalized negative affect may find its niche within the health domain; Lecci et al., 1996). This explanation would also account for the overlap with anxiety and depression, as both involve negative affect (e.g., Watson, Clark, & Tellegen, 1988). In this regard, we would expect to find that Bryan has always been a worrier; worrying about his grades in middle school, concerns over how his friends perceived him, and perhaps even some aspects of his health. As time passed and Bryan moved into adulthood, health concerns became more salient, giving rise to a large number of illness prevention pursuits that clearly reflected his hypochondriacal nature. Moreover, a consequence of the intense health focus is that Bryan's nonhealth projects were neglected. Not surprisingly, Bryan is now separated and his relationships with the children are likewise distant and strained. Thus, the young hypochondriac may have broad concerns that eventually manifest primarily (i.e., specialize) in the health domain, but the extensive nature of the adult hypochondriac's health focus ultimately results in broader disruptions that affect the entire project system. Of course, these developmental hypotheses are speculative and would require longitudinal data as well as the experimental manipulation of the variables of interest before any definitive causal conclusions could be drawn.

A second, and possibly parallel process, involves the development of automated behaviors that can reinforce and extend hypochondriacal thinking (Lecci & Cohen, 2002; see also Lecci & Cohen, 2004). Due to the absence of any association between hypochondriacal tendencies and measures of project self-efficacy and value (referred to as the directive function in self-regulatory theory), it can be concluded that some hypochondriacal behaviors are automated or, in the very least, well learned. Within a self-regulatory framework, the directive function (value and self-efficacy) is hypothesized to provide the willful component of any goal-type action (cf. Ford, 1987; Karoly, 1993). That is, personal projects should be undertaken if they provide either a sense of efficacy (mastery or accomplishment) or a sense of value (meaning) to the individual. In the absence of both efficacy and value (and because health projects are also experienced as aversive events for those evidencing hypochondriacal tendencies), it is suggested that volitional project striving should not occur, and would therefore be explained best by the existence of automated processes. Research also indicates that all effortful behavior, including project representations, can, with rehearsal, become automatic, effortless, and even preconscious (Bargh, 1990; Bargh & Chartrand, 1999; Freund, chap. 9, this volume). This might be expected for the more inveterate group of hypochondriacs, but the effect should be less evident in younger individuals if a developmental explanatory model is adopted (i.e., consistent with the changes in personal project content or endorsement). This conclusion would be consistent with the dominant models on illness belief acquisition that likewise suggest the role of automated (e.g., perceptual) mechanisms in the maintenance of such beliefs (e.g., Cioffi, 1991; Leventhal et al., 1997).

The Automaticity of Health Beliefs and the Role of Perceived Control

Obviously, Bryan is aware of the fact that he is concerned about his health, but he may be unaware of the extent to which he is consumed by it. By engaging in multiple, long-term health projects, there are subtle affective and cognitive changes that can reinforce the existence and pursuit of these projects. Consequently, Bryan is likely both unaware of and lacking control over at least some aspects of his health projects.

Several recent studies have clearly illustrated what can be termed the *automaticity* of health beliefs by exploring individual differences in illness vulnerability beliefs, response to an experimentally manipulated health threat, and the resulting perceptual bias (see Lecci & Cohen, 2002, 2004). In two of these studies, participants were randomly assigned to a health threat or no health threat condition and were then assessed with regard to their cognitive and affective response to this threat. A modified emotional Stroop task was employed where illness and control words were substituted for the color words and response latency was recorded. Consistent with the literature (e.g., Eckhardt & Cohen, 1997; Matthews & MacLeod, 1985), the data indicated that individuals who had experienced a health threat exhibited longer reaction times (RTs), but only for health words. However, this effect was dependent on stable individual differences in hypochondriacal tendencies (i.e., illness vulnerability beliefs). That is, longer RTs for health words were only observed when (a) individuals exhibited elevated hypochondriacal tendencies, and (b) individuals experienced a health threat. This finding, which was observed in two independent samples, illustrates the importance of both person and situation factors in the resulting perceptual bias associated with health (Lecci & Cohen, 2002).

The preceding findings were then replicated and extended in a follow-up study, where it was shown that experimentally manipulated control beliefs mitigate the observed perceptual effects. Specifically, by giving participants a relatively simple instruction that directed their attention to potentially controllable aspects of the health-threatening stimulus, hypochondriacal tendencies no longer resulted in longer response latencies for health-related words relative to neutral words, even when health fears were activated (Lecci & Cohen, 2004). In other words, although the actual threat (i.e., probability) of illness did not differ between the high and low control conditions, the perceptual consequences associated with the individual's response to the threat did.

One direction of inquiry that might be fruitful is to consider the manner by which personal projects are implicated in the perceptual biases associated with hypochondriacal tendencies (or illness vulnerability beliefs). Previous research indicates that there are qualitative differences between the health projects of those evidencing hypochondriacal tendencies and those not evidencing such tendencies, with those evidencing hypochondriacal tendencies being more likely to adopt illness avoidance projects as opposed to health promotion (approach) projects (Karoly & Lecci, 1993) as well as being more likely to endorse more serious (e.g., medically related) illness pursuits (Lecci et al., 1996). The key then is to determine whether the distinction in project content is related to differences in the activation of illness concern, to differences in the resulting control beliefs, or to both. If someone were to adopt Bryan's personal project system, would that person evidence a heightened sense of hypochondriacal thinking, a decreased sense of control over health projects, or both? Such a personal project-rooted investigation could lead to important advances in the treatment of hypochondriasis. For example, from an intervention standpoint, one might envision a reconceptualization of one of Bryan's health projects from "don't get sick" to "adopt a healthier lifestyle" and this approach-type project could almost instantaneously elevate perceptions of control as well as significantly decreasing both the automatic activation of illness concern and priming for the detection of physical symptoms.

There is some theoretical support for projects functioning as activators of illness concern. Researchers have argued that projects (or personal goals) are central to the regulation of attention and perception, functioning as perceptual guides for evaluating stimulus experiences (e.g., Klinger et al., 1981; Posner, 1988; Simon, 1994). In this regard, adopting numerous health-focused projects can serve as the direct antecedent of a heightened perceptual sensitivity for somatic cues. This can occur because projects provide the framework for the establishment of specific expectations and such expectations have been shown to increase symptom reporting and symptom sensitivity (e.g., Schmidt, Wolfs-Takens, Oosterlaan, & van den Hout, 1994).

Alternatively, health projects could provide a context to evaluate beliefs about the controllability of a health threat and these control beliefs can influence perception. Two studies have shown that individual differences in hypochondriacal tendencies are correlated with the appraisal of control associated with health (Lecci et al., 1996) and nonhealth projects (Karoly & Lecci, 1993). Research also indicates that all effortful behavior, including personal project (goal) representations, can, with rehearsal, become automatic, effortless, and even preconscious (Bargh, 1990; Bargh & Chartrand, 1999; Freund, chap. 9, this volume). The automaticity of this process underscores the possible link to control beliefs. Specifically, if a health project is more automated for those with elevated illness concerns, then such individuals might not perceive any control over the project's initiation and execution. Moreover, health projects could themselves function as both proximal and distal activators of illness concern that in turn result in perceptual biases. Finally, it would also be important to examine Bryan's nonhealth projects, and to ensure that they are sufficiently infused with meaning so that they, too, can compete for his attention on a micro (minute-to-minute) and macro (life-long) level. In this respect, personal projects are the centerpiece that maintains nonnormative illness beliefs, simultaneously having the potential to act as lynchpins for altering both automated and more willful health- and non-health-related action. Thus, there is hope for change for Bryan, but any interventions will need to consider his entire project system, and how each project sustains itself and influences other projects.

USE OF PPA IN PEOPLE WITH CANCER

In contrast to Bryan, for whom health projects unnecessarily assume a central role in the personal project system, Emily's visit to Dr. Jenkins is going to result in widespread disruption of her very full and mostly satisfying project system. In addition, it will be necessary for her to make an illness-related project a very high priority for an extended period of time. Dr. Jenkins tells Emily that the MRI shows a small growth in her brain. He does not know exactly what it is, but she will need to see a neurosurgeon to determine if it can be removed safely. If the growth is malignant, the surgery may be followed by chemotherapy, radiation therapy, or both. All in all, it appears that Emily is looking at weeks or months of doctor visits, medications, a hospital stay, and more tests. The last straw comes when Dr. Jenkins tells Emily that the episode yesterday was most likely a seizure and that she would not be able to drive for up to 6 months. She breaks down sobbing, asking him how she is supposed to take care of her children, her elderly mother, household chores, and her own work and hobbies if she cannot drive. Although sympathetic, Dr. Jenkins is quite firm about the potential dangers of getting behind the wheel. Emily calls her husband to pick her up and sits in the waiting room in shock.

A serious physical illness, such as cancer, has the potential to significantly disrupt many, if not all, of a patient's personal projects. Disease- and treatment-related symptoms, such as pain, fatigue, anxiety, and nausea, can make it difficult to carry out even basic self-care activities. The time required for treatments and other health-care visits may limit the extent of participation in work, family, or other important roles. The life-threatening nature of many cancers can affect the ability or willingness to plan for the future. Finally, priorities may shift in ways that profoundly affect the entire personal projects system in both negative and positive ways. The changes in the patient's personal projects might, therefore, provide a particularly meaningful and sensitive measure of the overall impact of disease and treatment from the patient's perspective. In fact, several authors have conceptualized health-related quality of life (QOL) as the effect of an illness on the realization of an individual's life plans or the ability to reach valued goals. Despite the existence of hundreds of QOL instruments designed to measure patient-reported outcomes of illness, until recently, none have incorporated PPA or any similar strategy.

The PPA methodology (Little, 1983, 1987) is ideal for examining numerous goal processes in people with chronic or life-threatening health conditions. To the extent that personal projects are a reflection of the major motivations in an individual's life, it may also shed light on some of the more perplexing and interesting questions about the significant individual variability in ability to successfully adapt to a deteriorating physical condition. Clinical experience suggests that a strong, but flexible, sense of self is at the root of that kind of adjustment. As has been discussed in other chapters in this volume, projects might be considered to be an observable, measurable representation of the self (see Little, 1993, for the original discussion). Empirical evidence is also suggestive, as flexibility in goals has been associated with less depression, greater life satisfaction, and higher self-esteem in older adult participants adjusting to retirement (Trepanier, Lapierre, Baillargeon, & Bouffard, 2001). In contrast, McGregor (chap. 6, this volume) provides an in-depth discussion of passionate project pursuit as compensation for personal uncertainty, mortality salience, and a loss of structure.

In this study, Peterman and colleagues (Peterman, Beaumont, & Rosenbloom, 2004; Peterman, Brady, & Cella, 2001; Peterman, Brady, Cella, & Chivington, 2003; Peterman, Brady, Hahn, & Merluzzi, 2000) first wanted to evaluate whether a PPA-based instrument would provide a psychometrically sound, individually meaningful measure of treatment burden that could be used in clinical trials or to guide treatment. Additionally, they wanted to obtain information that would increase our understanding of the responses that patients make to treatment-related interference and begin to identify when goal perseverance, shifting, and disengagement might be the most protective of the self.

There is little empirical work describing the actual process of engagement, disengagement, and shifting of actual goals in the face of illness or other major stressors (see Kuhl & Helle, 1986, for work on disengagement from pursuits in response to depression). Indirect support for the importance of these processes comes from research on positive expectancies, such as optimism and self-efficacy, as proxies for continued goal engagement (Scheier & Carver, 2001). For example, Jackson, Weiss, Lundquist, and Soderlind (2002) reported that optimists rated their personal projects as less stressful, more under control, and more meaningful than did pessimists. This suggests a greater level of engagement, at least in the face of ordinary life stressors. Optimism is also linked to reported expectation of a project's successful outcome, but not to reports of progress on a project (Little, 1996). A positive expectancy about a project's outcome or other dimensions clearly may be linked to decisions about engagement versus disengagement from goals when faced with obstacles, such as illness symptoms. In general, positive expectancies are linked with better psychological outcomes in medically ill populations (e.g., Friedman et al., 1992), including cancer patients (e.g., Carver et al., 1993). However, these general measures do not adequately describe the consequences of working on specific goals. For example, the emotional consequences for a patient with advanced cancer of hoping for a long life may be very different from those of hoping to have enough time for a personal visit with some old friends before death. In addition, a shifting from the former to the latter goal may also have significant negative or positive consequences. Wrosch, Scheier, and colleagues (Wrosch & Scheier, 2003; Wrosch, Scheier, Carver, & Schulz, 2003; Wrosch, Scheier, Miller, Schulz, & Carver, 2003) recently published theoretical and empirical work addressing the important self-regulatory function played by disengagement from unattainable goals and engagement or reengagement with alternative goals.

Data collection is wrapping up in Peterman et al.'s (2000) study of approximately 225 people with cancer. To maximize the likelihood that reported changes in personal projects would be due to cancer or treatment, participants were recruited to the study as they began their first chemotherapy treatment. Individuals were eligible if they had been diagnosed with cancer for the first time in the past 2 months or if they had a relapse or recurrence in the past 2 months and treatment for the previous diagnosis ended more than 2 years ago.

With Little's permission, his PPA methodology (Little, 1983, 1988, 1998) was adapted to meet the specific purposes of this study. PPA is both idiographic and nomothetic, allowing an individualized nomination of each participant's personally meaningful projects, as well as a means for the comparison of goal-related dimensions across subjects (Little, 1983). The PPA was chosen for its emphasis on behavioral projects that are most likely to be affected by disease and treatment conditions. It is designed to be supplemented with ratings of dimensions that are relevant to the particular project (Little, 1983, 1989), such as goal interference in this case.

On the first day of the first chemotherapy treatment, goal content is elicited in the typical way. Next, participants choose the "four projects that you most want to work on during the next 2 months while you are in chemotherapy." Although the PPA usually asks partcipants to rate all of the listed projects, it was important to minimize the questionnaire burden on the ill participants. Moreover, several studies have been able to identify important PPA variables using a limited number of projects (e.g., Lecci, MacLean, & Croteau, 2002). For each of the four chosen projects, the participants completed five questions, which we call the Goal Interference Scale (GIS), designed to assess the extent of cancer-related interference with progress on the project, as well as several other dimensions more commonly used in PPA (e.g., project meaning-fulness).[1] Several other items are used to assess patients' responses to the project (goal) interference. At each follow-up assessment, our participants were asked whether they were continuing to work on the projects they had named in the last assessment. Depending on the response, follow-up questions were asked to determine the status of that project and the others in the project system.

Preliminary Results: Descriptive and Psychometric Data

Given the cancer diagnosis, Peterman et al. were interested in the extent to which participants would list health-related projects. Out of 2,934 projects that were coded for content, almost 20% of them were oriented toward physical health. This is slightly greater than the 14% figure that was discussed earlier, indicating that these cancer patients currently undergoing chemotherapy may be understandably more concerned about their health. Of the remaining 80%, goals listed included everyday tasks ("keep house clean"), hobbies ("gardening,"), social connections

---

[1]As has generally been the case with the PPA, our participants reported very little difficulty completing the GIS. On a scale of 0 (*very easy*) to 5 (*very difficult*), the mean rating endorsed by participants was that the scale was *moderately easy* to fill out (score of 1, $SD = 1.3$), with almost half the sample rating it 0 (*very easy*). Participants commented: "It was easy to fill out," "there were no confusing questions," "questions are simple and to the point," and "it was self-explanatory." The only significant challenge to the feasibility and acceptability was when older cancer patients told us that they did not think that the examples that we gave were relevant to their age group. We remedied this by adding examples such as "visit my grandchildren," "find volunteer activities," and "enjoy my retirement."

("keeping relationship with my husband open during the cancer"), special activities ("prepare for a daughter's wedding," "plan a vacation"), new activities ("learn how to use e-mail," "become more active in politics"), spiritual activities ("set aside time to pray"), work activities ("prepare to return to work," "costing on computer for a company"), illness- or health-related activities ("start walking at least three times a week," "read more about my illness"), and abstract, self-enhancement goals ("find peace within myself," "do what makes me happy," "stay positive"). That 80% of participants' projects were not related to their health is a testament to the likely importance of remaining involved in multiple other aspects of life. All participants were able to answer the interference questions about their goals, even when their goals were abstract.

There were three questions that asked about the importance of each of the goals, with each question scored on a scale ranging from 0 (*not important at all*) to 5 (*extremely important*). The mean sum for these importance ratings was 12.3 (*SD* = 2.5) out of a possible total of 15, indicating that people were identifying goals that were very important to them. Furthermore, there was no difference in importance among the goals listed first, second, third, or fourth (*p* > .7), indicating that people considered all four listed goals to be very important.

Participants also answered the question "Did the questionnaire ask about things that were meaningful to you?" On a scale ranging from 0 (*not at all meaningful*) to 5 (*extremely meaningful*), the mean rating for this question was 3 (*moderately meaningful*; *SD* = 1.3), with a mode of 4 (*very meaningful*). Participants commented, "The questions are very meaningful because it is your life"; "The projects I listed are very important to me, so the questions about them are meaningful"; "They were meaningful because they applied to everyday life"; "Usually I don't like filling out forms, but I am glad I did this one. It was good for reflection."

We have also reported preliminary results to address the study's objectives. First, our effort to develop a psychometrically sound, individually meaningful measure of goal interference that can be used to quantify the burden of cancer and its treatment appears to have been successful (Peterman et al., 2001). The GIS, consisting of 20 interference-related questions (five for each of four projects), has a Cronbach's alpha of .89, indicating an excellent degree of internal consistency across questions and projects. The GIS is moderately correlated with well-validated measures of cancer-related QOL (.4 to .65 with the subscales and total score of the Functional Assessment of Cancer Therapy–General; Cella et al., 1993) and cancer-related symptoms. Known groups validity is also good, with greater goal interference reported by people with poorer functional status. These results suggest that the PPA-based GIS might be useful for documenting relative treatment burden in people with cancer.

Responses to Cancer-Related Goal Interference: Perseverance, Shifting, and Disengagement

As noted earlier, a central question of this study is one that arose repeatedly in clinical work with cancer patients: Which choices will maximize the well-being of someone whose cancer symptoms and treatment side effects are getting in the way of their important projects, goals, and activities? Carver and Scheier (1981, 1998) directly addressed the options in their behavioral theory of self-regulation. Let us return to Emily for a moment. Her neurosurgeon removes a small growth from her right frontal lobe and determines that it is, indeed, malignant. After a month or two of recovery from the surgery, she begins localized radiation therapy to attempt to kill any remaining cancer cells. The radiation causes a great deal of fatigue. Between the surgery and the radiation, Emily experiences significant interference with most of her personal projects. Specifically, she has great difficulty continuing her career as a software designer, the myriad activities to which she accompanies her 7-year-old son and 9-year-old daughter, her volunteer work serving meals in a homeless shelter, and her share of the many household tasks that are usually split between her and her husband. The great difficulty she has in carrying out these projects causes her to reevaluate both the importance of each project and her perception of likely progress on them. Both evaluations are likely to have consequences for the choice of whether or not to continue the project, such that she may be more likely to stop pursuing (disengage from) less important or more unattainable projects. For projects that are important, such as finishing a work project before the deadline, it may be possible to make adjustments in the desired rate of progress toward the goal (e.g., work fewer hours per week and extend the deadline) or to shift to a related goal that is important but more attainable (e.g., let a colleague take over that big project and focus on smaller ones that can be done at any time). Other times, it is possible or necessary to disengage from a particular goal and shift attention to new goals or increase attention paid to other existing, but more possible, goals.

This sort of reevaluation and reordering of projects and priorities has the potential to result in enhanced QOL and emotional well-being. In fact, it is one mechanism proposed by Tedeschi and Calhoun (Tedeschi, Park, & Calhoun, 1998) to account for posttraumatic growth. There is a great deal of interest today in exploring, understanding, and facilitating such growth in the wake of trauma or other negative life events. As described by Carver and Scheier (1981, 1998), interference with progress on projects or goals results in increased attention to those projects. This raises them from an automatic to a fully conscious level of awareness, which then makes it possible to make conscious decisions to continue or to stop participation in different projects that otherwise might be continued by sheer force of habit. However, the choices that will maximize Emily's physical and emotional well-being must be informed by many factors, which can make it rather difficult to determine the best courses of action (see Wrosch & Scheier, 2003).

The next step in the PPA and cancer study was a preliminary look at participants' responses to interference. In 121 participants with data at Time 1 (beginning of chemotherapy) and Time 2 (2 months later), 521 projects were reported as being important to work on over the 2-month period. Of these, 401 projects were still being worked on at Time 2: 38% of those were progressing at the same rate as previously. Of the other 62% that were progressing at a slower rate, participants reported feeling "OK" about that 80% of the time. For the minority of participants who had stopped work on a particular project, 77% of those projects had been replaced with another, equally important project. This appears to be an indication of adaptive goal shifting in the majority of cancer patients.

Clinical Implications. Our data suggest strategies for interventions to improve patient outcomes in the face of symptoms and side effects. For example, when confronted with goal interference, patients could be taught that they have various options for maintaining well-being; for example, they might be helped to identify new ways to achieve important goals, reduce their expectations for progress on existing goals, or shift their focus and energy to different, more attainable, goals (Schwartz, 1999). The goal interference measure would indicate (a) which patients are in need of the intervention (i.e., which are experiencing interference), and (b) salient goals to target and monitor. We hope to use the results of this study to plan and implement a practical and useful intervention for cancer patients facing disease or treatment-related interference with their important personal projects. One of the most important outcomes to monitor would be the sense of self that projects are believed to represent and support.

Personal Goals and Projects in People with Chronic Illness.   It appears that only a few other studies have examined the role of personal projects or goals in people with physical illness. One line of research has attempted to differentiate goal content based on whether health projects are self-selected or imposed (Karoly & Bay, 1990). In this research, the personal projects of children with Type I diabetes were shown to relate to physiological indicators, such that as health projects were more imposed then this was associated with metabolic control hemoglobin assays. The level of imposition may reflect the extent of parental involvement in the child's health project, which would, in turn, explain why more imposition (i.e., more parental involvement) is associated with better metabolic control. Apparently, however, this remains as one of the few published studies to examine the direct link between personal projects and a physical health outcome.

Using a different methodology, Rapkin et al. (1994) examined personal goals and goal-related activities among patients with HIV/AIDS, demonstrating a significant relation with health status, as measured by the Medical Outcomes Study SF-20 questionnaire. In addition, Rapkin et al. found that poor health generally, and symptoms of fatigue specifically, interfered with goal-directed activity: The number of goals not pursued due to illness had the strongest relation with the SF-20 subscales. Similarly, Affleck et al. (1998) demonstrated that pain and fatigue due to fibromyalgia interfered significantly with perception of progress made on a daily basis in social and health-related goals. Goal progress was also related to change in positive mood, such that it appeared that symptom changes had both a direct effect, and an indirect effect through goal progress, on positive mood. Therefore, it may be important to measure both symptoms and goal interference to obtain a complete picture of the path whereby disease and treatment affect well-being.

CONCLUSIONS AND DIRECTIONS FOR FUTURE RESEARCH

Research and theoretical formulations support the conclusion that one's physical health and, equally important, perceptions regarding one's current and future health, have a significant impact on the content of personal projects as well as the cognitive and affective appraisal of both health and nonhealth projects. It is also clear that there is convergent validity for a dual-process model of health beliefs, whereby both willful and automated health-related actions contribute to the perseverance of such beliefs. The emergent effects suggest that presumably static perceptual processes underlying the attention to health cues are in fact malleable, and might be influenced by simply altering one's construal of health projects from illness prevention to health promotion.

These findings foreshadow the potential utility of intervention tactics for nonnormative illness beliefs, which could occur at both the top-down and bottom-up levels. For example, perceptual interventions could involve the use of computerized tasks that foster habituation to illness-relevant stimuli through repeated exposure (see McKenna & Sharma, 1995). Habituation could result in making the individual less perceptually sensitive to detecting the stimulus, or it might reduce the negative affect associated with the perceptual experience (Cioffi, 1991). Project-based interventions would instead focus on the entire project system and how each project (health and nonhealth alike) sustains and interacts with all other projects (see Karoly, 1993), as well as how individuals subjectively appraise their health goals (e.g., reframing health projects as health promotion pursuits; see also Ewart, 1992, for a discussion of self-efficacy appraisals for the personal projects of patients). Recall that individuals who had experienced an illness concern induction were more likely to construe their health projects as illness prevention despite the fact that the surface content of the projects did not differ between the groups (e.g., goals like "exercise more," "lose weight," and "stay healthy" were cited equally by both groups). This highlights the fact that subjective appraisals, rather than real changes in project content, may underlie the motivational link to nonnormative illness beliefs (for a broader discussion of personal projects and treatment intervention see Karoly, 1999; Little, 1987). Importantly, the personal project approach provides an interpretation of illness beliefs that emphasizes normative and nonnormative life choices, rather than solely involving factors outside the individual's control (the latter view, when considered alone, is more consistent with a disease model).

Likewise, a personal project approach has a great deal to offer for the study of adaptation to the limitations and life disruption that are often imposed by cancer and other chronic or life-limiting illnesses. As we have demonstrated, the degree of disease- and treatment-related interference with project progress may be an excellent way to quantify illness impact. QOL measures are widely used in oncology clinical trials as a way to demonstrate that a treatment has a benefit to the patient. Inclusion of the GIS in an oncology clinical trial would be a logical next step if we elect to continue to think of it as a meaningful outcome measure. Is the measure sensitive enough to pick up differences between treatment arms? That is, does Treatment A or Treatment B result in higher scores (i.e. more interference) on the GIS?

There is a large literature on the relation of various cognitive appraisals of projects and types of projects to the experience of physical and psychological symptomatology. In our investigation, we plan to explore several related avenues. For example, we are coding the content areas of the goals (e.g., work, family, leisure) to explore whether cancer treatment creates greater interference in one dimension or another. We also consider which appraisal ratings might be included in our next project to more fully describe the project systems of people with cancer and the potential changes that might be important targets for interventions.

Finally, we are very excited about the possibility of designing an intervention to assist patients who are undergoing cancer treatment. Despite the myriad recent advances in symptom management, many people experience disease-related symptoms and treatment side effects that cannot be completely ameliorated. For example, bone pain is a common cancer symptom. Pain medication is often effective, but higher doses can result in an unacceptable level of sedation that makes it impossible to do anything but sleep. Many patients will learn to live with some pain just so that they can more fully participate in their lives. A PPA-based intervention could help such patients to identify their important projects, to consciously set realistic goals based on their pain level, and to titrate the medication such that the individual can explicitly make getting enough sleep a priority that she or he tries to meet every day. The therapist and participant could then monitor the balance between sleep and project progress. In addition, they can have an ongoing discussion about whether to try to shift strategies for pursuing a particular goal, shift the goals themselves, modify how much the patient is expecting from himself or herself, or alter the level of importance or meaning that he or she assigns to the goal. The next step will be a small, Phase-II-like trial of that type of intervention.

In conclusion, the PPA methodology is a flexible means of exploring people's perceptions of health and illness. It can guide interventions that are focused on modifying maladaptive beliefs (e.g., hypochondriasis; the Bryans of this world) or promoting adaptation to a changing physical condition (the Emilys of this world). We hope that this summary will motivate others to examine these exciting questions from the unique perspective of the personal projects that direct, reflect, and illuminate people's lives.

REFERENCES

Adler, A. (1927). *The practice and theory of individual psychology.* New York: Harcourt Brace.

Affleck, G., Tennen, H., Urrows, S., Higgins, P., Abeles, M., Hall, C., et al. (1998). Fibromyalgia and women's pursuit of personal goals: A daily process analysis. *Health Psychology, 17,* 40–47.

Bandura, A. (1988). Self-regulation of motivation and action through goal systems. In V. Hamilton, G. H. Bower, & N. H. Frijda (Eds.), *Cognitive perspectives on emotion and motivation* (pp. 37–61). Norwell, MA: Kluwer Academic.

Bargh, J. A. (1990). Auto-motives: Preconscious determinants of social interaction. In E. T. Higgins & R. M. Sorrentino (Eds.), *Handbook of motivation and cognition: Foundations of social behavior* (Vol. 2, pp. 93–130). New York: Guilford.

Bargh, J. A., & Chartrand, T. L. (1999). The unbearable automaticity of being. *American Psychologist, 54,* 462–479.

Barsky, A. J., Cleary, P. D., Sarnie, M. K., & Klerman, G. L. (1993). The course of transient hypochondriasis. *American Journal of Psychiatry, 140,* 273–283.

Cantor, N., & Zirkel, S. (1990). Personality, cognition, and purposive behavior. In L. A. Pervin (Ed.), *Handbook of personality: Theory and research* (pp. 115–164). New York: Guilford.

Carver, C. S., Pozo, C., Harris, S. D., Noriega, V., Scheier, M. F., Robinson, D. S., et al. (1993). How coping mediates the effect of optimism on distress: A study of women with early stage breast cancer. *Journal of Personality and Social Psychology, 65,* 375–390.

Carver, C. S., & Scheier, M. F. (1981). *Attention and self-regulation: A control theory approach to human behavior.* New York: Springer-Verlag.

Carver, C. S., & Scheier, M. F. (1998). *On the self-regulation of behavior.* New York: Cambridge University Press.

Cella, D. F., Tulsky, D. S., Gray, G., Sarafian, B., Lloyd, S., Linn, E., et al. (1993). The Functional Assessment of Cancer Therapy (FACT) scale: Development and validation of the general measure. *Journal of Clinical Oncology, 11,* 570–579.

Chen, E., Matthews, K., Salomon, K., & Ewart, C. K. (2002). Cardiovascular reactivity during social and nonsocial stressors: Do children's personal goals and expressive skills matter? *Health Psychology, 21,* 16–24.

Cioffi, D. (1991). Beyond attentional strategies: A cognitive-perceptual model of somatic interpretation. *Psychological Bulletin, 109,* 25–41.

Eckhardt, C. I., & Cohen, D. J. (1997). Attention to anger-relevant and irrelevant stimuli following naturalistic insult. *Personality and Individual Differences, 23,* 619–629.

Ellington, L., & Wiebe, D. J. (1999). Neuroticism, symptom presentation, and medical decision making. *Health Psychology, 18,* 634–643.

Elliot, A. J., & Sheldon, K. M. (1998). Avoidance personal goals and the personality–illness relationship. *Journal of Personality and Social Psychology, 75,* 1282–1299.

Emmons, R. A., & King, L. A. (1988). Conflict among personal strivings: Immediate and long-term implications for psychological and physical well-being. *Journal of Personality and Social Psychology, 54,* 1040–1048.

Ewart, C. K. (1992). Role of physical self-efficacy in recovery from a heart attack. In R. Schwarzer (Ed.), *Self-efficacy: Thought control of action* (pp. 287–304). Washington, DC: Hemisphere.

Feldman, P. J., Cohen, S., Doyle, W. J., Skoner, D. P., & Gwaltney, J. M., Jr. (1999). The impact of personality on the reporting of unfounded symptoms and illness. *Journal of Personality and Social Psychology, 77,* 370–378.

Ford, D. H. (1987). *Humans as self-constructing living systems: A developmental perspective on behavior and personality.* Hillsdale, NJ: Lawrence Erlbaum Associates.

Friedman, L. C., Nelson, D. V., Baer, P. E., Lane, M., Smith, F. E., & Dworkin, R. J. (1992). The relationship of dispositional optimism, daily life stress, and domestic environment to coping methods used by cancer patients. *Journal of Behavioral Medicine, 15,* 127–142.

Gray, J. A. (1987). *The psychology of fear and stress* (2nd ed.). New York: Cambridge University Press.

Jackson, T., Weiss, K. E., Lundquist, J. J., & Soderlind, A. (2002). Perceptions of goal-directed activities of optimists and pessimists: A personal projects analysis. *Journal of Psychology, 136,* 521–532.

Jemmot, J., Ditto, P., & Croyle, R. (1986). Judging health status: Effects of perceived relevance and personal relevance. *Journal of Personality and Social Psychology, 50,* 899–905.

Karoly, P. (1993). Mechanisms of self-regulation: A systems view. *Annual Review of Psychology, 44,* 23–52.

Karoly, P. (1999). A goal systems/self-regulatory perspective on personality, psychopathology, and change. *Review of General Psychology, 3,* 264–291.

Karoly, P., & Bay, C. (1990). Diabetes self-care goals and their relation to children's metabolic control. *Journal of Pediatric Psychology, 15,* 83–95.

Karoly, P., & Lecci, L. (1993). Hypochondriasis and somatization in college women: A personal projects analysis. *Health Psychology, 12,* 103–109.

Karoly, P., & Lecci, L. (1997). Motivational correlates of self-reported persistent pain in young adults. *The Clinical Journal of Pain, 13,* 104–109.

Kellner, R. A. (1986). *Somatization and hypochondriasis.* New York: Praeger.

Klinger, E., Barta, S. G., & Maxeiner, M. E. (1981). Current concerns: Assessing therapeutically relevant motivation. In P. C. Kendall & S. D. Hollon (Eds.), *Assessment strategies for cognitive behavioral interventions* (pp. 161–196). New York: Academic.

Kuhl, J. (1985). Volitional mediators of cognition–behavior consistency: Self-regulatory processes and action versus state orientation. In J. Kuhl & J. Beckmann (Eds.), *Action control: From cognition to behavior* (pp. 101–128). New York: Springer-Verlag.

Kuhl, J., & Helle, P. (1986). Motivational and volitional determinants of depression: The degenerated-intention hypothesis. *Journal of Abnormal Psychology, 95,* 247–251.

Lawton, M. P., Moss, M. S., Winter, L., & Hoffman, C. (2002). Motivation in later life: Personal projects and well-being. *Psychology and Aging, 17,* 539–547.

Lecci, L. (2004). An essential tool for the treatment and study of adult hypochondriasis [Review of the book *Hypochondriasis: Modern perspectives on an ancient malady*]. *Contemporary Psychology, 49,* 88–91.

Lecci, L., & Cohen, D. (2002). Perceptual consequences of an illness concern induction and its relation to hypochondriacal tendencies. *Health Psychology, 21,* 147–156.

Lecci, L., & Cohen, D. (2004). *Altered processing of health threat words as a function of hypochondriacal tendencies, perceived risk, and experimentally manipulated control beliefs.* Manuscript submitted for publication.

Lecci, L., Karoly, P., Ruehlman, L. S., & Lanyon, R. I. (1996). Goal-relevant dimensions of hypochondriacal tendencies and their relation to symptom manifestation and psychological distress. *Journal of Abnormal Psychology, 105,* 42–52.

Lecci, L., MacLean, M. G., & Croteau, N. (2002). Personal goals as predictors of college student drinking motives, alcohol use and related problems. *Journal of Studies on Alcohol, 63,* 620–630.

Leventhal, H. (1970). Findings and theory in the study of fear communications. In L. Berkowitz (Ed.), *Advances in experimental social psychology* (Vol. 5, pp. 119–186). New York: Academic.

Leventhal, H., Benyamini, Y., Brownlee, S., Diefenbach, M., Leventhal, E. A., Patrick-Miller, L., et al. (1997). Illness representations: Theoretical foundations. In K. J. Petrie & J. A. Weinman (Eds.), *Perceptions of health and illness: Current research and applications* (pp. 19–45). Amsterdam: Harwood.

Leventhal, H., Meyer, D., & Nerenz, D. (1980). The common sense representation of illness danger. In S. Rachman (Ed.), *Medical psychology* (Vol. 2, pp. 7–30). New York: Pergamon.

Leventhal, H., & Watts, J. C. (1966). Sources of resistance to fear-arousing communications on smoking and lung cancer. *Journal of Personality, 34,* 155–175.

Little, B. R. (1983). Personal projects: A rationale and method for investigation. *Environment and Behavior, 15,* 273–309.

Little, B. R. (1987). Personal projects analysis: A new methodology for counseling psychology. *Natcon, 13,* 591–614.

Little, B. R. (1988). *Personal projects analysis: Theory, method and research.* Ottawa, ON, Canada: Social Sciences and Humanities Research Council of Canada.

Little, B. R., (1989). Personal projects analysis: Trivial pursuits, magnificent obsessions and the search for coherence. In D. M. Buss & N. Cantor (Eds.), *Personality psychology: Recent trends and emerging directions* (pp. 15–31). New York: Springer-Verlag.

Little, B. R. (1993). Personal projects and the distributed self: Aspects of a conative psychology. In J. M. Suls (Ed.), *The self in social perspective: Psychological perspectives on the self* (Vol. 4, pp. 157–185). Hillsdale, NJ: Lawrence Erlbaum Associates.

Little, B. R. (1996). Free traits, personal projects and idio-tapes: Three tiers for personality psychology. *Psychological Inquiry, 7,* 340–344.

Little, B. R. (1998). Personal project pursuit: Dimensions and dynamics of personal meaning. In P. T. P. Wong & P. S. Fry (Eds.), *The human quest for meaning: A handbook of psychological research and clinical applications* (pp. 193–212). Mahwah, NJ: Lawrence Erlbaum Associates.

Little, B. R., & Chambers, N. C. (2004). Personal project pursuit: On human doings and well-beings. In W. M. Cox & E. Klinger (Eds.), *Handbook of motivational counseling: Concepts, approaches and assessment* (pp. 65–82). Chichester, UK: Wiley.

Mathews, A. M., & MacLeod, C. (1985). Selective processing of threat cues in anxiety states. *Behaviour Research and Therapy, 23,* 563–569.

McKenna, F. P., & Sharma, D. (1995). Intrusive cognitions: An investigation of the emotional Stroop task. *Journal of Experimental Psychology: Learning, Memory, and Cognition, 21,* 1595–1607.

Millar, M. G., & Millar, K. U. (1995). Negative affective consequences of thinking about disease detection behaviors. *Health Psychology, 14,* 1–6.

Ogilvie, D. M., & Rose, K. M. (1995). Self-with-other representations and a taxonomy of motives: Two approaches to studying persons. *Journal of Personality, 63,* 643–679.

Pennebaker, J. (1982). *The psychology of physical symptoms.* New York: Springer-Verlag.

Pervin, L. A. (Ed.). (1989). *Goal concepts in personality and social psychology.* Hillsdale, NJ: Lawrence Erlbaum Associates.

Peterman, A. H., Beaumont, J., & Rosenbloom S. (2004). Treatment-related goal interference mediates the relationship between symptoms and quality of life. *Psycho-Oncology, 13*(Suppl.), S219.

Peterman, A. H., Brady, M. J., & Cella, D. (2001). Goal Interference Scale: Evaluation of a new individualized health outcome measure. *Quality of Life Research, 10,* 197.

Peterman, A. H., Brady, M. J., Cella, D., & Chivington, K. (2003). Individualized QOL interventions: Maximizing adaptation to cancer-related goal interference. *Psycho-Oncology, 12,* S256.

Peterman, A. H., Brady, M. J., Hahn, E. A., & Merluzzi, T. (2000). Goal interference as a clinical outcome measure. *Psychosomatic Medicine, 62,* 113.

Pilowsky, I. (1978). A general classification of abnormal illness behaviors. *British Journal of Medical Psychology, 51,* 131–137.

Posner, M. I. (1988). Structures and functions of selective attention. In T. Boll & B. K. Bryant (Eds.), *Clinical neuropsychology and brain function* (pp. 171–202). Washington, DC: American Psychological Association.

Rapkin, B. D., Smith, M. Y., Dumont, K., Correa, A., Palmer, S., & Cohen, S. (1994). Development of the Idiographic Functional Status Assessment: A measure of the personal goals and goal attainment activities of people with AIDS. *Psychology and Health, 9,* 111–129.

Scheier, M., & Carver, C. (2001). Adapting to cancer: The importance of hope and purpose. In A. Baum & B.L. Andersen (Eds.), *Psychological interventions for cancer* (pp. 15–36). Washington, DC: American Psychological Association.

Schmidt, A. J. M., Wolfs-Takens, D. J., Oosterlaan, J., & van den Hout, M. A. (1994). Psychological mechanisms in hypochondriasis: Attention-induced physical symptoms without sensory stimulation. *Psychotherapy and Psychosomatics, 61,* 117–120.

Schwartz, C. E. (1999). Teaching coping skills enhances quality of life more than peer support: Results of a randomized trial with multiple sclerosis patients. *Health Psychology, 18,* 211–220.

Simon, H. A. (1994). The bottleneck of attention: Connecting thought with motivation. In W. D. Spaulding (Ed.), *Integrative views of motivation, cognition, and emotion* (Vol. 41, pp. 1–21). Lincoln: University of Nebraska Press.

Tedeschi, R. G., Park, C. L., & Calhoun, L. G. (Eds.). (1998). *Posttraumatic growth: Positive changes in the aftermath of crisis.* Mahwah, NJ: Lawrence Erlbaum Associates.

Trepanier, L., Lapierre, S., Baillargeon, J., & Bouffard, L. (2001). Tenacity and flexibility in the pursuit of personal projects: Impact on well-being during retirement. *Canadian Journal on Aging-Revue Canadienne Du Vieillissement, 20,* 557–576.

Watson, D., Clark, L. A., & Tellegen, A. (1988). Development and validation of brief measures of positive and negative affect: The PANAS scales. *Journal of Personality and Social Psychology, 54,* 1063–1070.

Watson, D., & Pennebaker, J. (1989). Health complaints, stress, and distress: Exploring the central role of negative affectivity. *Psychological Review, 96,* 234–254.

Weinstein, N. D. (1984). Why it won't happen to me: Perceptions of risk factors and susceptibility. *Health Psychology, 3,* 431–457.

Weinstein, N. D. (1987). Unrealistic optimism about susceptibility to health problems: Conclusions from a community-wide sample. *Journal of Behavioral Medicine, 10,* 481–500.

Wrosch, C., & Scheier, M. F. (2003). Personality and quality of life: The importance of optimism and goal adjustment. *Quality of Life Research, 12,* 59–72.

Wrosch, C., Scheier, M. F., Carver, C. S., & Schulz, R. (2003). The importance of goal disengagement in adaptive self-regulation: When giving up is beneficial. *Self and Identity, 2,* 1–20.

Wrosch, C., Scheier, M. F., Miller, G. E., Schulz, R., & Carver, C. S. (2003). Adaptive self-regulation of unattainable goals: Goal disengagement, goal reengagement, and subjective well-being. *Personality and Social Psychology Bulletin, 29,* 1494–1508.

13

Considering "The Optimality of Personality": Goals, Self-Concordance, and Multilevel Personality Integration

Kennon M. Sheldon

Consider somebody who really has it together. The different aspects of her personality seem to complement and harmonize with each other, she is well-liked by nearly everyone, and she is nearly always cheerful and happy. This does not mean that she is shallow—rather, she seems to have access to inner depths that sustain and nurture her. In addition, she is competent and efficient, and she is making excellent progress toward her life goals, with the prospects of an even better life ahead. How are we to understand this person, and to understand how to be more like her? Is it possible to quantify her "state of harmony," or to predict in advance her high level of functioning? This chapter focuses on these questions, and more generally, on positive personality integration and personal flourishing. What might it mean to say that a person has achieved optimality in personality?

THE SELF-CONCORDANCE CONSTRUCT

I approach these questions by focusing on my own self-concordance construct (Sheldon, 2002; Sheldon & Elliot, 1999; Sheldon & Houser-Marko, 2001). Self-concordance refers to the fit of personal goals with the striver's personality. The idea is that people have personality traits, needs, potentials, and talents that exist independently of their motivational lives. Our task, from this perspective, is to select self-appropriate strivings, projects, tasks, and goals that will allow us to express our traits and talents, to satisfy our needs and desires, and to maximize our potentials. However, self-knowledge is difficult (Wilson, 2002), and there are many factors that can cause us to misunderstand our own traits, needs, talents, and potentials, or to ignore them. Unfortunately, if we select the wrong goals or invest in the wrong projects we may waste much time and effort pursuing objectives that leave us no better off than we started. Of course, mistaken goals can sometimes be beneficial, as they may help people to learn necessary lessons, or go in unexpected but fortuitous directions. Still, the self-concordance model assumes that people are usually better off pursuing goals that fit their personalities, rather than goals that do not.

Considerable empirical data support this general assumption. For example, Sheldon and Elliot (1999) showed, in a semester-long study, that those who began the semester with self-concordant goal motivation were enabled to put sustained effort into the goals during the semester, rather than giving up as did many participants. As a result, self-concordant individuals better attained their goals. Goal attainment in turn predicted increased levels of global well-being from the beginning to the end of the semester. Finally, self-concordance interacted with attainment to influence well-being. That is, the more self-concordant the goals, the more attaining them produced enhanced well-being; in contrast, nonconcordant goals, even when attained, produced no new well-being. All of these effects were combined into a comprehensive longitudinal path model that fit the data well.

Next, Sheldon and Houser-Marko (2001) conducted a two-semester study to examine how the results of a first cycle of striving affected the subsequent cycle of striving. Replicating Sheldon and Elliot (1999), they showed that freshmen with self-concordant goals better attained their goals in their first semester of college, which led to enhanced well-being. Furthermore, Sheldon and Houser-Marko (2001) showed that first-semester attainment in turn led to increased self-concordance for the second semester's goals, which led to even higher levels of attainment in the second semester compared to the first, and finally, to even higher levels of well-being by the end of the year.

Did these positive changes last, or did high-performing freshmen eventually regress back to their 7starting points? Sheldon and Lyubomirsky (2004) recontacted these freshman during their senior year, and found that those who began their college career with self-concordant goals had succeeded in maintaining their first-year gains in well-being throughout college, and also had experienced outstanding academic and interpersonal success during that career. In short, the data suggest that starting a new situation with the right goals can have cascading positive effects for a person's life over time.

These and other findings (Sheldon & Elliot, 1998, 2000; Sheldon & Kasser, 1998, 2001) thus support the claim that self-concordance is a potentially important personality construct, with considerable dynamic influence on people's growth, achievement, and well-being. In the next section, I consider the conceptual background of the construct in greater detail. What does self-concordance really mean? Which aspects of personality is it most important for personal goals to fit or represent? Might some forms of self-concordance be less beneficial, or even harmful, for the individual? How is self-concordance to be measured? Are individuals able to assess their own self-concordance via self-report, or should implicit or peer-report measures of concordance be used instead?

THREE TIERS FOR PERSONALITY THEORY

To address these questions, we first need a structural framework for considering the relation of personal goals to the rest of personality (Little, 1996). A useful model was provided by McAdams (1995, 1996, 1998). The model proposes three levels or tiers of personality theory. Each represents an important area or branch of personality theory, branches that have traditionally been investigated in isolation from each other. However, McAdams argued that to thoroughly understand a person, we need independent information concerning his or her dispositional or habitual traits (Level I), his or her conscious goals and purposes (Level II), and his or her identities and self-stories (Level III).

Personality traits are stable dispositions to think, feel, and behave in certain ways. Trait constructs include the Big Five traits of extraversion, conscientiousness, neuroticism, agreeableness, and openness to experience; temperamentally based traits such as arousability and sociability; and many more specific traits, such as Machiavellianism, narcissism, self-consciousness, and self-monitoring. Goals and motives are the more or less conscious intentions that a person typically pursues. Goal constructs include people's personal projects, current concerns, and personal strivings; people's motivational styles and orientations (i.e., toward mastery, performance, or failure avoidance); and to some extent, people's behavioral skills and abilities. Identities and self-stories are the representations and beliefs that people have about themselves. They include the dominant self-characters that people live within, the unfolding stories and narratives that they tell about themselves, and the images of themselves in the future that help inform the selection of personal goals. Again, McAdams posited that traits, goals, and selves form three hierarchically adjacent tiers of organization within the personality system, which all need to be considered for complete understanding.

Concordance Between Goals and the Other Two Tiers

Now, let us return to the earlier question: What does it mean to be self-concordant so that one's personal goals correctly represent one's underlying personality? McAdams's three-tier system suggests two possible answers to this question: Self-concordance might involve consistency or coherence between (a) one's personal goals (at Level II) and one's selves and identities (at Level III), or (b) one's personal goals (at Level II) and one's personality traits and dispositions (at Level I).

What is the evidence that concordance of goals with each of the other levels of personality is conducive to well-being and positive outcomes? McGregor, McAdams, and Little (2004) showed that having personal goals that are concordant with one's personality traits is predictive of happiness. Similar results were reported by Diener and Fujita (1995) and Brunstein, Schultheiss, and Graessman (1998). At the self level of analysis, Sheldon and Emmons (1995) showed that having personal goals that are concordant with one's idiographic possible self-images provides personal benefits, as did Markus and Ruvolo (1989).

Is Level-Matching Always Beneficial? However, further reflection suggests that concordance between different levels of personality may not always be a beneficial state of affairs. What if the circumstances, contents, or conditions at a particular level are problematic for the individual? In such a case, he or she might be better off if there are inconsistencies between the other levels of personality and that level.

For example, consider a student in medical school, who is pursuing the goal of obtaining a surgical residency (Sheldon, 2004). This goal is dictated by a central image of himself in the future as a highly paid surgeon, and thus the goal is quite consistent with his sense of self. However, what if the goal conflicts with his personality traits? Suppose that he gets squeamish at the sight of blood, is discouraged by the lack of emotional contact that accompanies surgical activities, and is uncomfortable with the ego-centeredness of his surgically oriented peers. Suppose that he instead has a natural affinity for children, with an ability to make them laugh and to move toward health. Perhaps he should be pursuing the goal of obtaining a pediatric residency, rather than a surgical residency! Although a pediatrician goal would be inconsistent with the student's image of himself as a wealthy or famous surgeon, as is his father (at Level III), it would be consistent with his personality traits and dispositions (at Level I), and might perhaps be more personally beneficial in the long run.

As this example indicates, any two levels of personality could match each other, while simultaneously being inconsistent with the third level of personality. As McAdams (1996) suggested, it appears that all three levels of personality need to be considered together to derive a complete picture. McAdams's view also suggests that everything is fine as long as there is simultaneous matching among all three levels of personality.

However, further reflection suggests that even this may not always be true. What if a person has problems at all three levels of personality? Here, consistency between levels may still be disadvantageous. For example, suppose that the medical student's struggle to achieve the surgical residency and actualize the surgeon self-image creates much negative affect and anxiety, but he is also high in the Big Five trait of neuroticism. In fact, the distress evoked by the residency goal expresses and activates this trait. In one sense this might seem desirable, as the student has succeeded in selecting a goal that allows him to be true to his traits. Is this always a good thing? Maybe not—perhaps the trait of neuroticism should be contained, rather than expressed, for people to reach full maturity and happiness potential (McCrae et al., 2000). To further illustrate that perfect consistency among three levels of personality is not always beneficial, suppose that the student's trait of agreeableness is part of what led him to the surgical goal in the first place, as he has long been prone to unquestioningly accept his father's desires and demands for him. Once again, the three levels of the student's personality support each other, but still, he is not happy.

In sum, it appears that we must consider the content of a particular level of personality (i.e., the characteristics at that level, by which it differs from other personalities), before concluding that other levels of the personality should fit with and support that level. If the content of a particular level is problematic, then it may be more adaptive in the long run if the other levels are inconsistent with that level. Indeed, such inconsistency may provide a vital means of altering or changing that level. For example, by deciding to adopt the self-inconsistent goal of obtaining a pediatric residency, the medical student might succeed in modifying the problematic self-as-surgeon image, finally replacing it with the more trait-appropriate image of himself as a pediatrician.

On what basis should the medical student decide to change his goal; that is, how might he answer his father's objections, and also rule out the possibility that he is merely "copping out" on the surgeon goal, because the goal is more difficult than he first imagined? Are there any absolute criteria for telling which personality characteristics, and configurations of characteristics at different levels, are best overall—criteria that go beyond a person's traits, goals, and selves, but are influenced by them, and that in turn lead to positive performance and happiness outcomes for the individual?

Adding a Fourth Tier to McAdams's Hierarchy

The Need for a Foundational Tier. To address this question, let us return to McAdams's hierarchy. Notice that McAdams's three tiers focus only on aspects of personality that are thought to vary: people's differing traits, goals, and identities. However, might there be aspects of personality that are the same across people—fundamental processes or dynamics that exist for all persons alike? In other words, is there a prototypical or default human nature that characterizes all humans equally, on which individual differences rest? Many emerging data in evolutionary psychological perspective suggest that there is indeed a foundational human nature (Buss, 2001; Pinker, 2002); that is, a suite of specialized adaptations and social dispositions that is distinctive to human beings, as compared to beings of other species.

Thus, I suggest that we add a fourth level to McAdams's model, at the bottom of the hierarchy: the organismic foundations of personality.

Considering this level will give personality theory a way to achieve greater consilience (Wilson, 1998) with evolutionary and biological theory (see also Little, 1996). Also, by considering prototypical human needs and nature, we may gain a framework for understanding this chapter's primary question (i.e., the nature of optimal personality functioning) and the more general question of human flourishing addressed in this volume. To illustrate the potential value of this approach, consider that we would not expect to be able to understand a particular high-performing automobile without first understanding the functioning of a typical or generic automobile. Human personality may be the same way. Figure 13.1 illustrates the augmented McAdams hierarchy.

What types of invariant and foundational constructs should be located at the bottom tier of personality? There are a number of possibilities, including evolved social cognitive mechanisms (i.e., innate propensities for distinguishing between ingroup and outgroup members, for modeling others' states of mind, for detecting cheaters within social exchange relations, etc.), sociocultural universals (i.e., innate propensities to gossip, make music, form religions, or create art), and psychological needs (i.e., innate propensities to strive for and to enjoy certain experiences, such as those involving competence, connectedness, and self-esteem; see Sheldon, 2004, for further discussion of these different types of human universals).

Of the set just listed, I suggest that the psychological needs are the best construct to locate at the foundational level of personality (Sheldon, 2004). They are more directly personal than sociocognitive and sociocultural mechanisms, giving them powerful motivational and affective implications. Also, psychological needs may have important implications for individuals' personal flourishing and psychological well-being, depending on whether they are satisfied or not. Thus, they may offer absolute criteria for determining which personality character-

Self/Life -Story
+
Personality = Motives/Goals/Intentions
+
Traits/Individual Differences
+
Foundational Personality Processes

Figure 13.1.   Adding a fourth tier to McAdams's three tiers of personality.

istics, and configurations of characteristics, are ideal. Accordingly, I consider psychological needs in more detail here.

Psychological Needs as the Foundation of Personality. Psychological need constructs have a long history in psychology, beginning with Murray (1938) and continuing on through McClelland (McClelland, Atkinson, Clark, & Lowell, 1953), Maslow (1971), Jackson (Jackson & Guthrie, 1968), and Deci and Ryan (1985, 2000). Although some conceptions view needs as acquired individual differences in motivation that vary significantly between people, I suggest they are better defined as innate experiential requirements for thriving that are common to all persons. There are two reasons for this suggestion. First, if needs were found to vary significantly among people, then it would be hard to say that they are really needs, rather than mere preferences. If many people do not need it, is it really a need? Second, the experiential requirement definition can help us to understand the causes of human flourishing. Regardless of what a person is doing, if he or she is experiencing much need satisfaction, then presumably he or she is flourishing. To use an analogy, psychological needs can be viewed as "nutriments" that promote psychological growth and health, in the same way that satisfied needs for water, soil, and sunshine promote growth and health in plants (Ryan, 1995).

If we accept this definition, the next question becomes this: What are the basic, foundational, universal, or species-typical psychological needs that are common to everyone? Ultimately, this is an empirical question. For example, needs might be identified via the consistent relation of need satisfaction to many types of positive outcomes, in all persons, in all cultures (Baumeister & Leary, 1995). Indeed, this is exactly the approach taken by researchers in the self-determination theory (SDT) tradition. Deci and Ryan (1991, 2000) proposed that there are three basic psychological needs: for autonomy (the sense that one endorses and owns one's behavior), competence (the feeling that one is successfully completing tasks requiring skill and concentration), and relatedness (the feeling that one is close to, and contributing to, important others). There is now considerable research data supporting Deci and Ryan's proposal, data in which each of these three qualities of experience uniquely predicts a wide variety of performance and well-being outcomes (Filak & Sheldon, 2003; Reis, Sheldon, Gable, Roscoe, & Ryan, 2000; Sheldon, Ryan, & Reis, 1996) in a wide variety of cultures (Deci & Ryan, 2000).

But are autonomy, competence, and relatedness the complete set? Most SDT research has focused only on these three, without also considering the other possible needs that humans may have. To address this issue, Sheldon, Elliot, Kim, and Kasser (2001) tried to explain "what is satisfying about satisfying events." They evaluated 10 candidate psychological needs, derived from the prior psychological needs literature: autonomy, competence, relatedness, self-esteem, pleasure/stimulation, physical health, meaning/self-actualization, money/luxury, security/safety, and popularity/fame. In a series of studies, participants first described the most satisfying event that had occurred to them within the last month. They then rated the extent to which each of the 10 candidate needs was present during the event, as well as rating their positive mood during the event.

Across these studies, 4 of the 10 candidate needs consistently emerged as actual needs, by two different criteria: They manifested the highest mean levels within people's ratings of the satisfying event, as determined by within-subjects analyses of variance, and each uniquely predicted the positive mood associated with the event, as determined by simultaneous regression analyses. The four retained needs included SDT's proposed three (autonomy, competence, and relatedness), and also self-esteem. Sheldon et al. (2001) also showed that the same four needs emerged in a South Korean sample, supporting Deci and Ryan's claim that these are foundational aspects of personality that exist within every person within every culture.

Psychological Need Satisfaction as a Fourth Type of Matching. Notice that including psychological needs as a fourth, foundational tier within McAdams's hierarchy provides new ways of understanding which personality characteristics and configurations are optimal. Simply put, the optimal characteristics and configurations would be the ones that produced the greatest amount of psychological need satisfaction. To illustrate, let us return to the medical student. In pursuing the surgical residency goal (which is discordant with his traits but concordant with his dominant self-image), he experiences very little autonomy, and also less competence than he would like. He maintains relatedness with his father, but it is a low quality of relatedness, in which his own needs and nature are given insufficient consideration. His tendency toward neuroticism is given full expression, but this too fails to produce true need satisfaction. Meanwhile, his trait of relating well to and caring

for children is not being expressed. By these criteria, something is defi-
nitely amiss.

What if he switches to a pediatric residency goal? He will soon gain
much new autonomy and competence. It may come at the cost of relatedness with his father, but this may be mitigated in the longer term, as
he gains higher quality relatedness with his young patients and their
parents, and also gains the potential to transform his relationship with
his father. In addition, he gains the opportunity to express his more nurturing traits, and to keep his neuroticism in check.

In short, the quantity of psychological need satisfaction that an individual is experiencing in his or her life may provide an excellent criterion for evaluating the "optimality" of his or her personality. Indeed, the
degree of matching between the top three levels of personality and
foundational needs may turn out to be the most important form of
matching of all (compared to trait-to-goal, trait-to-self, and goal-to-self
matching). Where deficits of need satisfaction are found, one might
seek the causes by examining both the characteristics and the configurations of characteristics at the top three levels of that personality. Problematic elements might then be targeted for improvement or alteration.
Although personality change is difficult, it is also quite possible to bring
about, even at the genetically influenced trait level of analysis (McCrae
et al., 2000).

What if a person intentionally chooses discordant goals to achieve a
desired self-objective? For example, consider an introvert who chooses
the goal of running for political office, because her ideal self-image is of
a person who takes action to solve community problems. Although the
frequent social interactions required for attaining election are nonconcordant with her desire to avoid social stimulation, she chooses to pay
this cost to approach a highly valued future self. Is this a problem?
Maybe not. From the need-satisfaction perspective, the question is,
does this personality configuration produce satisfaction? By this criterion, domination of one level of personality by another level (here,
domination of traits by ideal self-images) may sometimes be very desirable. Of course, those who have ways of mitigating the costs of antitrait
activities would doubtless be better off than those who do not (see Little
& Joseph, chap. 14, this volume).

Two Higher Level Tiers Within Personality?   One further issue is
worthy of brief discussion here. Does personality stop at the level of the
self, or should we take account of the fact that personalities are always

nested within social relationships, and within the larger culture (Brandstätter & Lalonde, chap. 10, this volume; Little, 1999)? In other words, consistent with social interactionist and social ecological perspectives on personality, we might posit that there are two higher levels to personality, beyond the four tiers discussed so far: social relations and culture. Furthermore, one might extend the matching idea to these levels, to examine the concordance of a person's needs, traits, goals, and selves with the person's important personal relationships and with the dominant culture.

I believe that these upper two levels indeed supply independent and important information for determining the optimality of personality. Just as at the lower four levels, however, the desirability of consistency with the two higher levels would depend on the characteristics at those two levels. (Is the important relationship a negative and limiting one, as in the case of the medical student and his famous father? Is the cultural goal of achieving status and wealth an empty one, unworthy of pursuit?) Also, the ultimate criterion for determining optimality would remain the same: Do the characteristics and configurations produce psychological need satisfaction?

Before leaving this topic, it is important to point out that the quest for positive relations between self and others, and between self and culture, is not necessarily inconsistent with personal needs and happiness. In fact, such quests may actually be quite consistent with the psychological needs, in particular the need for relatedness. In other words, there is no necessary conflict between personal psychological need satisfaction and positive social and cultural relations. Indeed, psychological needs may be viewed as precisely the motivational systems that evolved to solve problems at every level of personality, including the social and cultural (Sheldon, 2004).

SELF-CONCORDANCE AND THE SIX TIERS
OF PERSONALITY

In this section I return to my own goal-based measure of self-concordance (Sheldon & Elliot, 1999; Sheldon & Houser-Marko, 2001), examining it in light of the preceding discussion. In fact, our typical measure of self-concordance does not directly address any of the five types of goal matching discussed already (i.e., goals-to-needs, goals-to-traits, goals-to-self, goals-to-social relations, or goals-to-culture). Instead, the measure employs SDT's concept of perceived locus of causality for behavior. The question is this: Do people feel that the causes of their own behavior are internal to the self, or do they feel that their behavior is caused by external, ego-alien factors (see Deci & Ryan, 1991, 2000, for further discussion)? Self-concordance is typically operationalized as the extent to which goals are pursued for intrinsic (for the enjoyment of it) and identified (because you believe in it) motivations, more so than for introjected (to avoid self-inflicted guilt) and external (to attain material rewards or to avoid social disapproval) motivations. According to SDT, these four motivations are located on a continuum of internalization ranging from high to low, with the former two being considered autonomous motivations, and the latter two being considered controlled motivations (Ryan & Connell, 1989). As can be seen, this measure defines the state of self-concordance in humanistic terms, as occurring when one feels much self-ownership and self-expression in one's behavior (Rogers, 1961).

Although my self-concordance measure does not directly assess the five types of goal matching described earlier, it may assess them indirectly. The aggregate self-concordance measure may itself be viewed as a measure of personal autonomy, one of the psychological needs specified by SDT (Deci & Ryan, 2000; Sheldon et al., 2001). Turning to the four subscales within the measure, intrinsic motivation seems relevant to the trait level of analysis, as intrinsic motivations are thought to reflect one's enduring interests and passions, dispositions that certainly vary across individuals. Identified motivation is relevant to the self level of analysis, as identified motivations are thought to reflect a person's conscious convictions and enduring self-images. Identified motivation is also relevant to the social interaction and cultural levels of analysis, as the ability to identify with a life goal requires considerable positive socialization and cultural support (Deci & Ryan, 1991). Introjected motivation may correspond to the personality trait of neuroticism, in which a person is chronically worried and anxious about what to do. External motivation does not seem to correspond directly to needs, traits, and selves. However, it may be representative of negative conditions at the social interaction or cultural levels of analysis, as external motivation is typically found in cases where optimal social and cultural supports for internalization are lacking (Deci & Ryan, 2000).

In short, by addressing (at least indirectly) the extent to which personal goals have positive relations with each of the other three levels of personality as well as with society and culture, and by also representing humanistic conceptions of optimal selfhood, Sheldon and colleagues' measurement approach may provide the best summary index of self-concordance to date.

Problems for Self-Report Measures of Self-Concordance?

Illusory Self-Concordance.   Still, a significant limitation of the measure may be the fact that it is based on self-report. Again, self-knowledge is uncertain (Wilson, 2002), and this may include the self-knowledge that is needed to report accurately on the consistency of one's goals with one's deeper personality. Notably, however, this may actually demonstrate an advantage to the measurement approach based in SDT. Rather than trying to directly address deep consistency, the measure instead approaches consistency indirectly, by focusing on interests, identifications, and the presence of guilt or extrinsic motivation within the person's goal system. I believe that these issues are relatively easy to report on (compared to reporting directly on goal-to-need, goal-to-trait, or goal-to-relationship matching), and also, that reporting on them is not especially fraught with social desirability. Many people have ambivalent relationships with their goals, and are thus readily willing to admit that they do not enjoy them, that they do not really believe in them, or that they feel some pressure in doing them. Thus, my self-concordance measure may correspond to actual self-concordance (i.e., the overall degree of matching between the various levels of personality) in most cases.

Still, it may be illuminating to consider the circumstances in which self-reported self-concordance is not correct; that is, cases when a person is self-deceived, and evidences illusory self-concordance. What is illusory self-concordance, according to this measure? It is the state of believing that one is not motivated by external forces and internal guilt, when one is; and also, believing that one is motivated by interest and identification, when one is not. It is to have false beliefs about the motivational sources of one's own behavior, beliefs that most other people who know one well would agree are inaccurate or biased.

Might Illusory Self-Concordance Sometimes Be Beneficial?   Motivations and one's construals of them are, of course, somewhat subjective. Indeed, to a considerable extent, people's relationships with their own goals and intentions are a matter of personal declaration (Sartre, 1965). Thus, this question arises: What if illusions of identification or incorrect beliefs that one is not externally motivated are actually positive things? Indeed, according to SDT, taking possession of one's motivations, and overcoming the feeling of being externally controlled by them, is an extremely important personality developmental process (Deci & Ryan, 2000). To illustrate the process, consider a young student who only does his schoolwork because he "has" to. However, when he is older and more mature he does it willingly, even when it is not enjoyable, because it is consistent with his self-endorsed values and goals. According to SDT he has fully internalized these motivations to his own benefit. Again, however, might some cases of internalization be problematic, because the person is actually self-deceived about the self-appropriateness of the goals he or she is pursuing?

Let us return to the medical student who has assumed, for as long as he can remember, that he will walk in his father's footsteps. When surveyed about the goal of becoming a surgeon, the student reports enjoying and identifying with the process of pursuing it, and also reports little external or introjected motivation. That is, the goal appears self-concordant, by self-report. However, those who know the student wonder about the goal's true appropriateness for him—again, he has a somewhat fastidious nature, and becomes squeamish at the sight of blood. His father is assertive and controlling, and his siblings think he secretly fears he will lose his father's love and respect if he does not follow in the father's footsteps. As noted, the student also has a natural gift for relating with children, and perhaps would be better suited to become a pediatrician. Perhaps his seeming self-concordance for the surgeon goal is a case of illusory self-concordance.

Distinguishing Between Two Types of Illusory Self-Concordance. This discussion suggests that there are at least two ways in which reports of high self-concordance may be wrong. The first way is when the exaggerated reports reflect the operation of a positive internalization process or process of "standing behind" one's motives. Here, the person is commendably taking existential responsibility for his goals, enhancing his own personal power. He is also actively creating consistency between the goal and self levels of analysis, or between Levels III and IV in the revised McAdams hierarchy. This type of illusory self-concordance may not be ideal, but it doubtless has benefits. The second way is when the exaggerated reports reflect denial, foreclosure, or a failure to recognize the unquestioned but maladaptive edicts that actually rule one's behavior. This type of illusory self-concordance may be symptomatic of real problems in the personality system. How can we tell the difference between these two states of affairs in which inflated goal self-concordance is either authentic or inauthentic?

I suggest that the best way to distinguish these is by considering the consistency of the goals with other levels of personality. In the case of the medical student, the surgeon goal clearly does not fit his personality traits and dispositions (except the trait of neuroticism, which we decided earlier should be restrained, not given full expression). Also, it does not seem to fit his psychological needs; as he pursues the surgical residency he feels a sense of pressure, tension, and anxiety (lack of autonomy), a sense of failing to perform surgically relevant tasks well (lack of competence), and a sense of failing to connect with his anesthetized patients (lack of relatedness). Based on this analysis, the counseling recommendation would be clear: Change your goal.

However, what if we consider the two proposed highest levels of analysis, of social and cultural relations? Again, the surgeon goal is consistent with the desires and expectations of his father, and with U.S. culture's emphasis on status and material success. Again, however, content matters; perhaps this personal relationship and this aspect of U.S. culture are themselves problematic, and thus, perhaps it is better if the other levels of personality do not concord with them. In the end, the counseling recommendation might remain the same: Change your goal.

Implicit Attitudinal Measures. Another potential route for measuring "true" self-concordance might be via indirect assessment methodologies, such as projective tests or the Implicit Attitude Test (IAT; Greenwald, Nosek, & Banaji, 2003). The IAT in particular has potential as a means of measuring a person's deeper feelings about his or her goals. The IAT asks participants to respond to various attitude or category objects, paired with either positive words or negative words. If a participant's responses are slowed down when the category is paired with positive words and speeded up when the category is paired with negative words, the participant is said to have a negative implicit attitude toward the category, regardless of how he or she says he or she feels about it. The IAT has been used to study many affectively charged issues, such as racism, sexism, and ageism because it provides a "pipeline," in principle, to the person's true feelings on the matter. Presumably, one could also assess people's true feelings regarding their goals in this way.

The potential advantage of using the IAT to access true self-concordance is that it may reveal instances when a person's goals are not aligned with his or her needs and traits (Levels I & II of his or her personality), even though the conscious self (at Level IV of his or her personality) is very aligned with the goals. Presumably, implicit negative attitudes toward goals are more likely to result when the self-avowed goals are nonconcordant with needs and traits. Because the goals lead a person to perform behaviors that are incongruent with his or her traits and dispositions and that do not produce psychological need satisfaction, the deep emotional assessment of them is less positive than his or her conscious assessment of them (see the construct of free traits discussed by Little & Joseph, chap. 14, this volume). Future research will be required to explore these interesting possibilities.

CONCLUSION

To summarize, we have been casting for ways to assess the optimality of personality based on the concept of self-concordance; that is, the degree of fit between personal goals and the other aspects of personality. To address these questions, we postulated that personality has at least four levels or tiers (needs, traits, goals, and selves), and perhaps two higher tiers as well (social relationships and culture). From this perspective, goal self-concordance might involve matching between personal goals and any of the other five levels of personality. However, we concluded that matching between personal goals and psychological needs may provide the most reliable criteria for establishing optimality because psychological needs are invariant features of human nature, the satisfaction of which (in theory) automatically promotes personal thriving (Deci & Ryan, 2000). As long as need satisfaction is occurring, mismatches between the other levels may be nonproblematic. Indeed, such mismatches may be the very means by which particular personality characteristics are altered, so that the person approaches even greater satisfaction in the future.

We also discussed Sheldon and colleagues' humanistically oriented measure of self-concordance, which is based on SDT's concept of internal versus external perceived locus of causality for behavior. We concluded that this measure indirectly assesses good fit between goals and the other levels of personality, and is also relatively straightforward to report on. Thus, it may provide the best measure of self-concordance to date. However, to pinpoint cases in which participants are maladaptively self-deceived regarding their true motivations for their goals, it may be necessary to directly consider the consistency of the goals with the other levels of personality, and in particular, the psychological needs. It may also be useful to measure people's implicit affective attitude regarding goals as a pipeline to the person's true feelings regarding his or her goals. Such research remains to be conducted.

What is the optimal personality, according to this suite of conceptual and measurement approaches? Simply a person who is self-concordant by self-report, and who also shows concordance between the goals and the other levels of his or her personality, as assessed both by self-report and by peer report. Also, it is a person who manifests positive implicit attitudes toward his or her goals, as well as positive explicit ones. It is a person whose goals provide many need-satisfying experiences along the way. To return one last time to the self-deceived medical student (who thinks he wants to be a surgeon, but really does not), if he allows himself to begin exploring the possibility of becoming a pediatrician instead, and begins experiencing much new autonomy, competence, and relatedness as a result, and if he lets these feelings be his guide, then he may be able to revise his inaccurate self-image and find a truly fulfilling career. He may thus become maximally self-concordant, as defined both in SDT's humanistic terms, and in terms of creating an optimal configuration among the different levels of his personality.

REFERENCES

Baumeister, R. F., & Leary, M. R. (1995). The need to belong: Desire for interpersonal attachments as a fundamental human motivation. *Psychological Bulletin, 117,* 497–529.

Brunstein, J. C., Schultheiss, O. C., & Grässman, R. (1998). Personal goals and emotional well-being: The moderating role of motive dispositions. *Journal of Personality and Social Psychology, 75,* 494–508.

Buss, D. M. (2001). Human nature and culture: An evolutionary psychological perspective. *Journal of Personality, 69,* 955–978.

Deci, E. L., & Ryan, R. M. (1985). *Intrinsic motivation and self-determination in human behavior.* New York: Plenum.

Deci, E. L., & Ryan, R. M. (1991). A motivational approach to self: Integration in personality. In R. Dienstbier (Ed.), *Nebraska symposium on motivation: Vol. 38. Perspectives on motivation* (pp. 237–288). Lincoln: University of Nebraska Press.

Deci, E. L., & Ryan, R. M. (2000). The "what" and "why" of goal pursuits: Human needs and the self-determination of behavior. *Psychological Inquiry, 11,* 227–268.

Diener, E., & Fujita, F. (1995). Resources, personal strivings, and subjective well-being: A nomothetic and idiographic approach. *Journal of Personality and Social Psychology, 68,* 926–935.

Filak, V., & Sheldon, K. M. (2003). Student psychological need-satisfaction and college teacher-course evaluations. *Educational Psychology, 23,* 235–247.

Greenwald, A. G., Nosek, B. A., & Banaji, M. R. (2003). Understanding and using the Implicit Association Test: I. An improved scoring algorithm. *Journal of Personality and Social Psychology, 85,* 197–216.

Jackson, D. N., & Guthrie, G. M. (1968). Multitrait–multimethod evaluation of the personality research form. *Proceedings of the Annual Convention of the American Psychological Association, 3,* 177–178.

Little, B. R. (1996). Free traits, personal projects and idio-tapes: Three tiers for personality psychology. *Psychological Inquiry, 7,* 340–344.

Little, B. R. (1999). Personal projects and social ecology: Themes and variation across the life span. In J. Brandtstdäter & R. M. Lerner (Eds.), *Action and self-development: Theory and research through the life span* (pp. 197–221). Thousand Oaks, CA: Sage.

Markus, H., & Ruvolo, A. (1989). Possible selves: Personalized representations of goals. In L. A. Pervin (Ed.), *Goal concepts in personality and social psychology* (pp. 211–241). Hillsdale, NJ: Lawrence Erlbaum Associates.

Maslow, A. (1971). *The farther reaches of human nature.* New York: Viking.

McAdams, D. P. (1995). What do we know when we know a person? *Journal of Personality, 63,* 365–396.

McAdams, D. P. (1996). Personality, modernity, and the storied self: A contemporary framework for studying persons. *Psychological Inquiry, 7,* 295–321.

McAdams, D. P. (1998). Ego, trait, identity. In P. M. Westenberg & A. Blasi (Eds.), *Personality development: Theoretical, empirical, and clinical investigations of Loevinger's conception of ego development* (pp. 27–38). Mahwah, NJ: Lawrence Erlbaum Associates.

McClelland, D., Atkinson, J., Clark, R., & Lowell, E. (1953). *The achievement motive.* New York: Appleton-Century-Crofts.

McCrae, R. R., Costa, P. T., Jr., Ostendorf, F., Angleitner, A., Hrebickova, M., Avia, M. D., et al. (2000). Nature over nurture: Temperament, personality, and life span development. *Journal of Personality and Social Psychology, 78,* 173–186.

McGregor, I., McAdams, D. P., & Little, B. R. (2004). *Personal projects, life-stories, and well-being: The benefits of acting and being true to one's traits.* Unpublished manuscript.

Murray, H. (1938). *Explorations in personality.* New York: Oxford University Press.

Pinker, S. (2002). *The blank slate: The modern denial of human nature.* New York: Viking.

Reis, H. T., Sheldon, K. M., Gable, S. L., Roscoe, R., & Ryan, R. (2000). Daily well being: The role of autonomy, competence, and relatedness. *Personality and Social Psychology Bulletin, 26,* 419–435.

Rogers, C. (1961). *On becoming a person: A therapist's view of psychotherapy.* Boston: Houghton-Mifflin.

Ryan, R. M. (1995). Psychological needs and the facilitation of integrative processes. *Journal of Personality, 63,* 397–427.

Ryan, R. M., & Connell, J. P. (1989). Perceived locus of causality and internalization: Examining reasons for acting in two domains. *Journal of Personality and Social Psychology, 57,* 749–761.

Sartre, J. P. (1965). *Being and nothingness: An essay in phenomenological ontology* (H. E. Barnes, Trans.). New York: Citadel.

Sheldon, K. M. (2002). The self-concordance model of healthy goal-striving: When personal goals correctly represent the person. In E. L. Deci & R. M. Ryan (Eds.), *Handbook of self-determination research* (pp. 65–86). Rochester, NY: University of Rochester Press.

Sheldon, K. M. (2004). *Optimal human being: Towards integration within the person and between the human sciences.* Mahwah, NJ: Lawrence Erlbaum Associates.

Sheldon, K. M., & Elliot, A. J. (1998). Not all personal goals are personal: Comparing autonomous and controlled reasons for goals as predictors of effort and attainment. *Personality and Social Psychology Bulletin, 24,* 546–557.

Sheldon, K. M., & Elliot, A. J. (1999). Goal striving, need satisfaction, and longitudinal well-being: The self-concordance model. *Journal of Personality and Social Psychology, 76,* 482–497.

Sheldon, K. M., & Elliot, A. J. (2000). Personal goals in social roles: Divergences and convergences across roles and levels of analysis. *Journal of Personality, 68,* 51–84.

Sheldon, K. M., Elliot, A. J., Kim, Y., & Kasser, T. (2001). What's satisfying about satisfying events? Comparing ten candidate psychological needs. *Journal of Personality and Social Psychology, 80,* 325–339.

Sheldon, K. M., & Emmons, R. A. (1995). Comparing differentiation and integration within personal goal systems. *Personality and Individual Differences, 18,* 39–46.

Sheldon, K. M., & Houser-Marko, L. (2001). Self-concordance, goal attainment, and the pursuit of happiness: Can there be an upward spiral? *Journal of Personality and Social Psychology, 80,* 152–165.

Sheldon, K. M., & Kasser, T. (1998). Pursuing personal goals: Skills enable progress, but not all progress is beneficial. *Personality and Social Psychology Bulletin, 24,* 1319–1331.

Sheldon, K. M., & Kasser, T. (2001). Getting older, getting better? Personal strivings and psychological maturity across the life span. *Developmental Psychology, 37,* 491–501.

Sheldon, K. M., & Lyubomirsky, S. (2004). *Achieving sustainable happiness: Change your actions, not your circumstances.* Unpublished manuscript.

Sheldon, K. M., Ryan, R., & Reis, H. T. (1996). What makes for a good day? Competence and autonomy in the day and in the person. *Personality and Social Psychology Bulletin, 22,* 1270–1279.

Wilson, E. O. (1998). *Consilience: The unity of knowledge.* New York: Knopf.

Wilson, T. D. (2002). *Strangers to ourselves: Discovering the adaptive unconscious.* Cambridge, MA: Belknap Press/Harvard University Press.

14

Personal Projects and Free Traits: Mutable Selves and Well Beings

Brian R. Little and Maryann F. Joseph

M arkus is a strange man. People see him as a bon vivant, a thrill seeker and an irrepressible extravert. He even sees himself that way, on occasion. But there are aspects of his daily behavior that puzzle him and those who know him well. He can be seen, more often than he may suspect, escaping the spotlight, seeking solitude, acting like a bona fide introvert.

Deborah is a scary woman. People describe her as tough, acerbic, and disagreeable to a fault. She agrees she is disagreeable and takes pride in this depiction of herself. But there have been times when she, too, has been caught in conduct that seems to contradict her reputation—acts of kindness and moments of tenderness that seem totally out of character.

Such inconsistency is not rare, nor is it especially noteworthy, particularly to those subscribing to the received view of traditional social psychology. Until recently (e.g., Robins, Norem, & Cheek, 1999), the essentially mutable nature of selves has been taken as a given. Sometimes Markus is monkish; sometimes Mark is maniacal. Deborah is a demon in staff meetings; at home with her family, Debbie is a delight. Both individuals act in accordance with the situations that impinge on them or that they elicit in their daily lives. These forces shape mutable selves to meet contextual requirements.

We accept this view, within limits. However, we propose that it is precisely in the interplay between enduring structures and dynamic processes, between inner processes and external contexts, that some of the most distinctive and intriguing features of being human are revealed (Little, 2005; Little & Chambers, 2004). In this chapter we propose a new theoretical framework for understanding some of the chimerical aspects of complex people and the apparently disingenuous features of people's lives. We explore the probable gains and possible costs that acting out of character might impose. In doing so, we touch on matters that deal with three potentially conflicting forms of fidelity: fidelity to one's biological propensities, to one's cultural prescriptions, and to one's core personal projects. Each of these is natural in its own compelling way and their choreography has important implications for human health and flourishing.

THREE WAYS OF BEING ONESELF: FIRST, SECOND, AND THIRD NATURES

Our everyday conduct can be seen as expressions of three different human natures. What we call *first nature* is *biogenic*: Its roots are genetic and its influence is primarily conveyed through neurophysiological and related mechanisms. It comprises the distinctive propensities that a Markus or a Deborah brings into the delivery room at birth. Although first natures involve both stable and dynamic features, we restrict our analysis here to relatively fixed traits, with a particular focus on extraversion and to a lesser extent on agreeableness. Fixed traits are difficult, but not impossible, to change, and they propel, guide, and constrain the developmental course of human lives.

Second nature is *sociogenic*: It arises in the course of socialization and exerts its influence through the rules and roles that govern how we think, feel, and act. Second natures, in a sense, predate our arrival into the world and influence conduct from the microlevel norms of dyadic interaction to the macrolevel functions of collective identity and cultural myths. They also propel, guide, and constrain personality across the life span.

Second nature influences may or may not be in conflict with one's first nature. A biogenic propensity to be audaciously idiosyncratic, casting oneself fearlessly into the daily fray, may conflict with a cultural prescription to blend in quietly or a maternal admonishment to grow up and stop embarrassing the whole family. In contrast, if that same biogenic propensity is lodged in a person raised in a family with a "Go for It!" sign over the fireplace, the result is less likely to be censure and conflict than frequent family high-fives.

The distinction between first and second nature may seem to be simply a restatement of the traditional distinction between nature and nurture, but we mean something quite different. There are several ways of dealing with the perdurable nature–nurture issue. One is to opt for an extreme view on either side of the nature–nurture divide. Another is to argue that the distinction should be abolished and that we should adopt only holistic models that avoid arbitrarily separating and contrasting genetics and environments. We take a rather different view. Instead of abandoning the concept of acting naturally, we wish to expand its conceptual range so that we have more nuanced ways of dealing with what is natural about individuals. To accomplish this, we need to take a further step and propose that humans have third natures (Little, 2000b).

Third nature is *idiogenic*: Its origin is personal, idiosyncratic, and singular. Third natures shape lives through the individual's pursuit of personal projects (Little, 1983, 1999b). To advance these projects people may sometimes adopt *free traits*, which we define as "culturally scripted patterns of conduct carried out as part of a person's goals, projects, and commitments, independent of that person's 'natural' inclinations" (Little, 2000a, pp. 92–93). Free traits may be strategically invoked in daily action, especially in pursuit of the core projects of our lives. Like the other two natures, third natures propel, guide, and constrain personality across the life span, but they also open up paths for human flourishing that are not afforded by genetic or cultural endowments. We propose that third natures are a distinctively, if not uniquely, human way of being and whether they are pursued effectively is critical for whether individuals and societies flounder or flourish (Little, 1996).

Unlike perspectives emphasizing the contrast between nature and nurture or genes and environment, we submit that both genetic and contextual features are active elements of all three natures. Before, during, and after birth, environmental factors influence genetic expression (e.g., Coll, Bearer, & Lerner, 2005; Gottlieb, 1991, 1998) and hence partially shape our first natures. Social and cultural influences emerged in the course of evolutionary development and were shaped through selection factors arising from our species' need to live in groups (e.g., Hogan, Jones, & Cheek, 1985). The pursuit of personal projects involves the orchestration of genetic, cultural, and personal forces that impinge on us daily. To adopt another metaphor, one we return to in our concluding comments, personal projects are actions that comprise the "developmental dance between biological process and social context" (Rende, 2004, p. 109).

Thus Mark, despite his own biological dispositions and his upbringing, may commit himself to projects that require him to act in a highly extraverted, outgoing fashion. In short, Mark needs to be, at times, what we call a pseudo-extravert to advance his core projects (Little, 1996). Such seemingly disingenuous action may be engaged in because of fleeting situational pressures or roles that he tries on every now and then. However, particularly if they are associated with an enduring core personal project, they may become essentially stable free traits—his pseudo-extraversion may be his most defining characteristic, the singular mark of Mark. His third nature project pursuits may feel as natural to him as responding to first nature biogenic needs or embracing second nature cultural norms, particularly if practiced readily and if they confer advantages to the projects about which he cares deeply. Yet they may still conflict with either or both of his first and second natures. Markus might well be paying a price for his conduct.

Deborah, too, may have a set of core projects that arise from her deep commitment to succeed in a senior management position. When she grew up in the 1960s, her mother encouraged and admonished her to set no limits to her career success. There was no conflict there. Today, however, at home with those she loves, the hard-nosed, hard-driving Deborah sometimes compromises her first nature propensities. Particularly after protracted periods of nurturing her family she needs to escape. She heads to the gym, puts on her boxing gloves, and steps into the ring. In that setting her reputation precedes her: Do not mess with Deb.

Acting Out of Character: Toward a Free Trait Agreement

Another way of putting this is to say that individuals may occasionally act out of character (Little, 1996, 1999a, 2000a). The polysemous nature of the phrase is intentional. In one sense of the phrase, to act out of character means to act against what others, and the actor, might see as typical. However, acting out of character also means acting in accordance with one's character—the term here referring to one's core beliefs or most vital projects. For a biogenic introvert to act in an extraverted way is to act out of character, in at least one sense of the phrase, and perhaps in both. Similarly when first nature agreeable people act in a decidedly unpleasant fashion it may be to advance a core project that matters deeply to them; perhaps to rectify an egregious wrong: a question, in short, of character. To understand these mutable selves and the natures underlying them we need to conjoin several different perspectives and research literatures in personality, social, and health psychology, which we selectively invoke later.

In so doing, we also find that we cross the boundary into the philosophical domain, particularly to key questions in moral and ethical philosophy. We need to confront issues concerning the claim that projects have in our lives and those of others, particularly when the internal and external constraints of our social ecology are impelling us or admonishing us to act in ways that subvert those projects.[1] As personality or developmental scientists, we have no particular warrant or training to adjudicate these issues. However, we do have the responsibility to provide evidence that could make such adjudications more sophisticated, more realistic, and more humane (Flanagan, 1991). In essence we are pointing the way toward a greater awareness of how and why individuals act out of character and the costs and advantages that this might incur both for the individuals and the environments in which they pursue their core projects. We make the case that what is needed at home, at work, and in our communities is reconciliation between individuals and within individuals whose multiple natures can make life complex and taxing. In short, we call for a free trait agreement.

A SOCIAL ECOLOGICAL THEORY OF FREE TRAITS: ASSUMPTIONS AND PROPOSITIONS

Little (2000a) presented some preliminary notes toward formalization of the foregoing theoretical concepts. We wish to modify and expand that model and then report empirical explorations of predictions derived from it. Essentially the model we discuss here is based on three assumptions and three propositions that comprise a free trait theory for personality and developmental science. As in the earlier publication, we focus on the domain of extraversion. Later, we address issues of generalizing to other traits.

Free trait theory comprises three assumptions and three explicit and testable propositions, two of which concern us in this chapter. We take

---

[1]See, in particular, Flanagan (1991), Lomasky (1984, 1987), and Williams (1981).

the assumptions to be generally uncontroversial, although the particular terminology used in formulating them is rather unconventional. These assumptions are as follows:

1. Individuals differ reliably in their biogenic disposition to extraversion.[2] These biogenic individual differences are conventionally referred to as *genotypic extraversion* and can be regarded as a core aspect of first natures (Little, 1996).

2. Individuals differ in the extent to which their typical observable behavior is regarded as extraverted. This is their *phenotypic extraversion*. It may derive directly from genotypic propensities or may represent cultural norms learned sufficiently well to have become second nature to them. Such conduct may also be required for the enactment of third nature personal projects. In short, phenotypic extraversion may be the result of first, second, or third natures.

3. Genotypic and phenotypic extraversion are partially independent, therefore in a given population some individuals exhibit a discrepancy or discordance between their genotypic and phenotypic extraversion. Although we view these as varying on a continuum, for expository purposes we refer to those for whom there is a notable discrepancy as *pseudo-extraverts* and *pseudo-introverts* or as engaging in *pseudo-extraverted* or *pseudo-introverted* behavior.

To these three assumptions we add three specific propositions that can be tested empirically:

4. Protractedly acting out of character (e.g., as a pseudo-extravert or pseudo-introvert) induces strain that can exact costs in emotional and physical well-being. The greater and more extended the discordance with biogenic first natures, the greater will be the strain. Costs will involve psychological discomfort at first; eventually they may result in stress, burnout, and finally compromised health and physical well-being.

5. The costs of acting out of character can be mitigated by the availability of *restorative niches* in which individuals have a chance to express or nurture their first natures.

---

[2]This may be due to differences in reactivity to neocortical stimulation, differences in dopamine levels, or several other plausible neurophysiological mechanisms (e.g., Eysenck, 1967; Eysenck & Eysenck, 1985; Stelmack, 1981; Zuckerman, 1987, 1991).

6. Environments differ in the extent that they afford niches where first natures can be enacted and restored and, to the extent they do, those environments will themselves be sustainable.[3]

In the following sections we (a) provide a more detailed and expanded treatment of the three assumptions underlying free trait theory by examining the biogenic, sociogenic, and idiogenic forms of extraverted conduct; (b) selectively review research that indirectly supports our two empirical propositions: that free traited behavior may exact costs and that various forms of restoration may mitigate these costs; (c) review empirical research directly based on the social ecological model of free traits; and (d) conclude with a research agenda that has both theoretical and applied implications for how we can understand and enhance human flourishing.

ELABORATING THE ASSUMPTIONS: BIOGENIC, SOCIOGENIC, AND IDIOGENIC EXTRAVERSION

Biogenic Extraversion: Arousal Explanations and Alternatives

There is some consensus in the personality literature that each of the Big Five traits of openness, conscientiousness, extraversion, agreeableness, and neuroticism may have a genetic base (e.g., Jang, McCrae, Angleitner, Riemann, & Livesley, 1998; Loehlin, McCrae, Costa, & John, 1998). Some quantitative behavioral genetics research estimates that 50% of the variance of traits such as extraversion are attributable to heredity. It is important to point out that this is based on population estimates and that such estimates are not applicable to the individual case. Although there is mounting evidence of polygenetic influences on personality, there is also considerable variability in the quantitative estimates of such influences. Estimates are influenced by the nature of the measures of personality (e.g., ratings of self vs. others), the age and gender of the population being studied, and contextual factors that may be present during assessment (Grigorenko, 2002).

Extraversion is one of the most extensively researched traits of the Big Five, and is routinely recovered as a major factor in studies of per-

---

[3]The sustainability would arise from such environmental settings being more likely to retain a critical mass of individuals who are themselves sustained by the environment (Little & Ryan, 1979). Proposition 3 goes beyond the direct scope of this chapter as it deals with aspects of the contexts within which projects are pursued. This theme is addressed, however, in the final chapter of this volume.

sonality in different cultures (e.g., McCrae & Costa, 1997). Plausible physiological mechanisms underlying extraversion have been identified, including low levels of neocortical arousal (Eysenck, 1967), relatively strong behvioral activation system activity (Gray, 1981), and differential activation of dopaminergic pathways (Zuckerman, 1991).

One of the earliest and most influential models was that of Eysenck (1967), who argued that differences in extraversion were related to neocortical arousal, with extraverts being chronically underaroused and introverts overaroused. Drawing on the classic Yerkes–Dodson (1908) and Hebb (1955) models of an optimal level of arousal, extraverts were posited as seeking out stimulation and introverts trying to avoid or reduce it. Although early evidence was largely consistent with this proposition, more recent evidence suggests that it is not that extraverts have low base levels of arousal, but rather, in the context of everyday levels of moderate environmental arousal, extraverts require more stimulation for optimal functioning, and introverts require less. Additionally, extraverts are less responsive to changes in environmental stimulation, whereas introverts are more so (e.g., De Pascalis, 2004; Geen, 1984).

Research continues to grow rapidly in this area; however, we take it that one relatively uncontroversial assumption about extraverts is that they seek out stimulation, and enjoy and benefit from arousing interactions with others. They also likely benefit from ingesting stimulants that activate various area of the neocortex. In contrast, introverts are more likely to avoid stimulation and arousing interactions, not necessarily because they do not value or enjoy them, but because their performance may be compromised by having their level of neocortical arousal rise over the optimal level. In short, if Mark is a first nature introvert, he should avoid coffee before bedtime or talking to a group of excited extraverts just before going on stage, which in itself will likely spike his arousal level.

Sociogenic Extraversion: Cultural and Contextual Factors

Bipolar factors of extraversion and introversion are routinely found in different countries (Church, 2000; McCrae & Costa, 1997). This entails that within cultures there will be, at the very least, phenotypic heterogeneity in this trait: Strongly introverted and extraverted individuals will appear wherever we might travel, or at least wherever people will fill out personality questionnaires. Moreover, there are also mean differences in extraversion between countries and such differences are likely to be part of the values transmitted within a culture. Such influences occur during the process of socialization throughout the life span. Perhaps this is most clearly seen in terms of dyadic interaction in which norms governing such features as how close one stands, the degree of touching deemed appropriate, and amount of eye contact varies considerably from culture to culture (Argyle, 1969).

Both role theorists and linguistic theorists (e.g., Sarbin,1986; Scheibe, 2000; Semin, Rosch, & Chassen, 1981) make strong cases that traits are socially constructed categories that we use to make sense of our own and others' behavior. Proponents of this view frequently charge biogenic approaches to traits with reifying concepts that are more appropriately seen as part of our cultural heritage. However, we do not see these as mutually exclusive approaches. It is possible to have biogenic propensities to engage in behaviors that are concordant with or discordant with conduct regarded as culturally appropriate and desired. Thus the United States, traditionally one of the most extraverted of countries in terms of mean levels and perceived value of extraversion, has its fair share of individuals who are biogenically disposed to introversion. If the claims of social norms are sufficiently strong then it may seem that conflict will almost certainly arise when an implacable biogenic introvert lives in an intransigent culture of extraversion. This view of an inevitable conflict between first and second natures is, we suggest, misguided. Third natures create a navigable space within which potentially conflicting natures can be harmonized, or at least harnessed to benefit selves and their societies. We turn now to discussing how third nature extraversion can achieve, at least for a while, a harmonization of competing natures.

Idiogenic Extraversion: Personal Projects and Free Traited Extraversion

Beyond the influences of temperamental and sociocultural factors, individuals may choose to adopt patterns of behavior that are phenotypically at odds with either or both of their biogenic or sociogenic natures. A biologically introverted woman from an introverted culture may have a consuming passion to be a front-line journalist covering dangerous and stimulating breaking events. Such strategic enactments are not fixed dispositions but free traits. We see these as idiogenic: Their origin lies neither in genetically rooted first nature, nor in peremptory pressures solely attributable to social roles and contextual pressures.

Rather, they are the personally constructed sets of action used strategically to advance goals and projects that matter to individuals. Although the trait-like scripts that are enacted derive from cultural learning, they are chosen and deployed, blended, and orchestrated by the individual. They are thus idiogenic in nature and, we submit, they are central to understanding some of the seemingly inexplicable aspects of daily life.

The foregoing distinctions might be illustrated by looking at a very different area in which the three natures are clearly reflected—the use of language. Our universal capacity for language is biogenic, which language we first speak is sociogenic, and what we choose to say is idiogenic. There may be subtle shadings that make differentiations among the natures difficult, such as the difference between local dialects and idiosyncratic speech patterns. The essential point is that in life as with language, there are three foundational aspects to the course it will take: those emanating from our biogenic legacy, those from our sociogenic heritage, and those freely constructed idiogenic accomplishments that we create for ourselves.

Returning to Markus and Deborah, we can suggest how idiogenic first natures can direct and give meaning to daily activity. Markus chooses, at times, to engage in behavior that others see as highly extraverted. He does this to advance core projects that require extraverted conduct, even though temperamentally such conduct might be out of character for him. He is a creative musician, but also an entrepreneur with five nightclubs and when he leaves the serenity of the studio where he composes, he opens the door and is immediately "on" as the extraverted, energizing but still decidedly "cool" impresario. Deborah is biologically disposed to negative affectivity: She is also quick to anger and does not suffer fools or phonies gladly. However, her commitment to be a fun and responsive parent, a core project for her, leads her to act at home in ways that most would see as not only agreeable but generous to a fault.

Although Markus and Deborah might regard themselves as acting rather disingenuously in some of their daily activities, they may be acting with a fidelity to projects that matter to them and often to others as well. That such behavior might extract a toll, both emotionally and physically, is something they may know only too well. However, it is more likely that they may be oblivious to the downside of acting in a free traited fashion. The costs of acting out of character are not a common theme in the everyday discourse of people who occasionally reflect on their personalities, nor is it a common topic of research in trait psychology, nor in the various goal and action theories that are currently being studied. It is precisely this neglect of idiogenic natures that free trait theory attempts to redress.[4]

Fitting In, Opening Up, and Getting Out: Relevant Evidence From Related Research Areas

Three research areas, although not explicitly concerned with free traits, bear centrally on its themes and can be invoked as providing indirect support for its empirical propositions.

The person–environment fit literature has long provided robust and consistent evidence that individuals benefit when they are engaged in occupations, roles, or settings that are concordant with their personalities (e.g., Kulka, 1979; Lerner, 1983; Pervin, 1968). McGregor, McAdams, and Little (in press), for example, demonstrated that university students who were socially oriented in their traits were happier if they were engaged in personal projects that were social in nature. If one is not fitting into a particular role or setting it is possible to change the environment by leaving or modifying it, or by changing one's own personal characteristics. For example, Roberts and Robins (2004) studied personality change in Berkeley students over 4 years as undergraduates and found that they became increasingly disagreeable but less neurotic as they progressed through their programs. In so doing, students had a better fit with an environment that was consensually evaluated as highly competitive and demanding. From a free traits perspective, the pressures to adopt the characteristics of the setting might induce real change in personality among some students, but also only apparent change in others. It is possible that some of these students were, by first nature, highly agreeable individuals who learned over time to turn off their agreeableness to attend to their core projects of academic achievement. In short, to "fit in" such individuals would engage in free-traited disagreeableness. We would predict that such individuals will pay a higher cost than those who had already entered with a resolve to hit the books and ignore the seductions of convivial social pursuits. Interestingly, it was precisely this trade-off between academic and interpersonal pursuits that was featured in a study of transitions during a shorter time

---

[4]In the field of sociology, there has been a long tradition of research on "emotion work" originally developed by Hochschild (1979). This research examines role-induced requirements for affective displays, such as mandatory smiling by flight attendants. Although free trait theory is not restricted to role-induced requirements to act disingenuously, this creative and now extensive literature is highly relevant to our own research.

frame—the first semester at college (Cantor, Norem, Niedenthal, Langston, & Brower, 1987). Students who initially gave priority to social tasks and then switched to giving priority to their academic tasks adapted better than those who were unable to make such a switch. It seems clear that personality change occurs during these transitional periods, although we would submit that this is likely to be a sociogenic accommodation to contextual demands or an idiogenic commitment to a core project of succeeding at university. In either case, striking a workable balance between flexibility and fidelity is required.

Another research literature has some important warnings for those who protractedly act in ways that involve suppressing aspects of their first natures or of not opening up about important aspects of themselves (Pennebaker, 1993; Wegner, 1989). There is now a substantial body of research confirming the importance of opening up about aspects of oneself that may have been kept secret. Those who do avail themselves of opportunities to open up, after an initial period of increased autonomic arousal, have shown declines from the base-rate levels of arousal. They also exhibit decreased frequency of physical problems and illness, likely mediated by enhanced immune system functioning (Pennebaker, 1993; Pennebaker & Beall, 1986).

We suggest that acting out of character, such as behaving in a competitive and unsupportive way when naturally disposed to agreeableness, will exact the same kind of costs as those demonstrated in the research on self-disclosure. Moreover, the explicit attempt to suppress natural personalities or fixed traits may lead, as Wegner's (1989) research would suggest, to hypervigilance, cognitive resource depletion, and the ironic reappearance of first natures with their attendant complexities. For example, Markus, when engaged in a fractious negotiation about a proposed act for one of his clubs, might display a slight leakage of introversion—an averted gaze, a momentary pause in his typical staccato patter. Deborah may find, despite her utter fidelity to the project of keeping the family happy, that she flames her older daughter in an e-mail she later wished she had not sent.[5]

A person who appears to fit in but does not really, and who is aware of the discrepancy but does not open up about it, may still take advantage

---

[5]The term *leakage* is taken from the intriguing research of Lippa (1976), who found some support for the notion that extraverts and introverts who are asked to act out the opposite personality type were more likely to "leak" what we would call their biogenic orientation if they were low in self-monitoring (Snyder, 1974). High self-monitors leaked less. Two other recent and highly relevant studies of the subtle links of roles, goals, and well-being are found in Sheldon, Ryan, Rawsthorne, and Ilardi (1997) and Fleeson, Malanos, and Achille (2002).

of what we call restorative niches in which one's first nature is indulged by simply getting away (Little, 1996, 2000a). Where they should get away to depends on their biogenic orientations and the sociogenic prescriptions of the discordant context. For example, students who have accommodated to the modal style of a demanding and competitive undergraduate life might find solace in the monthly visit home where their families fondly facilitate the expression of biogenic bubbly selves.

The importance of restorative environments has been an active area of research and there is clear evidence that they have important psychological and physical health benefits (Hartig, Mang, & Evans, 1991; Kaplan, 1983). Although closely related, restorative niches differ from restorative environments in one important sense. Restorative environments are postulated as applying to humans in general and are typically recreational or idyllic retreats found in pristine nature or gardens—places that are devoid of the chaos and contrivances of modern life. Restorative niches, on the other hand, take multiple forms, corresponding to the first nature traits that need restoration. Thus for an agreeable extravert, a restorative niche might well be an ear-splitting nightclub with loud and loopy friends bouncing off walls until breakfast. For a Sartrean introvert, such a place would be the very definition of hell.

Some of the predictions we might make of favored restorative environments are straightforward, but some are intriguingly complex. For example, there is evidence that disagreeable people actually feel positive affect when engaged in activities that are normally regarded as unpleasant, such as engaging in a quarrelsome interaction (Coté & Moskowitz, 1998; Moskowitz & Coté, 1995). If such a biogenically disagreeable person works in an environment where a norm of niceness prevails, being "on" as a pleasant and affirming individual should, under our view, extract costs. Respite for that person is not likely to be found in the calming influence of traditional restorative environments. Indeed, an idyllic escape may well exacerbate stress rather than restore that person's first nature. For the deeply disagreeable person it may be more salutary to volunteer at a debt-collection agency or engage in one of the less refined varieties of martial arts offered at Deborah's gym. In short, restorative niches are a variant of restorative environments that are optimally designed for individuals of differing biogenic personalities. In such niches individuals can recover their first natures for a while and in so doing mitigate the costs of acting out of character.

EMPIRICAL EXPLORATIONS OF FREE TRAIT THEORY: FREE TRAIT RISK AND WELL-BEING

Refinement and Elaboration of Free Trait Theory

An initial empirical study of free trait theory was briefly reported in Little (1996). It found evidence consistent with the overall thesis that engaging in free-traited behavior might exact a cost if not mitigated by the use of restorative niches. Although promising, the study was clearly exploratory and dealt with global trait ascriptions rather than on discrepancies between more enduring traits and those manifested in ongoing projects. Subsequently a more critical and comprehensive examination was undertaken (Joseph, 2002) and the following sections draw primarily on that research.

The assumptions and propositions of free trait theory were conceptualized in terms of risk factors of free-traited behavior and mitigation factors. We created a measure of *free trait risk* as a ratio, where the numerator was a set of risk factors associated with engaging in free-traited behavior and the denominator was a set of mitigating factors that could reduce the cost of such behaviors. We hypothesized that the greater the free trait risk, the more likely that subjective well-being would be compromised. Our assessment of well-being comprised measures of life satisfaction, satisfaction in different life domains, depressive affect, and measures of physical health symptoms and severity. Consistent with other studies in our laboratory, these disparate measures yielded three clear clusters of physical illness, life satisfaction, and depressive affect.[6]

Global and domain-specific life satisfaction scales (Palys & Little, 1983) were used to assess general satisfaction with life as a whole, as well as with particular life domains (academic life, social life, home life, emotional state, and physical health) as they are at present.

Several conceptual and assessment modifications were entailed to test this hypothesis, involving choice of participants, and elaboration and expansion of both risk factors and mitigating factors.

---

[6]Physical health symptoms were assessed using an adaptation of the Carleton Symptom Checklist (Little, 1988), which prompts individuals to consider a list of symptoms (e.g., headaches, heart problems). Points were summed to yield an overall severity of symptoms score. Psychological well-being was assessed with measures of both negative and positive affective states. The Center for Epidemiological Studies Depression Scale (Radloff, 1977) was used to evaluate depressive symptoms over the past week. Based on the two major components of well-being identified by McGregor and Little (1998), participants were asked to give an overall rating on an 11-point scale of how happy their lives are at present and how meaningful their lives are at present. Global and domain specific *life satisfaction* scales (Palys & Little, 1983) were used to assess general satisfaction with life as a whole, as well as with particular life domains (academic life, social life, home life, emotional state, and physical health) as they are at present.

Selection of Participants. We chose as research participants individuals who were old enough to have consolidated relatively stable, biogenic traits, but were also at a life stage where they might be called on to engage in projects that required acting out of character. Participants were 109 older undergraduate students and graduate students from a diversity of fields with a mean age of 35.09 years (*SD* = 9.09); 72.2% of the participants were female.[7]

Risk Factors: Assessing Genotypic and Phenotypic Extraversion. Free trait theory postulates that a major risk factor is the discrepancy between genotypic and phenotypic traits. Ideally, genotypic extraversion would involve neurophysiological measures and phenotypic extraversion would be obtained by consensual ratings by judges on how "extravertedly" a person acts in performing various projects. Our preliminary studies have not included such measures, but we have tried to develop appropriate proxy measures that might point to promising directions for more elaborate research. We assessed biogenic extraversion by augmenting an extraversion scale with items containing more somatic and biogenically based material (e.g., subjective effects of stimulants, sleeping patterns).[8] Phenotypic extraversion was measured by adapting personal projects analysis so that participants were asked "If a stranger could observe you during this project, would they likely assume that you are more extraverted or introverted because of your actions/behaviors?"[9] An individual's general phenotypic extraversion score was calculated by averaging these ratings across the individual's rated personal projects.

An important consideration incorporated into the revised theory was that daily life is full of demands to act against one's fixed traits. Indeed, as suggested earlier, inability to flex to such demands would in itself be suggestive of maladaptive rigidity. Thus it is expected that for many individuals, the effects of protracted free-traited action alone may not be sufficient to manifest costs to well-being. However, the presence of ad-

---

[7]For more details on the characteristics of the participants, see Joseph (2002). Neither age nor gender had a significant effect on any of the relationships reported here; therefore results pertain to the full sample.

[8]The scale used was Little's (1987) the Short Personality Assessment (SPA), Extraversion scale.

[9]Instructions asked the participant to use 10 if, while engaged in this project, you appear to be highly extraverted (outgoing, active, gregarious, or appearing easily bored), and 0 if you seem highly introverted (reserved, serious, or appearing to have little need for externally based excitement or sensory stimulation).

ditional life stress is likely to allow potential costs to precipitate out, and we included a brief measure of this in the study.[10]

We assumed that this combined general and free-trait-related stress may be sufficient to suppress immune functioning, and affected individuals are thus hypothesized to be more likely to experience physical health symptoms, even once potential confounds (health behaviors, negative affect, and age) are controlled.

Mitigating Factors. The principal mitigating factor in the original free traits model was the availability and use of restorative niches. In an exploratory study in our laboratory, Hotson (1997) found that when he asked participants to identify any restorative niches they used in their daily lives they frequently listed activities and projects rather than fixed places. Thus, instead of "bowling alley," the restorative activity or project of "go bowling" was as likely to be invoked. Accordingly, we adopted the term *restorative projects,* both to provide some continuity with previous research that had examined restorative features of projects (Howe, 1986) and to broaden the scope of restorative possibilities to include both covert and overt action. Beyond having niches in which to restore oneself, restorative projects include self-regulatory activities such as trying to change one's mood and engaging in action that is not restricted to a particular place or setting. Among the restorative projects engaged in by participants in this study were "drink tea in quiet room alone," and "attend the Godsmack (or Limp Bizkit) concert."

Drawing on Pennebaker's research (Pennebaker, 1993; Pennebaker & Beall, 1986; Petrie, Booth, & Pennebaker, 1998) on opening up (see also Jourard, 1964, on self-disclosure), we expanded free trait theory to include measures of whether respondents have access to other people with whom they could reveal their first natures and share personal information. We anticipated that this would serve as another mitigating factor reducing the costs of free-traited behavior.[11]

---

[10]We used two rationally derived (Burisch, 1984) items asking whether participants have been "experiencing any upheaval" in their lives over the past 6 months, and whether they have "felt really stressed over the past 6 months."

[11]For assessment purposes, four questions were asked concerning disclosure about one's true nature. These included (a) an estimate of the "number of people who really know the 'natural you'"; (b) the "proportion of people in your life who matter to you/whom you care about [who] know the natural you"; (c) whether "you have anyone you can talk to about your personality, your projects, your activities, and your feelings"; and (d) whether "you have anyone you can really 'be yourself' with." The three scores were averaged to yield a mean self-disclosure score.

These extended conceptions of risk and mitigating factors, together with the more sharply defined original set of free trait measures, were incorporated into the free trait risk index. This omnibus index now captures and quantifies both the discrepant action that can lead to costs when resources to adapt to stress are taxed and the restorative projects and self-disclosure that can mitigate such costs:

Free Trait Risk Index = $\dfrac{\textbf{Risk}}{\textbf{Mitigation}}$

Where: **Risk = Absolute Discrepancy (Phenotypic – Genotypic Extraversion × Stress)**
Mitigation = average (mean Restorative Projects + mean Self-Disclosure)

Free trait total risk index scores using this equation have a possible range of 0 (low theoretical risk for incurring costs to well-being) to 100 (high theoretical risk for incurring costs to well-being).

Results.   The results support the central propositions of the expanded free trait theory (Little, 2000a, Propositions 4 & 5). The free trait risk index was significantly related to poorer well-being unless mitigated by restorative projects and self-disclosure. The index correlated significantly with severity of symptoms ($R = .45, p < .001, n = 100$), life satisfaction ($R = -.38, p < .001, n = 102$), and depressive affect ($R = .44, p < .001, n = 102$).[12]
As anticipated, absolute genotypic–phenotypic extraversion discrepancy alone (i.e., without taking into account other stress or factors that mitigate costs) did not correlate significantly with the three outcome measures. Individuals seem to be able to deal with a certain level of stress without incurring physical or psychological costs. However, when the stress of discrepant behavior combines with other stress, a relation to costs becomes readily apparent.
In addition to testing the omnibus free trait prediction, we also examined another potential mitigator of acting out of character, based on our earlier distinction between idiogenic and biogenic extraversion. The *idiogenic fidelity* of projects was measured by adopting Sheldon and

---

[12]Age, health behaviors, and negative affect were not confounded with total risk, and do not compromise the relation between total risk and physical symptom severity.

Elliot's (1999) self-concordance project rating dimensions.[13] We reasoned that individuals who were acting in a completely trait-concordant fashion would be least likely to experience costs in well-being and that individuals who were acting in ways that were both biogenically discordant and lacked idiogenic fidelity would be most at risk. Contrast tests clearly supported this prediction. It was also found that of the two types of discrepancy, idiogenic discrepancy was significantly more likely to compromise each of the well-being indicators than was biogenic discrepancy. In short, although both extracted costs, acting out of character in projects that were not concordant with one's idiogenic nature were more taxing than acting out of character in projects that ran counter to one's biogenic nature.

FREE TRAITS: RESEARCH, POLICY, AND PERSONAL IMPLICATIONS

We have presented the assumptions, propositions, and initial empirical explorations of a theory of free traits and acting out of character. We turn finally to a research agenda that we hope will be explored by those finding these propositions of interest and offer some reflections on policy implications and on the relevance of the theory for personal reflections about our lives.

Research Implications

First, some caveats. Although we have adduced evidence from bodies of research in several fields that support the propositions of free trait theory, direct empirical evidence is still very preliminary. Although results are generally consistent with the general theoretical propositions, there are boundary conditions, particularly related to general stress, that may need to be taken into account for the postulated effects to be discernible. Moreover, it is critical to the fair test of free trait theory that we move beyond proxy measures and use more direct measures of biogenic traits and their phenotypic counterparts, and that we engage participants in our studies who are exposed daily to more demanding calls to act out of character than our students might have been. Our research agenda gives priority to increasing the power to detect effects that might

---

[13]The ratings differentiate between external, introjected, identified, and intrinsic reasons for engaging in a project. Using Sheldon and Elliot's (1999) formula, we averaged the intrinsic and identified ratings, and subtracted the averaged external and introjected rating.

have been obscured in preliminary investigations. Similarly, there are a number of potentially powerful risk and mitigating factors that have yet to be explored in this research program. Among the many factors that should enhance the likelihood of free-traited behavior occurring are high self-monitoring tendencies (Snyder, 1974, 1987), strong social and environmental pressures to act in a biogenically discordant fashion, clear scripts about how to act discordantly, and social reinforcement for successfully acting out of character. Among potential mitigating influences are resilience factors that represent radically different approaches to life—from a sense of humor that allows us to take our disparate selves a little less seriously to a sense of the ultimate significance of the projects we undertake, no matter what the cost.

Although free trait theory is intended to apply to any biogenically rooted trait, we have focused here on extraversion. Extraversion has characteristics that make it particularly appropriate for free trait theory. First, as a biogenic trait there are several plausible neurophysiological mechanisms subserving it and research in this area is burgeoning as new methods of studying brain activity in vivo are developed. Second, as a sociogenic trait it is clearly an everyday concept that people invoke to explain their own behavior, certainly in Western culture and most likely with equivalent concepts in other cultures. Third, as an idiogenic trait, being more extraverted is one of the most frequently invoked intrapersonal projects that people list when they complete a personal projects analysis (see Little & Gee, chap. 2, this volume). This suggests that extraversion is both normatively valued, at least in certain regions of North American and European culture, and that it requires some conscious, articulated planning to be developed and deployed. Finally, extraversion is distinctive in that it poses a double jeopardy for individuals who adopt it as a free trait. We assume that enacting any free trait exacts a cost in autonomic arousal, but introverts who are acting in a pseudo-extraverted fashion also increase their neocortical arousal, which is likely to compromise their performance. In contrast, a person acting as a pseudo-agreeable individual may incur a cost in terms of autonomic arousal but there is no reason to assume that there will be costs in terms of neocortical functioning. For these reasons, then, extraversion has been the trait of choice for those of us interested in the concept of free-traited behavior.

However, it is intriguing to consider the Big Five traits in terms of free trait theory and to examine both poles of these traits. Is it easier for an extravert to act introvertedly than vice versa? Can people who have been closed to experience for three decades mount a credible appearance of openness? Or, will they always seem to have had 1 year of experience repeated 29 times? Some everyday acts that seem perplexing take on new meaning when viewed as free traits. Although it seems likely that individuals will mount as free traits those that are socially desirable, their particular social ecology might create pressures for them to adopt traits that are congruent with their spouses or their roommates. Pseudo-neurotic behavior, for example, might occur when a biogenically stable person is living with a truly neurotic one. There are, we suspect, subtle social sanctions against students who do not "neurose" over upcoming examinations at college, and they may adopt expressions of concern and frustration that show sociogenic fidelity to friends but are not really reflective of the biogenic self. Individuals who occupy roles that demand high levels of agreeableness but who are biogenically not disposed to such behavior are likely to find the protracted enactment of pleasantness wearying.

Thus far we have been looking at free traits one trait at a time, although it is conventional to view traits as forming profiles of five (plus or minus two) traits. For free trait theory, this actually poses less of a problem than for orthodox conceptions of traits, where it becomes necessary to postulate mechanisms of which fixed trait becomes salient in what situation. Free trait theory assumes that there are styles of presentation that combine several components of basic traits into the service of a core project or valued role. Little (1989) suggested that one such pattern was a ubiquitous Professional International Elite (PIE) style shown among executives and professionals whether they hail from Hartford, Helsinki, or Hong Kong. In terms of the Big Five trait dimensions, it can be suggested that PIE embodies high openness, high conscientiousness, moderate extraversion, high initial agreeableness, and low neuroticism. With some of these traits there is a temporal dimension that is important. For example, agreeableness would be seen as a desirable initial stance, but if the interaction or task involves negotiations or debate, a shift away from easy compliance would be regarded as the more professional stance to take. The ability to shift from earnest conscientiousness at times is part of the flexible deployment of traits as project-linked resources. However, the considerable homogeneity one sees, for example, in executive-class air travel conceals the fact that many of these individuals might be acting out of character while being "on" as perspicuous professionals. Our roles and our projects entail us rising to occasions, but we do need to know that PIE in the sky may exact its costs.

Policy Implications

Although not examined empirically or extensively in this chapter, the sixth proposition of free trait theory is important when we consider implications for contextual analysis, whether it is in marital therapy, organizational analysis, or urban planning. There are policy implications of free trait theory. One implication is that restorative niches and projects need to be available in settings when the demands of acting out of character exceed the capacity of their occupants to cope. Beyond providing restorative niches, environments need to be responsive to biogenic, sociogenic, and idiogenic natures and to nurture them in ways that will lead to sustainable project pursuit. Biogenic natures, with their strong hereditary provenance, require contexts that afford such differences opportunities to thrive; sociogenic natures require meaningful, coherent traditions, scripts, and stories through which individuals are able to find shared meaning in their pursuits. Brandstätter and Lalonde (chap. 10, this volume) give a poignant illustration of how the destruction of cultural identities can shatter personal lives. Idiogenic natures, the deeply rooted proclivity to pursue personal projects, require the space within which such projects can be pursued with impunity. The provision of moral space in which project pursuit is protected is at the very heart of a philosophy of rights (Lomasky, 1984, 1987). That is, prudential concerns are sufficient to regulate individual lives in a Robinson Crusoe sense. However, in a world of other agents, when Friday comes along, and each person is committed to his or her own projects, questions of forebearance among individuals become critical. Prudence here is insufficient; morality becomes paramount in deciding how to live one's life.

Personal Implications

Free trait theory also allows us to reflect individually on our personal lives in ways that may be revealing and salutary. We might regard this as calling for a free trait agreement. This agreement is a simple one: I will be willing to act out of character to advance core projects that matter to others if they will grant me the respite of restorative niches in which I can regain my first nature on occasion. Whether this be an agreement struck with one's romantic or business partners, with one's children or parents, it is likely, if ratified, to redound to the benefit of all.

Finally, the most personal level of all—our self-reflections about the multiple "mini-mes" that we become in the pursuit of core projects—

can sometimes be disconcerting. We become aware of how disjointed our lives and our selves can be. The dance among the biological, social, and personal aspects of our all too human selves can seem more like random lurching than choreography. The pursuit of core projects may provide considerable value for ourselves and for others and it may leave a legacy, despite the disparate set of selves we have had to be to bring these projects to fruition. However, in acting out of character to advance core projects, we may well have to create dissonance, not reduce it, and enhance inner conflict, not assuage it. Flourishing may be fatiguing.

However, at the end of our days, whenever they come, one might hope for some reconciliation, a final dance with one's selves. An invitation to such a dance appears in the deeply moving final chapter of Flanagan (1996). This dance may be a solo performance: a Markus musing on his Marks and a Deborah reflecting on her Debs. We might also hope for similar dances of reconciliation with those with whom we have shared our lives—at least a pas-de-deux, and perhaps a community barn dance. Better still, it seems prudent to have these dances with self and others while we have both time and self-awareness to do so with lucidity. Human beings, at times, should be able to reconcile the strategic imbalances, the costly free traits, and the inevitable incongruities that emerge throughout our lives. They will make Markus less strange and Deborah less scary. Such intermittent reconciliations are likely to help triple-natured people be wise creatures and well beings. They will enhance our flourishing by helping us appreciate the subtle choreographies of catching our balance.

REFERENCES

Argyle, M. (1969). *Social interaction.* London: Methuen.

Burisch, M. (1984). Approaches to personality inventory construction: A comparison of merits. *American Psychologist, 39,* 214–227.

Cantor, N., Norem, J. K., Niedenthal, P. M., Langston, C. A., & Brower, A. M. (1987). Life tasks, self-concept ideals, and cognitive strategies in a life transition. *Journal of Personality and Social Psychology, 53,* 1178–1191.

Church, A. T. (2000). Culture and personality: Toward an integrated cultural trait psychology. *Journal of Personality, 68,* 651–703.

Coll, C. G., Bearer, E. L., & Lerner, R. M. (Eds.). (2005). *Nature and nurture: The complex interplay of genetic and environmental influences on human behavior and development.* Mahwah, NJ: Lawrence Erlbaum Associates.

Coté, S., & Moskowitz, D. S. (1998). On the dynamic covariation between interpersonal behavior and affect: Prediction from neuroticism, extraversion, and agreeableness. *Journal of Personality and Social Psychology, 75,* 1032–1046.

De Pascalis, V. (2004). On the psychophysiology of extraversion. In R. R. Stelmack (Ed.), *On the psychobiology of personality: Essays in honor of Marvin Zuckerman* (pp. 295–327). New York: Elsevier.

Eysenck, H. J. (1967). *The biological basis of personality.* Springfield, IL: Thomas.

Eysenck, H. J., & Eysenck, M. W. (1985). *Personality and individual differences: A natural science approach.* New York: Plenum.

Flanagan, O. (1991). *Varieties of moral personality: Ethic and psychological realism.* Cambridge, MA: Harvard University Press.

Flanagan, O. (1996). *Self expressions: Mind, morals and the meaning of life.* New York: Oxford University Press.

Fleeson, W., Malanos, A. B., & Achille, N. M. (2002). An intraindividual process approach to the relationship between extraversion and positive affect: Is acting extraverted as "good" as being extraverted? *Journal of Personality and Social Psychology, 83,* 1409–1422.

Geen, R. G. (1984). Preferred stimulation levels in introverts and extroverts: Effects on arousal and performance. *Journal of Personality and Social Psychology, 46,* 1303–1312.

Gottlieb, G. (1991). *Individual development and evolution: The genesis of novel behavior.* New York: Oxford University Press.

Gottlieb, G. (1998). Normally occurring environmental and behavioral influences on gene activity: From central dogma to probabilistic epigenesis. *Psychological Review, 105,* 792–802.

Gray, J. A. (1981). A critique of Eysenck's theory of personality. In H. J. Eysenck (Ed.), *A model for personality* (pp. 246–276). Berlin: Springer-Verlag.

Grigorenko, E. L. (2002). In search of the genetic engram of personality. In D. Cervone & W. Mischel (Eds.), *Advances in personality science* (pp. 29–82). New York: Guilford.

Hartig, T., Mang, M., & Evans, G. W. (1991). Restorative effects of natural environment experiences. *Environment and Behavior, 23,* 3–26.

Hebb, D. O. (1955). Drive and the C.N.S. (conceptual nervous system). *Psychological Review, 62,* 243–254.

Hochschild, A. (1979). Emotion work, feeling rules, and social structure. *American Journal of Sociology, 85,* 551–575.

Hogan, R., Jones, W. H., & Cheek, J. M. (1985). Socioanalytic theory: An alternative to armadillo psychology. In B. R. Schlenker (Ed.), *The self and social life* (pp. 175–198). New York: McGraw-Hill.

Hotson, H. (1997). *Free traits and restorative niches: Exploring some elements of a social ecological model of well-being.* Unpublished bachelor's thesis, Carleton University, Ottawa, ON, Canada.

Howe, N. (1986). *Depressive affect and personal projects: The role of "special projects."* Unpublished bachelor's thesis. Carleton University, Ottawa, ON, Canada.

Jang, K. L., McCrae, R. R., Angleitner, A., Riemann, R., & Livesley, W. J. (1998). Heritability of facet-level traits in a cross-cultural twin sample: Support for a hierarchical model of personality. *Journal of Personality and Social Psychology, 74,* 1556–1565.

Joseph, M. F. (2002). *Free traits, personal projects, and well-being: The social ecology of mutable selves.* Unpublished bachelor's thesis, Carleton University, Ottawa, ON, Canada.

Jourard, S. M. (1964). *The transparent self: Self-disclosure and well-being.* Princeton, NJ: Van Nostrand.

Kaplan, S. (1983). A model of person–environment compatibility. *Environment and Behavior, 15,* 311–332.

Kulka, R. A. (1979). Interaction as person–environment fit. In L. R. Kahle (Ed.), *Methods for studying person–situation interactions* (pp. 55–71). San Francisco: Jossey-Bass.

Lerner, R. M. (1983). A "goodness of fit" model of person–context interaction. In D. Magnusson & V. L. Allen (Eds.), *Human development: An interactional perspective* (pp. 279–293). New York: Academic.

Lippa, R. (1976). Expressive control and the leakage of dispositional introversion-extraversion during role-played teaching. *Journal of Personality, 44,* 541–559.

Little, B. R. (1983). Personal projects: A rationale and method for investigation. *Environment and Behavior, 15,* 273–309.

Little, B. R. (1987). *Short Personality Assessment (SPA) scales.* Unpublished manuscript, Carleton University, Ottawa, ON, Canada.

Little, B. R. (1988). *Personal projects analysis: Theory, method and research.* Ottawa, ON, Canada: Social Sciences and Humanities Research Council of Canada.

Little, B. R. (1989). Personality myths about leaders. *Leaders, 12,* 189–192.

Little, B. R. (1996). Free traits, personal projects and idio-tapes: Three tiers for personality research. *Psychological Inquiry, 8,* 340–344.

Little, B. R. (1999a). Personal projects and social ecology: Themes and variation across the life span. In J. Brandtstadter & R. M. Lerner (Eds.), *Action and self-development: Theory and research through the life span* (pp. 197–221). Thousand Oaks, CA: Sage.

Little, B. R. (1999b). Personality and motivation: Personal action and the conative evolution. In L. A. Pervin & O. P. John (Eds.), *Handbook of personality theory and research* (2nd ed.). New York: Guilford.

Little, B. R. (2000a). Free traits and personal contexts: Expanding a social ecological model of well-being. In W. B. Walsh, K. H. Craik, & R. Price (Eds.), *Person environment psychology* (2nd ed., pp. 87–116). New York: Guilford.

Little, B. R. (2000b, November). *Personal projects and free traits: Lives liberties and the happiness of pursuit.* Radcliffe Fellows Lecture presented at the Radcliffe Institute for Advanced Study, Harvard University, Cambridge, MA.

Little, B. R. (2005). Personality science and personal projects: Six impossible things before breakfast. *Journal of Research in Personality, 39,* 4–21.

Little, B. R., & Chambers, N. C. (2004). Personal project pursuit: On human doings and well beings. In M. Cox & E. Klinger (Eds.), *Handbook of motivational counseling: Concepts, approaches and assessment* (pp. 65–82). Chichester, UK: Wiley.

Little, B. R., & Ryan, T. J. (1979). A social ecological model of development. In K. Ishwaran (Ed.), *Childhood and adolescence in Canada* (pp. 273–301). Toronto: McGraw-Hill Ryerson.

Loehlin, J. C., McCrae, R. R., Costa, P. T., Jr., & John, O. P. (1998). Heritabilities of common and measure-specific components of the Big Five personality factors. *Journal of Research in Personality, 32,* 431–453.

Lomasky, L. E. (1984). Personal projects as the foundation of human rights. *Social Philosophy and Policy, 1,* 35–55.

Lomasky, L. E. (1987). *Persons, rights and the moral community.* New York: Oxford University Press.

McCrae, R. R., & Costa, P. T., Jr. (1997). Personality trait structure as a human universal. *American Psychologist, 52,* 509–516.

McGregor, I., & Little, B. R. (1998). Personal projects, happiness, and meaning: On doing well and being yourself. *Journal of Personality and Social Psychology, 74,* 494–512.

McGregor, I., McAdams, D., & Little, B. R. (in press). Personal projects, life stories, and happiness: On being true to traits. *Journal of Research in Personality.*

Moskowitz, D. S., & Coté, S. (1995). Do interpersonal traits predict affect? A comparison of three models. *Journal of Personality and Social Psychology, 69,* 915–924.

Palys, T. S., & Little, B. R. (1983). Perceived life satisfaction and the organization of personal project systems. *Journal of Personality and Social Psychology, 44,* 1221–1230.

Pennebaker, J. W. (1993). Putting stress into words: Health, linguistic, and therapeutic implications. *Behavior Research and Therapy, 31,* 539–548.

Pennebaker, J. W., & Beall, S. K. (1986). Confronting a traumatic event: Toward an understanding of inhibition and disease. *Journal of Abnormal Psychology, 95,* 274–281.

Pervin, L. A. (1968). Performance and satisfaction as a function of individual–environment fit. *Psychological Bulletin, 69,* 56–68.

Petrie, K. J., Booth, R. J., & Pennebaker, J. W. (1998). The immunological effects of thought suppression. *Journal of Personality and Social Psychology, 75,* 1264–1272.

Radloff, L. S. (1977). The CES–D Scale: A self-report depression scale for research in the general population. *Applied Psychological Measurement, 1,* 385–401.

Rende, R. (2004). Beyond heritability: Biological process in social context. In C. G. Coll, E. L. Bearer, & R. M. Lerner (Eds.), *Nature and nurture: The complex interplay of genetic and environmental influences on human behavior and development* (pp. 107–126). Mahwah, NJ: Lawrence Erlbaum Associates.

Roberts, B. W., & Robins, R. W. (2004). Person–environment fit and its implications for personality development: A longitudinal study. *Journal of Personality, 72,* 89–110.

Robins, R. W., Norem, J. K., & Cheek, J. M. (1999). Naturalizing the self. In L. A. Pervin & O. P. John (Eds.), *Handbook of personality* (pp. 443–477). New York: Guilford.

Sarbin, T. R. (1986). *Narrative psychology.* New York: Praeger.

Scheibe, K. E. (2000). *The drama of everyday life.* Cambridge, MA: Harvard University Press.

Semin, G. R., Rosch, E., & Chassen, J. (1981). A comparison of the common-sense and "scientific" conceptions of extroversion–introversion. *European Journal of Social Psychology, 11,* 77–86.

Sheldon, K. M., & Elliot, A. J. (1999). Goal striving, need satisfaction and longitudinal well-being: The self-concordance model. *Journal of Personality and Social Psychology, 76,* 482–497.

Sheldon, K. M., Ryan, R. M., Rawsthorne, L. J., & Ilardi, B. (1997). Trait self and true self: Cross-role variation in the big-5 personality traits and its relations with psychological authenticity and subjective well-being. *Journal of Personality and Social Psychology, 73,* 1380–1393.

Snyder, M. (1974). The self-monitoring of expressive behavior. *Journal of Personality and Social Psychology, 30,* 526–537.

Snyder, M. (1987). *Public appearances, private realities: The psychology of self-monitoring.* New York: Freeman.

Stelmack, R. M. (1981). The psychophysiology of extraversion and neuroticism. In H. J. Eysenck (Ed.), *A model for personality* (pp. 38–64). Berlin: Springer.

Wegner, D. M. (1989). *White bears and other unwanted thoughts.* New York: Viking/Penguin.

Williams, B. (1981). *Moral luck.* Cambridge, UK: Cambridge University Press.

Yerkes, R. M., & Dodson, J. D. (1908). The relation of strength of stimulus to rapidity of habit-formation. *Journal of Comparative Neurology and Psychology, 18*, 459–482.

Zuckerman, M. (1987). A critical look at three arousal constructs in personality theories: Optimal levels of arousal, strength of the nervous system, and sensitivities to signals of reward and punishment. In J. Strelau & H. J. Eysenck (Eds.), *Personality dimensions and arousal* (pp. 217–232). New York: Plenum.

Zuckerman, M. (1991). *Psychobiology of personality.* New York: Cambridge University Press.

V

The Continuing Pursuit:
Conclusion and Future Directions

15

The Sustainable Pursuit of Core Projects: Retrospect and Prospects

Brian R. Little and Adam M. Grant

Personal *Project Pursuit* has been an invitation to think about human personality and development in terms of the personal projects that people are pursuing and the goals and action that such projects conjoin. Some chapters have proposed that human flourishing is contingent on the sustainable pursuit of core projects. The volume itself has been a core project for us and we hope it will have an impact after its completion. Whether it does so will depend on whether the RSVPs it sends out are returned affirmatively. If people decide to come over to this perspective, or at least stop in for a while, it will auger well for personal projects analysis as a sustained and continuing pursuit. Whether they will come depends on the perceived value of the completed projects reported here and on the possible projects that it might stimulate. The intent of this final chapter, therefore, is to highlight the value and the promise of project analytic inquiry particularly for understanding human well-being and flourishing.

To achieve this, we take a Janusian view throughout this chapter, looking backward at the issues emerging from the foregoing chapters and looking forward at possibilities for future endeavors. We do not summarize each chapter, but rather seek common themes that emerge as we progress through the volume as well as implications for further development. Our prospective look is not restricted to those fields that are the major disciplinary allegiances of contributors to the volume, but incorporates recent research from other areas of scholarly and professional practice.

We begin by highlighting the distinctive stance that personal projects researchers take toward their research participants, a stance that facilitates access to the idiosyncratic internal and external factors determining the course and consequences of project pursuit. We then address the social ecological contexts (temporal, spatial, and sociocultural) within which pursuits are conceived and enacted, emphasizing the integrative value of accessing these contexts. We proceed to highlight the relevance of the volume to selected core issues in the fields of personality, motivational, and developmental science. Finally, we address the important and complex issue of human flourishing. We offer an alternative to current approaches and outline an agenda for continuing research that will lead, we hope, to better understanding of the quality of lives and greater facility in enhancing them.

PERSONAL PROJECTS METHODOLOGY: WHAT'S UP? WHY DO YOU ASK? WHERE ARE WE GOING?

As detailed by Little and Gee (chap. 2, this volume), personal projects analysis (PPA) is a distinctive methodology that serves as an integrative alternative to other techniques and assessment approaches currently used in the personality, motivational, developmental, and related fields. PPA begins by asking questions, but in a rather different way than in traditional assessment techniques. The answers to these questions allow us to understand the idiosyncratic pursuits in which a person is engaged as well as how they are proceeding. As we believe the sustainable pursuit of projects is a critical aspect of human well-being and flourishing, the substance of the questions and of the answers is critical. So, too, is our style of asking these questions and the stance we take toward those we study.

Asking Them: The Credulous Stance and Its Limits

One of the most distinctive features of PPA is the approach that it takes with respect to our research participants. This stance is what Kelly

(1955) characterized as both credulous and reflexive; that is, initially accepting the respondents' accounts of events, and using the same constructs to explain the conduct of the scientist and the participants (Little, 1983). The former relates to how much credence we give to the accounts of our participant collaborators; the latter allows us to use the same theoretical constructs to view both the participants we are trying to understand and our own projects as scientists.

Based on our conviction that individuals have specialized knowledge about their pursuits and the value they accord them, we adopt a position in which we are effectively asking "What's up?" to which the participants provide listings of personal projects. We then ask "What do you think about what you're doing?" and "How do you feel about what you're doing?" to which participants respond by providing ratings on the appraisal matrices. Personal goal researchers in this volume similarly go through a process of goal elicitation and appraisal with various modular matrices. These approaches are very much in the Kellian spirit. PPA assumes, for example, that there are not two epistemic solitudes, that of the researcher and that of the participant, but rather an interactive exchange in which the understandings of complex lives are coconstituted and integrated. It starts with the supposition that if we wish to understand the nature of people's concerns and pursuits, we should ask them, and they might just tell us (Allport, 1958; Kelly, 1958).

Of course they may not tell us, or may deliberately mislead us. However, such a response suggests, at least in basic research, that the relationship between the researchers and the respondents may be rather problematic. Implicit in such resistance is an unvoiced question—"Why do you ask?"—to which there is a clear answer from those using project analytic techniques for basic research: "Because we are fascinated by what you are doing." Indeed, this may be where there is the greatest conceptual divide between those who use PPA as a methodological procedure and those who use more experimental techniques, particularly those examining goal pursuit from a social psychological perspective.[1] Experimental researchers often explore goals that have been randomly assigned rather than being personally elicited and would view a credu-

---

[1]Those using assessment devices for selection or placement purposes would adopt such a credulous approach with justified trepidation. We are primarily concerned here with basic research. A more subtle issue involves whether we are primarily concerned with variable-centered or person-centered measurement. The short answer is both (Little & Gee, chap. 2, this volume).

lous approach as compromising experimental rigor because different styles of engagement with participants would be employed by different researchers. As we have seen in this volume, the move from using experimentally created goals to using personal goals as the unit of analysis (or combinations of both strategies) has been an important shift in methodology and a tilt, we feel, in the direction of a more credulous approach.

That said, we are very much aware of the dangers of excessive credulity in the human sciences. After all, the conventional definition of the term *credulity* suggests a degree of naivete, even gullibility, in matters rightly deserving greater skepticism. We wish to make two points regarding this issue. First, the methodologies used throughout this volume are not asking individuals about issues that are irrelevant to them or to form judgments about abstract representations of social topics about which they may have relatively little interest or limited convictions. In PPA, for example, we are asking them about the most salient features of their daily lives, which may include their major concerns and commitments. Because they are highly personal and already articulated projects, they are less likely to evoke mindless responding. Second, to our experimental colleagues who may be incredulous about credulity, we would like to note that such a stance toward participants, even in experimental research, was advocated by Festinger, a paragon of rectitude for generations of experimental social psychologists. When asked how to explain some inexplicable behavior by participants in an experiment, Festinger replied, "Just ask them" (Piliavin, 1989).

We see a credulous approach as essential at the beginning stages of human assessment, particularly for the elicitation of the units of analysis, the personal projects or goals, which then serve as the building blocks of subsequent inquiry. However, even if participants want to cooperate and are able to accurately convey the general nature and appraisal of their personal projects, they may be unable to resist the pull of implicit biases and illusory beliefs about more subtle aspects of themselves and their undertakings. At times, and for certain types of questions, we find it necessary to probe the project pursuer to determine influences that might escape the attention of even the most perspicuous of probands. Indeed, that is a message of several of the chapters in this volume (e.g., McGregor, chap. 6; Peterman & Lecci, chap. 12). As detailed by Little (chap. 1, this volume), personal projects began as an attempt to capture people who were essentially missing in action and required that we ask and listen carefully to their privileged accounts about what they thought they were doing. However, with active agents back in full view in contemporary psychology, we are intrigued by and strongly encourage incorporating experimental techniques that tap the implicit motives and preconscious guides that shape project construal and pursuit. Freund (chap. 9, this volume) and Sheldon (chap. 13, this volume) remind us of the importance of these issues and McGregor (chap. 6, this volume) warns us, with both expository zeal and experiments, that passionate project pursuits may well be compensatory convictions designed to subvert the terror of deep uncertainty.

Modular Flexibility and Integration: Assessment as Strategic Crafting

Another distinguishing feature of PPA and related methodologies is their flexibility and modular nature. This makes their use more a creative crafting than a mechanical test administration. For basic research this may be aimed at uncovering basic processes of goal construal, action, and project pursuit. For applied research this means that we can shape the assessment process to meet the distinctive requirements of the problem facing us. As seen in applied research concerned with quality of life, whether in clinical, health, or broader developmental contexts, PPA affords us the opportunity to use ad hoc assessment dimensions, and to adapt other modules in ways that directly assess the concerns of the participants and the investigators.

In chapters in this volume, personal project and personal goal methods were adopted to assess the subtle links between personal and cultural identity (Brandstätter & Lalonde, chap. 10), to measure successful transitions across the life course (Freund, chap. 9; Salmela-Aro & Little, chap. 7), and to assess the core personal projects that underlie (and can undermine) formal organizational projects (Grant, Little, & Phillips, chap. 8). PPA was used in conjunction with alternative units of analysis, but with its own idiosyncratic twist. Little and Joseph (chap. 14), for example, examined traits not only as the fixed features of conventional trait personality but also as strategic acts—free traits—that help advance core projects.

In terms of traditional research design, personal projects can be regarded as interdependent variables that can be used with equal justification as independent or dependent variables. Project dimensions used as vector scores treated normatively may be used as independent variables in experimentation and as predictor variables in applied correlational research. Under this research strategy, project dimensions of stress or enjoyment can be used in just the same way as one would use facet scales from the NEO–PI–R (Costa & McCrae, 1985) or other traditional trait or state assessment instruments. However, personal projects appraisals may also be used as dependent variables (Grant et al., chap. 8, this volume; Little, Lecci, & Watkinson, 1992; McGregor, chap. 6, this volume). Omodei and Wearing (1990) showed that personal project scores rated on the basic Murrayan needs serve as effective proxy variables for quality of life. Thus, whether as true dependent variables in experimental design or as quasi-dependent variables in correlational designs, personal projects offer idiosyncratically phrased, contextually relevant units of analysis. Indexes derived from PPA may also be treated as mediating variables that serve to link units such as traits with outcome measures relating to satisfaction or adaptation (e.g., Peterman & Lecci, chap. 12, this volume).

As evidenced by Salmela-Aro and Little (chap. 7, this volume), contemporary research also finds personal projects to be natural units of analysis for hierarchical and growth modeling and as providing a way of examining intraindividual change nested within persons during developmental sequences. Sheldon (chap. 13, this volume) demonstrates how personal goals are central to empirical research providing multilevel integration in personality, motivation, and developmental studies.

In short, this volume has demonstrated that researchers using PPA and related methodologies take a distinctive stance toward people participating in their studies and they deploy it in a flexible manner to assess factors conceived as predictors, mediators, and outcomes in both experimental and correlational designs, and as natural units for incorporation in the currently influential growth modeling and hierarchical analysis research designs.

A question that both research participants and researchers may and do ask is "Where are we going?" with projects methodology. For participants, the experience of doing PPA can help clarify, sometimes in unanticipated ways, the nature of their daily pursuits and many of them find the assessment process itself an enjoyable and valuable exercise (Omodei & Wearing, 1990; Phillips, Little, & Goodine, 1996). Therefore we give high priority to exploring new creative ways of feeding data back to individuals for purposes of self-understanding. The further development of multimedia and Web versions of PPA advances this goal considerably (see Little & Gee, chap. 2, this volume, for some early developments in these areas). It should also be mentioned that some individuals seem naturally to structure their days around projects in the rather conventional sense of deeds to be done and they may be predisposed to entering into this type of assessment exercise. Ironically, it may be those whose lives are less structured by explicit project pursuit but more by the ephemeral gusts of things that come along who may benefit most from sitting down and looking at the days of their lives. Research on the factors disposing individuals to get engaged in and benefit from the methodologies used throughout this volume would be intriguing.

For researchers, PPA is clearly different in its foundational assumptions from other assessment approaches (Little, 2000, 2005; Little & Gee, in press). Its openness to modular innovation means that PPA can be adopted to address new substantive problems, both theoretical and applied. It would be valuable to do longitudinal examinations of single core projects, large-scale endeavors that give meaning to people's lives over a longer stretch of time than those typically found in studies on project and goal pursuit. We see each of the lines of inquiry just reviewed being pursued vigorously in coming years and increased attention paid to some of the psychometric issues posed by PPA. Several of these have been addressed in past research (Little & Gee, in press) but there is a great deal of psychometric research needed to ensure that the data generated by PPA and related methodologies are both rich and reliable and as valid as measures of dynamic project pursuits can be. This will be both a continuing challenge and priority for the future.

As detailed in the opening chapters in this volume, the data gathered on personal projects have been archived in SEAbank, the social ecological analysis data bank that now contains holdings, including longitudinal studies, dating back to the 1970s. One of the goals of establishing this archival data bank is that it serves as a resource in the formulation of social policy regarding people's most cherished goals and in opening up paths to project pursuit that might facilitate flourishing, or at least a better chance to muddle through the perplexities of living.

PERSONAL PROJECTS IN PLACE, TIME, AND CULTURE: PERSONALIZATION AND INTEGRATION

The chapters in this volume have dealt with a diversity of contexts within which projects are pursued. In this section we wish to stand back and provide a somewhat more synoptic view of the social ecological features of goals, action, and personal projects, particularly the spatial, temporal, and sociocultural contexts that help shape project formulation and action (Little, 2000; Little & Ryan, 1979).[2] Each context poses important questions about the conditions necessary for successful project pursuit and the meaning that such pursuit provides in the lives of individuals and the larger community. Each also provides critical information for how sustainable project pursuit might be enhanced.

Projects in Place: The Physical Environmental Context

As described by Little (chap. 1, this volume), although the original conception of personal projects was envisioned primarily as a contribution to personality psychology, the earliest full theoretical and methodological treatment of it was published in a journal with closer links to environmental psychology and was shaped to emphasize that link (Little, 1983). Relatively little of the physical environment has figured in this volume, although there are glimpses of it when we talk about restorative niches and environments in Little and Joseph's chapter (chap. 14, this volume) on free traits. The physical milieu plays a subtler role in chapters such as Brandstätter and Lalonde's (chap. 10, this volume) exploration of projects as linking cultural and personal identities.

Studies on the physical context of project pursuit have appeared elsewhere however. Wallenius (1999, 2004) presented important research on the interdependencies of places and projects. She found that perceived supportiveness of the environment for one's personal projects predicts greater efficacy in project pursuit and higher life satisfaction and that noise stress and personal project stress interact to predict lower levels of self-reported health and higher somatic symptoms, independent of trait neuroticism.

Environmental settings both generate projects and facilitate or frustrate their pursuit. Canadian and Finnish winters provide compelling invitations to take on "shovel snow" projects as well as more exciting pursuits like skiing or at least artful slipping. Recent research in Scotland has explored the supportiveness of the physical environment on the outdoor pursuits of older persons. Researchers at the Edinburgh College of Art have adapted PPA to examine the desired outdoors projects of the elderly and the affordance provided by the immediately surrounding environment, from curb heights and cobblestones to local

---

[2]An intriguing discussion of the spatial-temporal nature of projects and their utility as units of analysis for the study of sexual differentiation is found in Binhammer, Henderson, and Moyes (1993).

lighting and transportation (Sugiyama & Ward Thompson, in press). What is important to note about such research is that the information about projects and places is local and personal. For basic research, data can be aggregated and used to test general hypotheses about spatial characteristics of goal and project pursuit. For applied purposes, however, it truly puts projects in their place with all the concrete immediacy of slippery sidewalks and rattling windows.

Projects in Time: The Temporal Context of Project Pursuit

Little (chap. 1, this volume) discussed personal projects as ways of capturing what Murray had originally envisaged with his concept of serials—temporally extended sets of salient action. Projects develop over time, although the temporal range is considerable. A personal project may be as short as a wink, which, unlike a blink, can launch a thousand joint projects between the winker and the winkee. A personal project may also be a lifelong calling ceasing only in death and, if the project pursuer has been sufficiently generative, perhaps not even then. Temporal features were a central concern in the original formulation of personal projects (Little, 1983)—indeed the article was organized around the major stages of project inception, planning, action, and termination, each with several substages.[3] These major stages are briefly discussed in this volume (Salmela-Aro & Little, chap. 7) in the context of looking at how relational issues arise at different stages in formulating and acting on projects. Ironically, and reflexively, a separate chapter on the temporal context on project pursuit was originally planned for this volume, but had to be abandoned due to the exigencies of the temporal context on project pursuit!

Chambers (chap. 5, this volume) is also deeply concerned with temporal issues, albeit primarily in the context of the linguistic formulation

---

[3]The four stages of personal project pursuit are inception, planning, action, and termination, each of which is comprised of a series of substages. The inception phase includes substages that take us from awareness (recognizing the possibility of the project), through identification, preevaluation, and acceptance (the decision to take on the project). The planning stage involves preparation for and management of the project, and comprises substages of proposal, administrative management, recruitment, and scheduling. The action stage (carrying out the activities relevant to completing the project) includes substages of engagement, control/continuity/motivation, and postevaluation. Finally, in the termination stage of completing and disengaging from the project, the substages involve end signaling, exit-barrier removal, conclusion, publication (making public the accomplishments of the project), compensation, and shutdown. Details on feedback loops and examples are provided in Little (1983).

of projects. However, his dissertation and subsequent research offers a highly sophisticated treatment of temporality from a project analytic perspective (Chambers, 2001). With some notable exceptions discussed later, the temporal aspects of personal projects have not been studied extensively and the substages have been completely ignored.

In studies of Type A personality and cardiovascular risk, the modular flexibility of PPA has been exploited by showing that, although time adequacy for projects is modestly predictive (in a negative direction) of risk, time pressure is more strongly related (in a positive direction) with such risk (Collette, 1985; Mickelson, 1984). Mavis (1981) used another imaginative temporal dimension relating to subjective age with middle-aged men. He found that men felt older in administrative projects such as "doing my tax return" and younger than their real age when engaged in sports (in those days we did not count poker as an athletic event).

One of the most extensive programs of research looking at temporal features of personal projects has been concerned with procrastination (e.g., Lay, 1986; Pychyl, 1996; Pychyl & Little, 1998; Szawlowski, 1987). In his dissertation research, Pychyl (1996) found that procrastination was a pervasive and pernicious presence in the lives of doctoral students. His highly productive Procrastination Laboratory is notable for its blend of basic and applied research (see http://http-server.carleton.ca/ ~tpychyl/). Pychyl and colleagues have explored the self-regulatory functions underlying procrastination (e.g., Blunt & Pychyl, 2005) as well as evaluating the effectiveness of counseling procedures for those who chronically put off that which was due yesterday (Pychyl & Binder, 2004). As part of that research program, Blunt and Pychyl (2000) published one of the few studies of personal project stages, showing that there are clear appraisal differences on project dimensions depending on where the project is situated on the timeline between inception and completion.

In short, the temporal contexts within which goals and projects are enacted play a critical role in determining whether they will be successful. The sustainable pursuit of core projects depends on individual differences in temporal orientation, the differential motivational impact of different stages of projects, the urgency posed by certain tasks, and the shifting horizon of project pursuit as one ages.[4]

---

[4]When we go beyond PPA methodology and examine temporal aspects of goal pursuit more broadly, several influential examples can be noted. There is an active network of researchers who have been concerned with future time perspective (e.g., Nurmi, 1991; Nuttin & Lens, 1985). Gollwitzer, Heckhausen, and colleagues have studied deliberation versus implementation mindsets in goal striving, showing that the two mindsets yield different processes, levels, and experiences of reflectiveness, memory, control, and commitment (e.g., Gollwitzer,

Although these examples attest to the considerable activity on the temporal unfolding of personal goals, such research might benefit from the detailed substage model originally formulated in personal projects research (Little, 1983), particularly in its emphasis on the joint influence of both stable personality factors on successful negotiation of substages and the orchestration of feedback from the social ecology in enhancing the likelihood that projects will be sustained or abandoned. Again, as with the spatial ecology, a highly personalized temporal ecology is revealed by the adoption of PPA and related assessment tools. Moreover, place and time can be conjoined and integrated within this procedure. It is possible to see, in the individual case, what the interrelations are between the location of one's projects and the temporal load they entail. Martennson (1977), for example, showed how well-being is inversely related to the geographical distance between places where one's daily projects are undertaken, a finding that will be all too recognizable by those who commute between homes, day care centers, and work places in a daily dash of dutiful projects.

Projects in Cultural Context: Sociogenic Influences Revisited

Many of the chapters in this volume have been concerned with how our personal goals and projects are deeply influenced by other people. Interpersonal aspects of project pursuit were reviewed (Salmela-Aro & Little, chap. 7) and found to have a pervasive effect on the formulation and enactment of goals and projects. A similar point was made in the organizational chapter (Grant et al., chap. 8) where personal projects were posited as vital links between individuals and organizations. In this section we reach beyond dyads and groups and look at the larger social systems and cultural factors within which projects are embedded. Little and Joseph (chap. 14, this volume) suggested that there is a sociogenic human nature, a set of culturally transmitted pathways through which our projects are created and channelized. What is the impact of those channels for the pursuit of projects and human well-being?

1999; Gollwitzer, Heckhausen, & Steller, 1990; Gollwitzer & Kinney, 1989). Maes and Karoly (2005) discussed three different phases of the self-regulation of personal goals: (a) selection, setting, and representation; (b) pursuit; and (c) attainment, maintenance, and disengagement. Cochran (1992) conceptualized the career as a personal project comprising a series of life tasks, which are in turn composed of action phases including preparing, goal setting, skill refining, actualizing, and completing. Finally, Carver, Scheier, and colleagues (e.g., Carver & Scheier, 1990, 1998, 2003) have studied self-regulation in goal pursuit, examining processes such as attainment (Lawrence, Carver, & Scheier, 2002) and disengagement (Wrosch, Scheier, & Miller, 2003).

Much of goal and project pursuit is sociogenically driven; that is, it arises from cultural and societal prescriptions and proscriptions about what projects to undertake and when to undertake them (Cantor, 1994; J. Heckhausen, 1999). Freund (chap. 9, this volume) is particularly convincing on the need to consider the impact of social goals as a separate and important source of influence on the life course.

We suggest that one key role of sociogenic forces is in providing what Antonovsky (1979) called a sense of coherence (Little, 1989). A sense of coherence is the belief that one's society and culture are intact and provide significance, predictability, meaning, and stability in daily life. Antonovsky postulated that a sense of coherence is salutogenic; that is, health-inducing, serving as a generalized resistance resource. He also found that a sense of coherence is lowest in transitional communities, those that have neither the predictability of traditional communal life nor the individual control afforded by modern urban society (Antonovsky, 1979). A sense of coherence, measured at the individual level should be reflected in one's everyday personal projects. Consistent with this prediction, Little (1989) reported significant relations between scores on Antonovsky's sense of coherence scale and greater meaning, community, and efficacy in personal projects and lower stress.

Two chapters in this volume can be interpreted as dealing with the impact of a sense of coherence on well-being. Brandstätter and Lalonde (chap. 10, this volume) poignantly demonstrate the costs of a loss of cultural continuity and meaning among Canadian Aboriginal youth. They emphasize the importance of personal projects as vehicles through which cultural and personal identity can be interleaved and the vital role of such a linkage for those who, like the majority of Aboriginal youth, adopt a narrative rather than essentialist view of the self. McGregor's (chap. 6, this volume) vivid description of the effects of variations in certitude between different historical epochs also implies that a lack of sociocultural coherence puts a considerable strain on individuals. We might expect that when cultures are in a state of rapid change, there will be deleterious effects on well-being, mediated by a lack of coherence and a corresponding tentativeness in one's personal project pursuits. McGregor's chapter adds an intriguing twist, however. He would expect the loss of coherence to lead some individuals, particularly those with implicit low self-esteem, to engage in compensatory passionate project pursuit. To add another twist, they might engage in a great deal of compensatory drinking.

Since its inception, personal projects research has explored questions of cultural and social influences on project pursuit. We have been particularly interested in the difference between Asian and Western countries in terms of how personal projects are constructed and pursued. For example, Xiao (1986) found that mainland Chinese students, compared with a closely matched sample of Canadian students, enjoyed their projects more. They also were considerably less likely to have initiated their projects. As one might expect from a collectivistic culture, Chinese students' projects were more likely to have been generated by their cadre or group. Richardson (2002), in exploring similarities and differences in the personal projects of Finnish, French, and Canadian students found that, although personal project dimensions were predictive of well-being in each country, the linkages were particularly strong for students in Finland. Interestingly, Haanpää (2002) also found that, whereas Russian and Finnish adolescents' personal project appraisals predicted well-being, the effects were stronger in the Finnish sample. Elliot and Friedman (chap. 3, this volume) discuss how sociocultural influences play out with respect to avoidance goals, showing that they are negatively related to subjective well-being in the United States, but unrelated in South Korea and in Russia. Recently an adaptation of PPA methodology has been used to explore the images of young women in Burkina Faso in sub-Saharan Africa. They were asked to sketch (in drawings) their personal project dreams for their futures as part of an evaluation of an international development program in the region. The resulting imagery is striking and represents the kind of creative use of PPA in contexts where we seek an understanding of project pursuit that literally has significance beyond words.[5]

Just as having space and time in which to pursue one's core projects are important factors in sustainable project pursuit, so too is living in a sociocultural context within which some degree of coherence exists that provides coherent paths along which such projects are viewed as meaningful enterprises. PPA and related methodologies allow each of these contexts to come into view and to be conjoined together within the single case. In this respect, they are person centered as well as variable centered. They are both personalized and integrative.

---

[5]This is a joint research project undertaken with Dr. Brenda Gail McSweeney of the Women's Studies Research Center/Brandeis University and Scholastique Kompaoré, Gender and Poverty Specialist/Consultant. We are grateful to Professor Phillip Stone at Harvard, who first noticed the possibilities for adapting PPA in this context.

RELEVANCE TO CORE ISSUES IN PERSONALITY, MOTIVATIONAL, AND DEVELOPMENTAL SCIENCE

This volume includes contributions from researchers who have disciplinary allegiances to three fields in particular: personality, motivational, and developmental psychology. Each of these fields is currently flourishing, partially because of major substantive and methodological advances within each field, but also because they are establishing collegial links with allied disciplines. Drawing on insights from molecular genetics to historical analysis, all three fields will serve to advance theoretical and applied goals. We believe that personal projects and related units help advance this interdisciplinary agenda (Little, 2005). We wish to examine, selectively, three areas of personality, motivational, and developmental science in which concepts featured in this volume are having an influence or could have in future research.

Contributions to Personality Science: Stability, Change, and Adaptive Flexibility

As discussed elsewhere in this volume, one of the central debates of personality science concerns the degree of stability and change in personality (for reviews, see Caspi, Roberts, & Shiner, 2005; Funder, 2001; Mischel, 2004). The Big Five personality traits, in particular, have been conceived of as dispositions that remain largely stable and consistent across the life course. We believe that the chapters in this volume shed new light on the issue of stability and change in personality.

First, several of the chapters adopt a more complex and multidimensional view of personality than those offered in dominant perspectives in the field. Rather than conceiving of each individual as occupying a single position along a continuum of personality dispositions—such that some individuals are relatively introverted and others more extraverted, for example—both Sheldon (chap. 13) and Little and Joseph (chap. 14) propose that individuals can occupy multiple positions along each continuum of personality dispositions. Sheldon argues that personality is comprised of needs, traits, goals, selves, social relations, and culture, and that individuals can organize the more labile of these levels of personality, such as personal goals, to achieve integration with the more stable of the levels, such as needs and culture. His perspective suggests that individuals can act to exercise agency over the degree of stability versus change in some levels of their personalities, whereas other levels are more biologically and socially constrained. Freund's (chap. 9, this volume) levels of goal representation theory, although not dealing with trait units as such, similarly conceives of different capacities to change depending on the degree of constraint imposed by the level of goal pursued. Automatic, nonconscious goals are particularly interesting in that they are evoked by repeated situational associations and may give rise, particularly in old age, to an evoked consistency all too familiar to others, but perhaps not to oneself (Bargh & Ferguson, 2000).

Little and Joseph (chap. 14, this volume) propose that the biogenic, sociogenic, and idiogenic natures of humans create possibilities for considerable inconsistency. An individual born in China may be a biogenic extravert due to high levels of cortical reactivity to stimulation, a sociogenic introvert due to internalizing cultural norms and values through socialization, and an idiogenic ambivert to adapt to the varying expectations of people encountered during a voyage around the world. Noteworthy about this perspective is that it also specifies varying degrees of mutability accordingly for each of the three natures. Biogenic natures, due to their strong genetic and intrauterine origins, are likely to be highly stable. Sociogenic natures, due to their origins in early socialization experiences, are likely to be relatively stable but subject to change based on internalization of a different set of cultural norms and values. Idiogenic natures, due to their distinctively personal origins, are most likely to change according to the commitments, life events, and even eccentricities of the individuals enacting them. These perspectives suggest that personality scientists may broaden and deepen their understandings of personality change by conceptualizing personality in terms of multiple natures with varying degrees of stability. In this respect, project analytic research offers a middle-level bridge between the higher level stabilities explored in trait research and the increasingly influential social cognitive learning models that explore microlevel stabilities or distinctive signatures of individuals in situations (Cervone, 2004; Mischel, 2004).

Some chapters in this volume move beyond the consistency theories that dominate both personality and social psychology toward an understanding of individuals as willing to cope with, and even seek out, inconsistency to advance personal projects that truly matter to them. For example, Little and Joseph (chap. 14, this volume) explicitly invoke the notion of acting out of character, which entails engaging in free traits that are incongruent with one or more natures. Cognitive dissonance theorists would remind us that such a condition is deeply discomforting and there will be strong efforts to reduce such dissonance (e.g., Elliot & Devine, 1994; Festinger, 1957). Although one might expect conative dissonance to be even more noxious than cognitive dissonance, acting in a free-traited manner to advance a core project is dissonance inducing. Yet people choose to act in free-traited ways despite the likely increase in discomfort entailed. In pursuit of core personal projects that provide meaning in their lives, character might trump consistency.

Brandstätter and Lalonde (chap. 10, this volume) also deal with consistency and change in an original way, positing differences in beliefs about the persistence of self by those holding narrativist or essentialist views and that these orientations are deeply influenced by one's culture. Indeed, their chapter brings a distinctive perspective both to studies of personality development and to issues in both cross-cultural and cultural psychology where units such as personal projects may illuminate issues that are less clear when viewed through the lens of traits (see Church, 2000).

Several of the chapters in this volume suggest that particular characteristics of project or goal systems are more salutary than others regardless of the traits of the individual enacting the projects, whereas other chapters advocate a "fit" perspective in which the effects of project system characteristics are moderated by the traits of the individual. For example, Elliot and Friedman (chap. 3) and Chambers (chap. 5) assert that avoidance goals are detrimental to well-being, whereas Peterman and Lecci (chap. 12) contend that avoidance goals are conducive to well-being for hypochondriacs. As a second example, Salmela-Aro and Little (chap. 7) report evidence that pursuing a high proportion of interpersonal, social, and relational projects is conducive to well-being, whereas Little and Joseph (chap. 14) review findings that such projects facilitate well-being for extraverts but undermine well-being for introverts. Clearly, specification of the boundary conditions pertaining to both main effects and domain effects need to be part of our continuing research agenda. There will no doubt be some cases where simple moderator variables are needed to detect a posited effect; in other cases we might find evidence relating to different levels of aggregation, where the main effects of project system characteristics at one level may be attenuated or even reversed by relevant personality traits at another level, an example of Simpson's paradox (Little, 2005).

Perhaps the most central theme sounded throughout the book on issues related to personality stability and change is the adaptive flexibility of human personalities as viewed through the perspective of the goal and project pursuit. Both resolute stability and chimerical change are detectable as we track people and their projects over time. The stability may be the result of biogenic or evolutionary pressures or it may derive from consciously formulated and cherished goals—idiogenic imperatives that will not be compromised. Similarly, the flexibility may be a biologically rooted easy-going nature, a sociogenic accommodation to the pressures of the moment, or a later life commitment to bring comfort and joy to one's very surprised family.

Contributions to Motivational Science: Self-Regulation and Affect

Many of the chapters in this volume contribute to research on self-regulation and affect in motivational psychology. Next, we briefly discuss the contributions of the chapters to research on approach–avoidance orientation in self-regulation, one of the old but tasty chestnuts in motivation. We also examine metamotivational states and affect in reversal theory, one of the newer perspectives that deserves chewing on.

Approach–Avoidance Orientation in Self-Regulation. Several of the chapters focus on how an understanding of the self-regulatory dynamics of approach–avoidance motives can advance current understandings of personal goal and project pursuit. Elliot and Friedman (chap. 3, this volume) and Chambers (chap. 5, this volume) generally agree that approach and avoidance motives are mutually exclusive (see also Ogilvie & Rose, 1995; Ogilvie, Rose, & Heppen, 2001). On the other hand, McGregor (chap. 6, this volume) proposes that motives to avoid uncertainty and anxiety may lead individuals to adopt and pursue projects with passionate approach motives. In his view, avoidance motives may give rise to approach goals and projects. How might these conflicting perspectives be resolved?

A personal projects perspective highlights that approach and avoidance motives for project pursuit may not be mutually exclusive. For example, when pursuing the project of "rebuild my relationship with my wife," an individual likely has an ideal positive outcome in mind that he is approaching (e.g., a loving marriage) and a feared negative outcome in mind that he is avoiding (e.g., a divorce). Whether he articulates the project in terms of approach or avoidance motives is likely influenced by both individual differences and contextual factors (e.g., Higgins, 1997, 1998). We suggest then that although most people phrase their projects in terms of either approach or avoidance motives, there are usually both sets of motives embedded within any pursuit. The concern is not whether an approach or avoidance motive guides the pursuit, but rather which motive is more influential in guiding the pursuit. Motives, like goals and projects, are organized into hierarchical systems guided by basic values (e.g., Schwartz & Bardi, 2001) and possible selves (e.g., Markus & Nurius, 1986), and most goals and projects are composed of smaller goals and projects and nested in constellations of larger goals and projects. We thus expect that individuals often carry both approach and avoidance motives for a given pursuit, with one set of motives temporarily or chronically more salient than another.

Researchers may therefore gain new insights into the dynamics of approach and avoidance project pursuit by focusing on approach and avoidance as separate motives instead of opposite poles of one continuum of motives. They may do so by asking participants to rate their projects on separate approach and avoidance dimensions, which would allow for the examination of the independence of, and interactions between, approach and avoidance motives from the actor's perspective (see Little, 1983; Riediger, chap. 4, this volume, for an identical treatment of measuring the positive and negative impact of projects).[6]

Metamotivational States and Affect in Reversal Theory. In addition to self-regulation research, a personal projects perspective can also inform and be informed by reversal theory (Apter, 1984, 2001), which may be a strong candidate for providing an organizing framework for the motivational and affective dimensions of personal project appraisals. Reversal theory is based on two core assumptions: (a) that peo-

---

[6] Researchers might find value in a 2 × 2 project pursuit scheme in which approach motives are coded as high or low and avoidance motives are coded as high or low. The low–low cell may involve the absence of a project, and the low–high and high–low cells represent the current focus of research. The high–high cell, in which individuals are pursuing their projects based on both approach and avoidance motives, has received little attention in motivation research. The presence of strong approach and avoidance motives may signal high project importance and commitment, where the individual is deeply concerned about the consequences of both success and failure, and motivation is reinforced by attention to potential benefits and costs. At the same time, these multiple motives may be overwhelming to the individual (e.g., Kiviniemi, Snyder, & Omoto, 2002). We believe a consideration of the role of multiple approach and avoidance motives in influencing goal and project pursuit represents a promising direction for further research, one that might guide researchers toward a return to early research on approach–avoidance conflict (e.g., Miller & Kraeling, 1952) and more recent research on variations in levels of action identification (Vallacher & Wegner, 1987) and misperceptions of approach and avoidance motivation (Miller & Nelson, 2002).

ple experience a basic, finite set of metamotivational states that drive their cognitions, emotions, and actions; and (b) that these states exist as opposing pairs, and contextual and personal factors can generate switches, or reversals, from one pole to the other.

The most extensively studied pair of metamotivational states is *telic–paratelic*. In telic states, individuals are goal oriented and serious minded in pursuit of an important purpose. In paratelic states, individuals are activity oriented and playful, engaged in the activity for its own sake (see also Ryan & Deci, 2000). Each state is associated with a different experience of emotions. Telic states result in anxiety when arousal is heightened through threats or demands, and relaxation when tasks are completed successfully. Paratelic states result in boredom when stimulation is low and pleasant excitement when stimulation is high. The other pairs of states are *autic–alloic* (self-focused vs. other-focused), *conformist–negativistic* (compliance-focused vs. independence-focused), and *mastery–sympathy* (taking and yielding by experiencing the world in terms of power and control vs. giving and receiving by experiencing the world in terms of giving and receiving).

By specifying that the emotions experienced in project pursuit depend on the metamotivational state of the individual, reversal theory is promising as a framework for organizing the affective experience of personal projects. Reversal theory suggests that affective experiences of personal projects can be both organized and predicted by a consideration of the four pairs of metamotivational states. Appraisals of personal projects according to telic–paratelic, autic–alloic, conformist–negativistic, and mastery–sympathy metamotivational states are likely to provide explanatory accounts of why particular motivational orientations and emotions are experienced in particular projects. Initial studies of the linkages between measures derived from reversal theory and personal project measures have been very encouraging (see, e.g., Chambers, 2001).

At the same time, a project analytic perspective has the potential to advance reversal theory and further our understanding of the affective experience of project pursuit. In the service of core personal projects, individuals may be required to enact multiple metamotivational states simultaneously or at the very least in rapid alternating saccades. For example, a professor seeking to engage his or her students may engage in "serious play," using humor to convey an important lesson and enacting both goal-oriented and activity-oriented states. A mother may carry out the personal project of spending more time with her son with the intention of simultaneously enriching her own life and her child's, enacting both autic and alloic states.

Reversal theory makes the strong claim that pairs of metamotivational states are phenomenologically exclusive and oppositional. We are more inclined to see these states as orthogonal modes that can exist in separation or in synergy.[7] Individuals may thus experience telic and paratelic states in tandem, focusing on enjoying both a process and an outcome. They may be enjoined by their projects to enact both autic and alloic states, focusing on self-interest and other interest. They may be both compliant and seeking to achieve independence, or simultaneously taking and yielding and giving and receiving. We hope that future research will apply reversal theory to the affective realm of personal project pursuit and examine how project commitment may yield synergies between the proposed poles of metamotivational states.

Contributions to Developmental Science: Projects Across the Life Course

Many of the contributions to this volume were written by developmental researchers with a strong life course perspective (see in particular Freund, chap. 9; Riediger, chap. 4; Salmela-Aro & Little, chap. 7; Wiese, chap. 11). A central theme of these chapters is how individuals navigate the transitions between developmental stages. Both goals about one's personal future and projects that anticipate and bridge transitions have been studied. We wish to highlight, by way of illustration, three stages of life, two involving life transitional periods and one final stage of life, by way of both emphasizing common themes and stimulating further research in developmental science.

New Life: The Transition to Parenthood. The first transition and one whose success or failure will ramify throughout one's life is, of course, one's birth, which is simultaneously a transition for the parent or parents. We have seen how expectant parents whose projects flexibly shift to concerns about parenthood are predictive of greater well-being after the transition to this onerous new state is completed (see Salmela-Aro & Little, chap. 7, this volume). Clearly, parental well-being is likely to be salutary for the newborn child. A study involving measures

---

[7]It should be noted that Apter himself explored cognitive synergies as underlying domains as disparate as humor and transcendental experience. However, he saw such synergies as applying to the perception of external events rather than experiencing internal states.

of successful birthing, including physical measures of successful delivery, showed that a critical factor was the emotional support provided by the spouse (McKeen, 1984).[8]

A recent doctoral dissertation (Churchill, 2005) has cast further light on this transition period by creatively adapting PPA to address the theoretical debate over the adaptive significance of optimism. Churchill presented strong evidence for constructive realism during pregnancy, finding that women who thought about both the positive and negative aspects of delivery and subsequent mothering had higher levels of well-being and more adaptive restructuring of personal projects 3 months postnatal than did mothers with either a positive or negative orientation. This was especially so when the transition was accompanied by unexpected negative surprises. Her findings are supportive of one of the key propositions of the social ecological model of personal projects (Little, 1999, 2000; Little & Ryan, 1979), which postulates that a sense of control is adaptive to the extent that it is based on an accurate reading of ecosystem resources and constraints.

Adolescence: Parents, Peers, and Project Pursuit.   The study of adolescents has been a major focus of project analytic research since its inception (Little, 1987). We have consistently found that project dimensions for this group, relative to older groups, were more negative, with a greater degree of stress and lower degrees of enjoyment in their daily projects. In attempting to clarify this, we examined the project appraisals as broken out by different content categories. One of the most interesting findings in this set of studies was that the projects in which adolescents felt most themselves were projects that involved others, including projects involving team sports, romantic relationships, and—highest of all—community projects, such as volunteering. To be clear, volunteering projects were not high in frequency, but for those who were engaged in them, such pursuits were extremely high in terms of self-expression. It raises the question of whether individualistic self-identity and communitarian engagement with others, often regarded as competitive claims on the developing self, may in fact be more closely linked. Perhaps, instead of needing to consolidate an identity before moving on to more intimate exchanges with others, identity and inti-

---

[8]In a fascinating convergence of findings across disparate domains, Dowden (2004) discovered precisely the same project variable, emotional support by others, as a critical factor for entrepreneurs giving birth to their new ventures. A priority research topic is precisely how people convey emotional support for new ventures, be they new creatures or new companies.

macy are coconstituted in projects that involve feelings both of being needed and of having something to give. Much more research is needed to determine if this is a replicable and robust effect and whether new forms of project pursuit (e.g., computer chat rooms) are serving a similar function.

A comprehensive and compelling study of young adolescent project pursuit was carried out by Wilmut (1997), who was particularly interested in examining the role that parents and peers played in the projects of students. Whereas prior research had used a dimension of "others' view of importance" of each project, Wilmut created separate columns for peers and parents. The research was carried out prior to the much publicized research claiming the relative unimportance of parental influence, relative to peer influence, during this period of development (Harris, 1995). Wilmut showed that well-being was higher if these adolescents felt their projects were viewed as important by their peers, but even more so if viewed as important by their parents. It is possible that this privileging of parental support over peer support is restricted to project pursuit and would not be picked up by other units of analysis, and it is hard to know to what extent the results are generalizable. However, it illustrates the way in which the modular flexibility of PPA can be used to explore, in a more fine-grained fashion, issues of development that have both theoretical and public policy implications of considerable importance.

Several chapters in this volume take an explicitly life-span developmental perspective, with strong representation by scholars affiliated over the years with the Max Planck Institute for Human Development in Berlin (Freund, Riediger, Salmela-Aro, Wiese). Their distinctive contribution has been to demonstrate how the selection, optimization, and compensation (SOC) model can be tested and expanded by the use of personal goal constructs (e.g., Freund & Baltes, 2000). A particularly important aspect of this model, exemplified by (Freund, chap. 9, this volume) is the importance of age-related institutional structures that set up expectations about when one should be engaged in certain tasks and projects. Higher well-being has been consistently found in those who are flexible and able to adjust their goal priorities in anticipation of upcoming developmental transitions.

Rather than seeing developmental transitions as the inevitable progression of epigenetic stages or as the product of simple social learning, the perspectives represented in this volume see developmental progressions as intimately tied to the balancing of the same multiple demands that we saw as essential to studying personality. Thus biogenic factors of hormonal changes, the sociogenic impact of both peer and parental expectations. and the idiogenic choices of desired possible selves need to be orchestrated by adolescents in transition to adulthood.

However, life-span theorists point to an additional and distinctively important feature and constant accompaniment to this orchestration—the unrelenting beat of the developmental clock. The well-being of adolescents en route to adulthood is enhanced if their projects are orchestrated so that both social expectations and developmental deadlines are met, a skill that will serve them well in later years (Heckhausen, 2002; Heckhausen & Schulz, 1999).

Personal Projects in Old Age: Selectivity and the Self. It is difficult to talk about the transition to old age, particularly as the current cohort of baby boomers are enjoying greater health and longevity than previous generations and have virtually redefined the possible projects, probable selves, and social expectations of what one can and should be doing in the later stages of life. However, it is clear that there are two life-span developmental trajectories that need to be considered—one of general growth and one of general decline—and that as aging progresses the relative rate of decline increases (Labouvie-Vief, 1981). In contrast with earlier perspectives (e.g., Havighurst, 1963) that viewed aging as primarily an adaptation of the individuals to a given context, both the Max Planck Institute contributors to this volume and those of us working within the social ecological perspective emphasize the balance between personal competencies and contextual affordances (see Freund, chap. 9, this volume, in particular).

Such balance is achieved not only by reacting to change but, as Murray argued almost seven decades ago, by proactive selection of goals and projects that are valued by the individual (Labouvie-Vief, 1981). Many of these goals will be attempts to deal with the loss of resources, both internal and external, that predictably accompany aging. However, the compensatory component of the SOC model is particularly helpful in understanding the nature of project pursuit in later age. For example, the reduction of social network size as one gets older is not simply a matter of passively observing the demise of friends, the dispersal of family, or the decline of flirtatiousness as a self-defining feature. Carstensen's (1992) socioemotional selectivity theory makes a strong case that as one gets older there is an explicit narrowing of the focus of interpersonal relations to a smaller number of special people. The reduction in network size as one gets older is not simply a matter of biogenic introversion kicking in, although it is not unlikely that sensitivity to overstimulation may play a role, but an explicit selection of goals and roles designed to advance core projects that may be centered on a few key people in one's life.

Such selective optimization and compensation helps explain one of our earliest studies with personal projects. In a multiple-cohort, longitudinal investigation we examined how projects were rated by three different groups, averaging in their 20s, 40s, and 60s (Little, Carlsen, Glavin, & Lavery, 1981). One of the most striking findings was that the personal projects of the oldest group were consistently more meaningful, manageable, efficacious, supported, and less stressful than the projects of the other groups.

At the time, these results seemed to run counter to the stereotypes of aging (although it is noteworthy that today we would not regard the 60s as old as we did 30 years ago). We looked closely at the content of the projects of this older group to determine what they were engaged in that appeared to have a salutary effect on their lives. The common element appeared to be that they had scaled down their projects. At first we thought this was a kind of accommodation to inevitable decline; instead, it seems more consistent with the view expressed earlier about the active shaping of one's commitments and selective optimization and compensation. For example, one woman who had been an author in her middle years and had wanted to write the "great Canadian novel" moved on to another project, "give workshops to young women on the craft of writing." In talking about this shift in her projects, she suggested that now she may be sowing the seeds for multiple great Canadian novels and this was fine with her. Such compensatory projects are not simply ways of dealing with personal decline, but potential vehicles for generativity, enhancing the capacities of a new generation of aspirants to the creative life (e.g., McAdams & de St. Aubin, 1998).

What is the relation of the features of personal projects to well-being across the life span? Two meta-analyses have examined this, one focusing on subjective well-being (Wilson, 1990), the other on depressive affect (Little et al., 2005). Although there were not noticeable differences in the factors influencing well-being at different ages, these samples were heavily tilted toward younger individuals. What was very clear, however, was that the same features of personal projects that predict positive aspects of well-being are virtually identical (in reverse direction) to those predicting depressive affect. As reported elsewhere in this volume (Little, chap. 1), being engaged in meaningful, manageable, supported projects that are not too stressful is conducive to subjective well-being and a deterrent to depressive affect.

Although personal project appraisals in old age might predict both positive and negative features of mood and perceived quality of life, the type of projects engaged in may be differentially associated with positive affect. Lawton, Moss, Winter, and Hoffman (2002), in a study of the personal projects of 600 community residents aged 70 or older, discovered six major types of project pursuit: activities of daily living, active recreation, other-oriented activities, intellectual activities, home planning, and spiritual moral activities. They reported that most indexes of personal projects were associated with positive affect and valuation of life, but only one was associated with depression. Recent clinical work has confirmed the utility of using personal project appraisals to predict vulnerability to bipolar disorder (Meyer, Beevers, & Johnson, 2004), so it is likely that the inclusion of appraisal dimensions with an older sample might predict both positive and negative affect in old age.

In an address by Coleman (Blitheway & Coleman, 1997), a longitudinal study of aging was reported in which participants were invited to form a narrative construction about the major themes and sense of personal continuity in their lives over a 20-year period. Most were able to find coherence in their life's stories (McAdams, 1993) and for those over 80 there was a greater sense of continuity than discontinuity in their lives over time. However, there was a subgroup, primarily women, who were not able to see their past lives as narratives but more as a series of scattered events beyond their control. Interestingly, for some of these women, growing older was a positive experience because, for the first time, they had a sense of control over their lives. This finding is intriguing on two counts. First, we have found that studies of personal narratives can be enhanced by starting with personal projects from the past, as a kind of narrative seed, and then having individuals trace through, retrospectively, the stories that may link the projects. In short, there may well be a narrative, albeit a rather more fragmentary one that can be stimulated by reflecting on the origins and consequences of deeds done and projects pursued in one's past. Second, the subset of women for whom old age brings a greater chance of authorship in their own narratives is, for us, an example of how idiogenic natures may, with age and circumstance, have a chance to displace the life-long claim of sociogenic natures.

In chapter 1 there was a footnote about the members of our Personal Projects interest group and it included a reference to Ai-Li S. Chin, who, in her mid-80s, has been grappling with precisely these issues. In discussions, she has mentioned how, in her own development in later life, she has been able to emerge out of the "cocoon of Confucianism" that had channeled her identity and action for so many years. Coleman's research and Chin's reflections are of particular significance to the first author. Coleman was a young student of Little's at Oxford in the late 1960s, and is now a senior professor writing about seniors; Chin is a valued new student of personal projects who is instructing her juniors about the experience of seniors. This is a strangely satisfying semisymmetry.

HUMAN FLOURISHING

As discussed in chapter 1, the personal projects perspective has been concerned, since its inception, with well-being, happiness, and the quality of lives. It has been informed by philosophical scholarship that has been concerned with issues of the quality of life and human flourishing and has been explicitly linked to the development of data banks that can serve as social indicators for decision makers (Little, chap. 1, this volume; Little & Ryan, 1979).

Human Flourishing and Positive Psychology

We conceive of human flourishing as comprising three important functions: a sense of personal well-being, the sustainable pursuit of core projects, and having impacts that enhance the well-being of others (see Salmela-Aro & Little, chap. 7, this volume, for a discussion of this in the context of interpersonal relations). In this concluding section, we revisit several of these issues and draw together what we have learned about the positive aspects of the human condition. Phrased this way, it is appropriate to link this volume with the burgeoning positive psychology movement and with closely related work in positive organizational scholarship. The focus of this movement is on understanding and enhancing the flourishing of individuals, groups, and institutions (for reviews, see Cameron, Dutton, & Quinn, 2003; Gable & Haidt, 2005; Linley & Joseph, 2004; Seligman & Csikszentmihalyi, 2000; Snyder &

Lopez, 2002). The movement has been sufficiently important to have attracted critical commentary.[9] Regardless of whether one is enthusiastic, contrarian, ambivalent, or neutral about positive psychology, it has clearly generated considerable interest from academics, practitioners, and laypersons. We should also point out that six of the contributors to this volume are actively involved in the positive psychology movement. Sheldon, for example, has been one of the generative figures in the field (see Sheldon & King, 2001). Other contributors would be best characterized as agnostic on the movement.

On balance, the positive psychology movement has the potential to make valuable contributions to the study of personal projects and the social ecological model of well-being. One example of such a contribution derives from the growing body of research on positive emotions (e.g., Fredrickson, 1998, 2001), which indicates that positive emotions both broaden individuals' momentary thought and action capabilities and build enduring physical, social, and psychological resources conducive to flourishing. The "broaden and build" model suggests that positive emotions may lubricate transitions between project stages and substages, increase capabilities for the awareness and identification of multiple possible projects, and enable disengagement from stressful personal projects.

A second example is drawn from recent research on the health benefits of writing about personal goals. Whereas prior research assumed that the physical and psychological health benefits of writing accrued through the mechanisms of catharsis and insight, research from a positive psychological perspective advances a different perspective: Writing about one's personal goals and projects can improve subjective well-being by enabling individuals to visualize and experience efficacy in enacting desirable possible selves (King, 2001). This evidence suggests that merely appraising one's personal projects may enhance flourishing by enabling the inception and planning of projects that are associated with a favorable personal identity, as well as constructive action in service of achieving these projects.

At the same time, this volume has the potential to make important contributions to positive psychology and to positive organizational scholarship. The most central contribution is the very creation of a unit

---

[9]For example, criticisms have been levied against positive psychology, including accusations of ideological bias, false dichotomies of good and bad, methodological weaknesses, and insufficient attention to the historically, temporally, and culturally contingent nature of positive (e.g., George, 2004; Guignon, 2002; Held, 2004; Lazarus, 2003a, 2003b; Sandage & Hill, 2001).

of analysis for predicting, explaining, and enhancing the flourishing of individuals and social collectives. The personal project, by serving as a personally salient unit at a middle level of analysis, enables researchers to study how both individuals and groups select, construe, pursue, and flourish in their activities and their lives. Moreover, as most of the chapters in this volume demonstrate in some way, the nature of personal project and goal pursuit has direct implications for understanding and for enhancing human flourishing.

Flourishing as Sustainable Project Pursuit

We have organized the volume to bring together contributions concerned with internal (conative, self-regulatory) processes, with external, contextual forces, and with the diverse ways in which well-being and flourishing can be conceived. As stated at the outset, we are fully aware that these are rather arbitrary divisions because of the interpenetration of conative and contextual features in everyday lives. Yet it will be helpful, if only as a thematic template, to highlight the relevance of each of these sections and the light they may shed on human flourishing. Part I provides a historical overview of how personal projects research and the study of well-being have been conceptual partners for decades and how the methodology is designed to incorporate new theoretical constructs into our empirical examinations of flourishing as individual well-being, as sustainable pursuit, and as social goods.

Internal Dynamics of Project Pursuit. In Part II, the common focus is on the internal, self-regulatory factors that lead to successful project formulation prior to throwing oneself fully into action. Elliot and Friedman (chap. 3) show that avoidance-focused personal goals can be detrimental to psychological and physical health. Similarly, Chambers (chap. 5) demonstrates that doing-focused phrasings of projects may enhance well-being, whereas trying-focused projects may actually undermine it. Riediger (chap. 4) warns us of the benefits of having projects that are mutually facilitative, particularly with older people. Whereas both Chambers (chap. 5) and Elliot and Friedman (chap. 3) highlight the costs of avoidance projects, McGregor (chap. 6) suggests that such projects may indirectly have beneficial implications for flourishing. He examines how avoidance-focused concerns in one domain of life may motivate individuals to adopt approach-focused projects in another domain of life to cope with or avoid personal uncertainty, and thus enhance their well-being. Together, these chapters suggest that approach-focused projects tend to be more facilitative of well-being than avoidance-focused projects, although there may be important boundary conditions that attenuate this relation. McGregor's (chap. 6) example of the passionate pursuit of the building of the St. John's basilica highlights that projects that may begin as compensatory, self-regulatory ways of enhancing individual-level well-being may result in concrete cultural products that endure and delight. His chapter provides the natural segue to considerations about the outside world of churches and chat rooms and the social ecology of project pursuit: from flourishing as personal well-being to flourishing as social relations. From a philosophical perspective, this represents a shift from seeing project pursuit as requiring prudential virtues that enhance one's own well-being to requiring moral virtues in which one's projects are evaluated in terms of the social good that may accrue as a result of their successful pursuit.

External Dynamics of Project Pursuit. In Part III, the external, social ecological factors that can facilitate and frustrate project and goal pursuit are highlighted. Salmela-Aro and Little (chap. 7) emphasize that personal projects are not merely individualistic pursuits, but are interlaced with interpersonal themes, from their very inception to their being completed or forestalled. Just as Riediger (chap. 4) looks at the formulation of goals to optimize mutual facilitation within persons, Salmela-Aro and Little look at the same process in terms of mutual facilitation between persons. The same theme emerges in the organizational chapter by Grant et al. (chap. 8) who propose that work may be more effectively redesigned to enhance well-being at the level of the project than the job, recommending that architects of work redesign interventions explore the value of assessing and altering employees' personal projects. The point here is not just that work environments need to be humanized or detoxified, a core theme of positive organizational scholarship, but that it is essential to understand the nature of the personal projects people are pursuing to help shape higher levels of mutual goal pursuits in organizations. Freund (chap. 9) adopts a comprehensive model of levels of goals in which a key theme is concordance between personal goals and personal and social expectations throughout the life span. Her perspective is particularly important in reminding us of the importance of concordance between projects and social ecologies in promoting well-being. This includes the possibility that some of the most important types of personal goals may be operating tacitly and yet shape daily action in unexpected ways, particularly in later adulthood. Brandstätter and Lalonde (chap. 10) make a very strong case for the pivotal role of projects in providing vehicles for interweaving personal identity and cultural identity. Although they show the tragic consequences of the loss of cultural identity among some Aboriginal peoples, they also raise a central point that we expand on later, the importance of that word *some*—of the need to avoid overgeneralizing about groups of people when we are formulating conceptions of human flourishing at the societal level.

Varieties and Vicissitudes of Flourishing.   In Part IV, on the varieties of well-being, several of the foregoing themes are revisited. Wiese (chap. 11) addresses this question: Is it goal attainment or goal pursuit that makes us happy? She challenges the common assumption that the successful completion of a personal project is beneficial to well-being. She suggests that successful completion of projects enhances subjective well-being when progress is faster than expected, when the individual attributes success to internal rather than external factors, and when projects are congruent with one's identity and with sociocultural expectations. Peterman and Lecci (chap. 12) treat projects as dependent variables indicative of well-being, suggesting that individual well-being suffers when mental and physical illnesses such as hypochondriasis and cancer interfere with project pursuit.

The topics of illness and disability are particularly relevant to our conception of human flourishing and deserve special comment here. When one is seriously ill or has suffered a sudden injury, the saliency of one's core projects can often become painfully clear. Such insights may have both a negative effect in terms of difficulties in therapeutic compliance but, ironically, they may also have a salutary effect when individuals restructure their project systems to both accommodate treatment and give priority to core projects. This insight about the vicissitudes of flourishing has been particularly important in research and practice in the rehabilitation fields, especially in occupational therapy and in the occupational science undergirding it. Christiansen, in particular, has been an articulate advocate for the use of a project analytic framework in rehabilitation, occupational science, and general health promotion (e.g., Christianson, Backman, Little, & Nguyen, 1999; Christiansen, Little, & Backman, 1998). Indeed, occupational therapists and related professionals are among the most active of researchers using personal projects as analytic units.

An especially interesting example of how awareness of core projects can be helpful in structuring rehabilitative activities has been provided by research practitioners in the United Kingdom. Hill and Aspinall have been working with patients suffering from macular degeneration and other "low vision" problems (e.g., Aspinall, 2005). In planning rehabilitative exercises with these patients, they experimented with using PPA to identify patients' most important concerns. They then created an index of which projects might serve as the most effective entry point for rehabilitative activity. The index combined the patient's ratings on several projects and the therapist's ratings of the likelihood that visual rehabilitative techniques might actually improve functioning in that domain. Those projects with the highest multiplicative ratings, a utility index, served as the targets for intervention. For example, one woman whose core projects centered on social entertaining had subsidiary projects that involved both shopping and cooking. On the basis of their intervention index, the therapist focused on the latter project, redesigning the cooking area of the kitchen to accommodate to the visual challenges experienced by the patient. This is a fine illustration of how meaning in one's life, in terms of core projects, can be discovered in the context of disability as well as being promoted by highly targeted intervention.[10]

The two final chapters in Part IV are explicitly concerned with questions of well-being, flourishing, and the role of goals and projects in promoting those states. Sheldon (chap. 13) argues that projects that are congruent with multiple levels of personality—needs, traits, goals, selves, social relations, and culture—are facilitative of well-being. Little and Joseph (chap. 14) propose a tripartite conceptualization of personality comprising biogenic, sociogenic, and idiogenic natures, and suggest that the pursuit of personal projects incongruent with each nature can be costly for psychological and physical well-being, yet serve to provide and sustain a sense of meaning. Together, these chapters highlight the complexity of human natures and personalities, and underscore that the pursuit of personal projects has the potential to enhance or undermine well-being, depending on whether one's projects are congruent or incongruent with one's natures and personalities. There are both commonalities and differences in these two perspectives. Both empha-

---

[10]Details of this procedure emerged from conversations between the first author and Hill and Aspinall in Edinburgh in 2004. We are indebted to them for allowing us to refer to their research here, but we should underscore that it is still in its preliminary stages. That said, it serves as a fine example of the imaginative adaptation of PPA for rehabilitation.

size that there are core, evolutionary aspects to project pursuits, that there are cultural factors that channelize them, and that there are idiosyncratic features that make project pursuit truly personal.

One apparent difference lies in the extent to which congruency, coherence, and concordance are regarded as the ultimate criteria for defining human flourishing. Here, Sheldon (chap. 13, this volume) appears to be on the "yes" side. Little and Joseph (chap. 14, this volume) are more ambivalent. In their model, strategic imbalance in project pursuit, where physical costs are willingly incurred to advance a core project that matters deeply, can be counted as evidence of flourishing. Of course it might also be counted as evidence of incipient perishing, which raises the perdurable question of which, if any core projects are worth dying for. We do not attempt to answer that question, nor are we sure that we can do so adequately without a platoon of philosophers yelling instructions at us.

There are two remaining issues that need to be addressed to round out our project on personal project pursuit: an examination of the public policy implications of the perspectives presented in this volume, and some caveats about how to advance research and practice in this area without falling into some dangerous traps.

POLICY IMPLICATIONS OF PERSONAL PROJECT PURSUIT

With rare exceptions, the ability to flourish is supported and sustained by multiple others. These supporting actors include not only family and friends, but also those explicitly mandated to intervene in lives and communities so as to better the human condition and enhance human flourishing. These agents include voluntary and philanthropic organizations that aim to create more vibrant communities and governments that have responsibility for implementing public policies so as to benefit entire cities and nations. When we move up to intervention at this scale, does the study of personal goals and projects have anything to contribute to the development of more effective public policy?

We would respond with a definitive yes, on several levels. An obvious response takes us back to where we started, with the distinctiveness of the methodology. Using a personal projects lens for the development of public policy would impel policymakers to start with a political conception of people that takes them seriously as agents, as Sen (1985) advocated in his capability approach, as do feminist perspectives on public policy. Such a conception involves inquiring into what people think they are doing and what facilitates and frustrates the realization of their goals and projects. When formulating public policy on a national scale, exhaustive research on individuals' projects and the differences among them is impractical. What is practical is participatory research and means of engaging a sufficient number of citizens from a particular community or population group to learn how a proposed program or policy might affect their lives. In short, the policy process would reflect the logic of personal projects methodology by asking people directly. They may just tell us something that we did not already know based on logic models, theoretical stances, or ideological orientations. To the extent that existing databanks, such as SEAbank, already contain information about the personal projects of different communities and their effect on well-being, policymakers are better able to ask the right questions of citizens. More than having good data, however, a projects perspective on policy speaks to the need for fair procedures and for being broadly inclusive in engaging citizens to capture the real nature of agency (Peter, 2003).

A second-order response is that public policies and programs could be built on a better understanding of the potential substitutability or compensatory nature of projects. As the contributors to this volume working with the SOC model have illustrated so well, underlying goals are achieved in different ways as people age. The goal may stay the same while the pursuits or the means of achieving it are reinvented as needed by declining capabilities. When the age of a population, lack of financial resources (on the part of individuals or public authorities), or other factors constrain certain pursuits, what alternatives might be provided that would have more or less the same impact? Although the concept of substitutability has long been applied in occupational therapy and recreational planning, the use of personal projects as an analytical focus allows it to be extended to many other fields, such as urban design and social and cultural programs.

A third level to our response points to the capacity of personal projects analysis to connect personal identities and projects with cultural identities and projects. As Brandstätter and Lalonde (chap. 10, this volume) illustrate, successful pursuit of the community project of self-governance for indigenous peoples is reflected in lower suicide rates and enhanced pursuit of an individual's projects. As they note, we could not explain why Aboriginal communities that have gained greater control over local services and over their own self-determination have higher indicators of well-being by using the usual methods of program evaluation. If we focused, as program evaluation so often does, on attitudes toward the acquisition of fire-fighting equipment or a local police force, we would clearly miss the point. A projects approach should also provide a caution against being too enthralled with the current popularity of outcome measurement that collects population health or related indicators and that assesses programs by their impact on these high-level indicators.

Finally, the contribution to public policy of a personal projects perspective lies not only in the focus on project pursuit but on social ecologies. Choices about individual goals and action are made in the context of a social ecology that both facilitates and constrains choice. For this reason, a personal projects perspective could not be seen as inherently ideological. It would not necessarily favor certain degrees of state intervention or particular political orientations. Indeed, a project analytic framework could be used to support a liberal, even a libertarian approach to policy that views the appropriate role of the state as staying out of an individual's personal project space, thereby expanding individual choice (Lomasky, 1984, 1987). Alternatively, it is compatible with communitarian or social justice approaches that see government as having a key role in creating the conditions that allow rights to be converted into achievable projects (Sen, 1985) and in shaping social ecologies so that individual choice can be effectively exercised (Phillips, 2004).

CONCLUSIONS AND CAVEATS: TOWARD THE SUSTAINABLE PURSUIT OF CORE PROJECTS

In different ways, and using closely linked but not identical terminology, the contributions to this volume have this in common: They have elucidated the conditions under which goal and project pursuit can go well and contribute to human flourishing or can go awry and make lives miserable.

One of its novel contributions, in Part I, is the detailed introduction to personal projects theory and methodology, including an analysis of the relation of this to goals research. Theoretical and research articles on personal projects have appeared regularly over the past quarter-century, but other than in technical reports, theses, and dissertations, there has not been a conveniently accessible introduction to PPA methodology. We hope that the more comprehensive introduction provided in this volume will stimulate researchers and practitioners alike to adopt and adapt PPA, as well as to build on the many creative adaptations of it in other chapters of this volume.

Our central theoretical proposition, broad enough we feel, to subsume both project analytic and more purely goals-based research, is that well-being is contingent on the sustainable pursuit of goals and projects that are accorded vital importance in our lives. In Part II we examined some of the internal, self-regulatory factors that can militate against sustainable pursuit, including the problematic nature of an overabundance of avoidance goals, unnecessarily complex and trying ways of talking about our projects, conflict between pursuits that matter, and the deadening effect of a loss of certitude in a complex world. However, the tone of each chapter is nuanced. Avoidance goals are not universally problematic; sometimes "just doing it" can get us into trouble depending on what "it" is. Conflict between projects can occasionally lead to greater integrative complexity; the terror of uncertainty can launch passionate pursuits that may be indescribably cruel or utterly redeeming. For those wishing simple main effect statements on how to lead better lives, a better location would be found on the second floor (the pop psych section) of McGregor's bookstore, not here.

In Part III we examined some of the social ecological, contextual factors that can promote or frustrate the pursuit of goals and projects. We explored the vital role played by other people and organizations in bringing projects to fruition, the equally vital role of culturally created developmental channels along which our projects may be compelled to proceed, and the personal costs of cultural annihilation and the role of projects in linking our pasts with our futures. Yet here again, the conclusions to be drawn need to be nuanced. Other people can be loving partners in projects pursuit, but they can also suck the life out of our personal undertakings; lack of cultural cohesion can be deadly, but it can also serve as the stimulant for massive cultural change and restoration.

In Part IV, where we explicitly examine the linkages among goals, projects, and well-being, we find some commonalities, but also some differences. The commonalities revolve around the desirability of coherence—whether it is in the concordance of goal achievement with one's values, with the increased saliency of one's core projects occasioned by physical illness, or among levels of selves or among diverse natures.

In this final chapter we have sought to summarize the subtle ways in which goals and projects can be shaped by one's internal volitional dynamics, by the surrounding social ecology, and by the political systems that can facilitate the sustainable pursuit of core projects in ways that benefit all or some or can create conditions in which personal project pursuit is proscribed or punished.

Four caveats are in order. This volume started out as a very different project than it has ended up becoming. This is hardly surprising in academic publishing, but there is a nice degree of reflexive relevance and it seems appropriate to let the reader know how the project has mutated. When we began this project a few years ago, European and North American researchers were far less integrated than they now are. We originally saw the book as an opportunity to bring researchers from two different traditions together and that was a major goal. The folly of that goal becomes clear when one realizes that a large proportion of the researchers have changed continents between the inception and conclusion stage of this project (some of them twice)! So, the conjoining of European action and goal theory with North American projects research, a key aspiration for this volume, rapidly disappeared. The reality is that we are so commingled as a research community it is misleading to perpetuate the illusion that we are bringing strangers together for a novel wedding. In fact, we have been living together for a number of years.

A second caveat, or perhaps reminder, is that we have been particularly mindful of the role of the participants in the research we report in this volume. We have been aware of them as singular individuals. Broad generalizations about project pursuit and human flourishing are aesthetically pleasing but often wrong. Even our own early research on Asian versus North American differences in the relative impact of internal dispositions and external situations on daily conduct seems coarse and misleading. We need to know which Asian, which North American, of which particular ethnic group, of what age, with what strengths and frailties, and living in what conditions, before venturing to appraise that person's capacity for flourishing. However, by understanding the most cherished goals and core projects of that singular creature we will have taken an important step in understanding what it is we wish to sustain, to amplify, and to preserve inviolate. That step is essential before flourishing can be understood and enhanced.

Third, it is critical to remember that the sustainable pursuit of core projects is not simply a matter of individuals maximizing, in a prudential fashion, the utility and progress of their own projects. If, in the act of sustaining one's core projects, the supportive ecological network is compromised, the project will not be sustainable (Little & Ryan, 1979). Gains in project pursuit may not be sustainable if the local ecology, be it human or physical, is taxed beyond capacity. Prudential project pursuit may be a necessary condition of flourishing, but it is not a sufficient condition. Concern for others and respect for the conditions that enable one's own pursuits to be successful are also necessary for sustained pursuit and flourishing.

Finally, it would be misleading to conclude that human flourishing is contingent only on the rational pursuit of clearly articulated goals and projects. The tenacious pursuit of goals and core projects may bring a measure of pleasure and success in one's life. However, such pursuit might also blind us to possibilities to which we are utterly oblivious. Indeed, the wisdom of framing one's future through the resolute pursuit of life goals has been challenged in a convincing fashion by Larmore (1999), who concluded that such pursuit may often blind us to the unexpected good of unplanned events. This is not to say that we should be indiscriminately hedonistic and lurch from project to project in the hope of short-term delight. It does mean, however, that in addition to focal commitment to valued projects, human flourishing may require a sensitivity to what might be happening just around the corner. Acuity of peripheral vision may also be a necessary component of a flourishing life.

REFERENCES

Allport, G. W. (1958). What units shall we employ? In G. Lindzey (Ed.), *Assessment of human motives* (pp. 239–260). New York: Rinehart.

Antonovsky, A. (1979). Health, stress, and coping. San Francisco: Jossey-Bass.

Apter, M. J. (1984). Reversal theory and personality: A review. *Journal of Research in Personality, 18,* 265–288.

Apter, M. J. (2001). *Motivational styles in everyday life: A guide to reversal theory.* Washington, DC: American Psychological Association.

Aspinall, P. A. (2005). *On quality of life.* Unpublished manuscript, School of the Built Environment, Heriot Watt University, Scotland.

Bargh, J. A., & Ferguson, M. J. (2000). Beyond behaviorism: On the automaticity of higher mental processes. *Psychological Bulletin, 126,* 925–945.

Bem, D. J. (1972). Self-perception theory. In L. Berkowitz (Ed.), *Advances in experimental social psychology* (Vol. 6, pp. 1–62). New York: Academic.

Binhammer, K., Henderson, J., & Moyes, L. (1993, Winter). Introduction. [Feminist(s) Project(s)/Projets (des) feminists]. *Tessera, 15,* 6–13.

Blitheway, B., & Coleman, P. G. (1997). *Exploring the experience of ageing: An overview.* Adelaide, Australia: World Congress of Gerontology.

Blunt, A. K., & Pychyl, T. A. (2000). Task aversiveness and procrastination: A multidimensional approach to task aversiveness across stages of personal projects. *Personality and Individual Differences, 28,* 153–167.

Blunt, A. K., & Pychyl, T. A. (2005). Project systems of procrastinators: A personal project-analytic and action control perspective. *Personality and Individual Differences, 38,* 1771–1780.

Cameron, K., Dutton, J. E., & Quinn, R. E. (Eds.). (2003). *Positive organizational scholarship: Foundations of a new discipline.* San Francisco: Barrett-Koehler.

Cantor, N. (1994). Life task problem solving: Situational affordances and personal needs. *Personality and Social Psychology Bulletin, 20,* 235–243.

Carstensen, L. L. (1992). Social and emotional patterns in adulthood: Support for socioemotional selectivity theory. *Psychology and Aging, 7,* 331–338.

Carver, C. S., & Scheier, M. F. (1990). Origins and functions of positive and negative affect: A control-process view. *Psychological Review, 97,* 19–35.

Carver, C. S., & Scheier, M. F. (1998). *On the self-regulation of behavior.* New York: Cambridge University Press.

Carver, C. S., & Scheier, M. F. (2003). Self-regulatory perspectives on personality. In T. Millon & M. J. Lerner (Eds.), *Handbook of psychology: Personality and social psychology* (Vol. 5, pp. 185–208). New York: Wiley.

Caspi, A., Roberts, B. W., & Shiner, R. L. (2005). Personality development: Stability and change. *Annual Review of Psychology, 56,* 453–484.

Cervone, D. (2004). The architecture of personality. *Psychological Review, 111,* 183–204.

Chambers, N. C. (2001). Time and personal action: Tenses and aspects of project pursuit (Doctoral dissertation, Carleton University, 2000). *Dissertation Abstracts International, 62*(2B), 1130.

Christiansen, C. H., Backman, C., Little, B. R., & Nguyen, A. (1999). Occupations and well-being: A study of personal projects. *American Journal of Occupational Therapy, 53,* 91–100.

Christiansen, C. H., Little, B. R., & Backman, C. (1998). Personal projects: A useful approach to the study of occupation. *American Journal of Occupational Therapy, 52,* 439–446.

Church, A. T. (2000). Culture and personality: Toward an integrated cultural trait psychology. *Journal of Personality, 68,* 651–703.

Churchill, A. C. (2005). *Hoping for the best while preparing for the worst: Constructive realism, personal projects and the transition to motherhood.* Unpublished doctoral dissertation, Carleton University, Ottawa, ON, Canada.

Cochran, L. (1992). The career project. *Journal of Career Development, 18,* 187–197.

Collette, D. (1985). *Personal projects analysis: An index of individual differences moderating the effects of life stress.* Unpublished bachelor's thesis, Carleton University, Ottawa, ON, Canada.

Costa, P. T., Jr., & McCrae, R. R. (1985). *The NEO Personality Inventory manual.* Odessa, FL: Psychological Assessment Resources.

Dowden, C. E. (2004). *Managing to be "free": Personality, personal projects and well-being in entrepreneurs.* Unpublished doctoral dissertation, Carleton University, Ottawa, ON, Canada.

Elliot, A. J., & Devine, P. G. (1994). On the motivational nature of cognitive dissonance: Dissonance as psychological discomfort. *Journal of Personality and Social Psychology, 67,* 382–394.

Festinger, L. (1957). *A theory of cognitive dissonance.* Evanston, IL: Row, Peterson.

Fredrickson, B. L. (1998). What good are positive emotions? *Review of General Psychology, 2,* 300–319.

Fredrickson, B. L. (2001). The role of positive emotions in positive psychology: The broaden-and-build theory of positive emotions. *American Psychologist, 56,* 218–226.

Freund, A. M., & Baltes, P. B. (2000). The orchestration of selection, optimization and compensation: An action-theoretical conceptualization of a theory of developmental regulation. In W. J. Perrig & A. Grob (Eds.), *Control of human behavior, mental processes, and consciousness: Essays in honor of the 60th birthday of August Flammer* (pp. 35–58). Mahwah, NJ: Lawrence Erlbaum Associates.

Funder, D. C. (2001). Personality. *Annual Review of Psychology, 52*, 197–221.

Gable, S. L., & Haidt, J. (2005). What (and why) is positive psychology? *Review of General Psychology, 9*, 103–110.

George, J. M. (2004). Review of the book *Positive organizational scholarship: Foundations of a new discipline. Administrative Science Quarterly, 49*, 325–329.

Gollwitzer, P. M. (1999). Implementation intentions: Strong effects of simple plans. *American Psychologist, 54*, 493–503.

Gollwitzer, P. M., Heckhausen, H., & Steller, B. (1990). Deliberative and implemental mind-sets: Cognitive tuning toward congruous thoughts and information. *Journal of Personality and Social Psychology, 59*, 119–127.

Gollwitzer, P. M., & Kinney, R. F. (1989). Effects of deliberative and implemental mind-sets on illusion of control. *Journal of Personality and Social Psychology, 56*, 531–542.

Guignon, C. (2002). Hermeneutics, authenticity and the aims of psychology. *Journal of Theoretical and Philosophical Psychology, 22*, 83–102.

Haanpää, I. (2002). Adolescents' personal projects and well-being. In Joensuu and Petrozavodsk. *Psykologia, 37*, 221–229.

Harris, J. R. (1995). Where is the child's environment? A group socialization theory of development. *Psychological Review, 102*, 458–489.

Havighurst, R. J. (1963). *Successful aging, process of aging: Social and psychological perspectives* (Vol. 1, pp. 299–320). New York: Atherton.

Heckhausen, J. (1999). *Developmental regulation in adulthood: Age-normative and sociostructural constraints as adaptive challenges.* New York: Cambridge University Press.

Heckhausen, J. (2002). Transition from school to work: Societal opportunities and the potential for individual agency. *Journal of Vocational Behavior, 60*, 173–177.

Heckhausen, J., & Schulz, R. (1999). Selectivity in life-span development: Biological and societal canalizations and individuals' developmental goals. In J. Brandtstädter & R. M. Lerner (Eds.), *Action and self-development: Theory and research through the life span* (pp. 67–103). Thousand Oaks, CA: Sage.

Held, B. S. (2004). The negative side of positive psychology. *Journal of Humanistic Psychology, 44*, 9–46.

Higgins, E. T. (1997). Beyond pleasure and pain. *American Psychologist, 52*, 1280–1300.

Higgins, E. T. (1998). Promotion and prevention: Regulatory focus as a motivational principle. In M. P. Zanna (Ed.), *Advances in experimental social psychology* (Vol. 30, pp. 1–46). New York: Academic.

Kelly, G. A. (1955). *The psychology of personal constructs.* New York: Norton.

Kelly, G. A. (1958). The theory and technique of assessment. *Annual Review of Psychology, 9*, 323–352.

King, L. A. (2001). The health benefits of writing about life goals. *Personality and Social Psychology Bulletin, 27*, 798–807.

Kiviniemi, M. T., Snyder, M., & Omoto, A. M. (2002). Too many of a good thing? The effects of multiple motivations on stress, cost, fulfillment and satisfaction. *Personality and Social Psychology Bulletin, 28*, 732–743.

Labouvie-Vief, G. (1981). Proactive and reactive aspects of constructivism: Growth and aging in life-span perspective. In R. M. Lerner & N. A. Busch-Rossnagel (Eds.), *Individuals as producers of their development: A life-span perspective* (pp. 197–230). New York: Academic.

Larmore, C. (1999). The idea of a life plan. In E. F. Paul, F. Miller, Jr., & J. Paul (Eds.), *Human flourishing* (pp. 96–112). New York: Cambridge University Press.

Lawrence, J. W., Carver, C. S., & Scheier, M. F. (2002). Velocity toward goal attainment in immediate experience as a determinant of affect. *Journal of Applied Social Psychology, 32,* 788–802.

Lawton, M. P., Moss, M. S., Winter, L., & Hoffman, C. (2002). Motivation in later life: Personal projects and well-being. *Psychology and Aging, 17,* 539–547.

Lay, C. H. (1986). At last, my research article on procrastination. *Journal of Research in Personality, 20,* 474–495.

Lazarus, R. S. (2003a). Does the positive psychology movement have legs? *Psychological Inquiry, 14,* 93–109.

Lazarus, R. S. (2003b). The Lazarus manifesto for positive psychology and psychology in general. *Psychological Inquiry, 14,* 173–189.

Linley, P. A., & Joseph, S. (2004). *Positive psychology in practice.* New York: Wiley.

Little, B. R. (1983). Personal projects: A rationale and method for investigation. *Environment and Behavior, 15,* 273–309.

Little, B. R. (1987). Personal projects and fuzzy selves: Aspects of self-identity in adolescence. In T. Honess & K. Yardley (Eds.), *Self and identity: Perspectives across the life span.* London: Routledge & Kegan Paul.

Little, B. R. (1989). Personal projects analysis: Trivial pursuits, magnificent obsessions, and the search for coherence. In D. M. Buss & N. Cantor (Eds.), *Personality psychology: Recent trends and emerging directions* (pp. 15–31). New York: Springer.

Little, B. R. (1999). Personality and motivation: Personal action and the conative evolution. In L. A. Pervin & O. P. John (Eds.), *Handbook of personality theory and research* (2nd ed.). New York: Guilford.

Little, B. R. (2000). Free traits and personal contexts: Expanding a social ecological model of well-being. In W. B. Walsh, K. H. Craik, & R. H. Price (Eds.), *Person–environment psychology: New directions and perspectives* (2nd ed., pp. 87–116). Mahwah, NJ: Lawrence Erlbaum Associates.

Little, B. R. (2005). Personality science and personal projects: Six impossible things before breakfast. *Journal of Research in Personality, 39,* 4–21.

Little, B. R., Carlsen, N., Glavin, G. Y., & Lavery, J. (1981). *Personal projects analysis across the life span.* Unpublished report, Social Sciences and Humanities Research Council of Canada, Ottawa, ON, Canada.

Little, B. R., Dowden, C., Chambers, N. C., Hunt, J., Richardson, K., Hargrave, A., et al. (2005). *Personal projects and depressive affect: A meta-analysis.* Unpublished manuscript, Social Ecology Laboratory, Carleton Univeristy, Ottawa, ON, Canada.

Little, B. R., & Gee, T. L. (in press). Personal projects analysis. In N. Salkind (Ed.), *Encyclopedia of measurement and statistics.* Thousand Oaks, CA: Sage.

Little, B. R., Lecci, L., & Watkinson, B. (1992). Personality and personal projects: Linking big five and PAC units of analysis. *Journal of Personality, 60,* 501–525.

Little, B. R., & Ryan, T. J. (1979). A social ecological model of development. In K. Ishwaren (Ed.), *Childhood and adolescence in Canada* (pp. 273–301). Toronto: McGraw-Hill Ryerson.

Lomasky, L. E. (1984). Personal projects as the foundation for basic rights. *Social Philosophy and Policy, 1,* 35–55.

Lomasky, L. E. (1987). *Persons, rights and the moral community.* New York: Oxford University Press.

Maes, S., & Karoly, P. (2005). Self-regulation assessment and intervention in physical health and illness: A review. *Applied Psychology: An International Review, 54,* 267–299.

Markus, H., & Nurius, P. (1986). Possible selves. *American Psychologist, 41,* 954–969.

Martennson, S. (1977). Childhood interaction and temporal organization. *Economic Geography, 53,* 99–115.

Mavis, B. (1981). *Personal projects as indicators of change in men at mid-life.* Unpublished master's thesis, Carleton University, Ottawa, ON, Canada.

McAdams, D. P. (1993). *The stories we live by: Personal myths and the making of the self.* New York: Morrow.

McAdams, D. P., & de St. Aubin, E. (Eds.). (1998). *Generativity and adult development: How and why we care for the next generation.* Washington, DC: APA Press.

McKeen, N. A. (1984). *The personal projects of pregnant women.* Unpublished bachelor's thesis, Carleton University, Ottawa, ON, Canada.

Meyer, B., Beevers, C. G., & Johnson, S. L. (2004). Goal appraisals and vulnerability to bipolar disorder: A personal projects analysis. *Cognitive Therapy and Research, 28,* 173–182.

Mickelson, W. P. (1984). *Personal project systems and health status.* Unpublished master's thesis, Carleton University, Ottawa, ON, Canada.

Miller, D. T., & Nelson, L. D. (2002). Seeing approach motivation in the avoidance behavior of others: Implications for an understanding of pluralistic ignorance. *Journal of Personality and Social Psychology, 83,* 1066–1075.

Miller, N. E., & Kraeling, D. (1952). Displacement: Greater generalization of approach than avoidance in a generalized approach–avoidance conflict. *Journal of Experimental Psychology, 43,* 217–221.

Mischel, W. (2004). Toward an integrative science of the person. *Annual Review of Psychology, 55,* 1–22.

Nurmi, J. -E. (1991). How do adolescents see their future? A review of the development of future orientation and planning. *Developmental Review, 11,* 1–59.

Nuttin, J., & Lens, W. (1985). *Future time perspective and motivation: Theory and research method.* Hillsdale, NJ: Lawrence Erlbaum Associates.

Ogilvie, D. M., & Rose, K. M. (1995). Self-with-other representations and a taxonomy of motives: Two approaches to studying persons. *Journal of Personality, 63,* 633–679.

Ogilvie, D. M., Rose, K. M., & Heppen, J. B. (2001). A comparison of personal project motives in three age groups. *Basic and Applied Social Psychology, 23,* 207–215.

Omodei, M. M., & Wearing, A. J. (1990). Need satisfaction and involvement in personal projects: Toward an integrative model of subjective well-being. *Journal of Personality and Social Psychology, 59,* 762–769.

Peter, F. (2003). Gender and the foundations of social choice: The role of situated agency. *Feminist Economics, 9*(2–3), 13–32.

Phillips, A. (2004). Defining equality of outcome. *Journal of Political Philosophy, 12,* 1–19.

Phillips, S. D., Little, B. R., & Goodine, L. A. (1996). *Organizational climate and personal projects: Gender differences in the public service* (Research Paper No. 20). Ottawa, ON, Canada: Minister of Supply and Services.

Piliavin, J. A. (1989). When in doubt, ask the subject. A solicited response to Egan, J. M. "Graduate school and the self: A theoretical view of some negative effects of professional socialization." *Teaching Sociology, 17,* 208–210.

Pychyl, T. A. (1996). Personal projects, subjective well-being and the lives of doctoral students. *Dissertation Abstracts International, 56*(12), 7080B. (UMI No. NN02961)

Pychyl, T. A., & Binder, K. (2004). A project-analytic perspective on academic procrastination and intervention. In H. C. Schouwenburg, C. Lay, T. A. Pychyl, & J. R. Ferrari (Eds.), *Counseling the procrastinator in academic settings* (pp. 149–165). Washington, DC: APA Books.

Pychyl, T. A., & Little, B. R. (1998). Dimensional specificity in the prediction of subjective well-being: Personal projects in pursuit of the Ph.D. *Social Indicators Research, 45*, 423–473.

Richardson, K. (2002). Personal projects analysis and well-being: Cultural explorations (Masters thesis, Carleton University, Ottawa, Canada, 2001). *Masters Abstracts International, 40*, 1630.

Ryan, R. M., & Deci, E. L. (2000). Self-determination theory and the facilitation of intrinsic motivation, social development, and well-being. *American Psychologist, 55*, 68–78.

Sandage, S. J., & Hill, P. C. (2001). The virtues of positive psychology: The rapprochement and challenges of an affirmative postmodern perspective. *Journal for the Theory of Social Behaviour, 31*, 241–260.

Schwartz, S. H., & Bardi, A. (2001). Value hierarchies across cultures: Taking a similarities perspective. *Journal of Cross-Cultural Psychology, 32*, 268–290.

Seligman, M. E. P., & Csikszentmihalyi, M. (2000). Positive psychology: An introduction. *American Psychologist, 55*, 5–14.

Sen, A. (1985). *Inequality reexamined.* Cambridge, MA: Harvard University Press.

Sheldon, K., & King, L. A. (2001). Why positive psychology is necessary (foreword to the special section). *American Psychologist, 56*, 216–217.

Snyder, C. R., & Lopez, S. J. (Eds.). (2002). *Handbook of positive psychology.* London: Oxford University Press.

Sugiyama, T., & Ward Thompson, C. (in press). Environmental support for outdoor activities and older people's quality of life. *Journal of Housing for the Elderly, 19*, 3–4.

Szawlowski, S. (1987). *Procrastination from a project analytic perspective.* Unpublished bachelor's thesis, Carleton University, Ottawa, ON, Canada.

Vallacher, R. R., & Wegner, D. M. (1987). What do people think they're doing? Action identification and human behavior. *Psychological Review, 94*, 3–15.

Wallenius, M. (1999). Personal projects in everyday places: Perceived supportiveness of the environment and psychological well-being. *Journal of Environmental Psychology, 19*, 131–143.

Wallenius, M. (2004). The interaction of noise stress and personal project stress on subjective health. *Journal of Environmental Psychology, 24*, 167–177.

Wilmut, K. (1997). *Personal projects, well-being, and the social ecology of early adolescence.* Unpublished master's thesis, Carleton University, Ottawa, ON, Canada.

Wilson, D. A. (1990). *Personal project dimensions and perceived life satisfaction: A quantitative synthesis.* Unpublished master's thesis, Carleton University, Ottawa, ON, Canada.

Wrosch, C., Scheier, M. F., & Miller, G. E. (2003). Adaptive self-regulation of unattainable goals: Goal disengagement, goal reengagement, and subjective well-being. *Personality and Social Psychology Bulletin, 29*, 1494–1508.

Xiao, B. L. (1986). *A comparison of personal projects between Chinese undergraduates and Canadian undergraduates.* Unpublished manuscript, Social Ecology Laboratory, Department of Psychology, Carleton University, Ottawa, ON, Canada.

Author Index

Subject Index